PRAISE FOR THOMAS CLAIRE'S *BODYWORK*

"*Bodywork* is definitely 'The Bible' of our time in the field of bodywork. I highly recommend this book for both the layman and the professional."

—OHASHI

"An excellent resource."

—DR. BERNIE SIEGEL, AUTHOR OF *LOVE, MEDICINE & MIRACLES*

"*Bodywork* is the best source of information about a wide variety of exciting therapeutic modalities that I have seen. Every chapter is a clear, in-depth description—a gold mine of trustworthy information for anyone seeking a kind of bodywork appropriate for their wants and needs. Practitioners as well as clients will find it invaluable. Thomas Claire has dispelled much of the confusion about the different styles and strengths of the many forms of bodywork in America, and has helped to define bodywork's rightful place in health care."

—DEANE JUHAN, AUTHOR OF *JOB'S BODY: A HANDBOOK FOR BODYWORK*

"Today the field of bodywork is so rich and varied that it can be overwhelming. Thomas Claire's excellent book, *Bodywork*, is the perfect guide into this wonderful world."

—DEBORAH CAPLAN, M.A., P.T., AUTHOR OF *BACK TROUBLE: A NEW APPROACH TO PREVENTION AND RECOVERY BASED ON THE ALEXANDER TECHNIQUE*

"I would highly recommend Thomas Claire's *Bodywork* as a clear and concise comprehensive guide. Claire's unique way of explaining the 'feel' of a typical session is especially informative and meaningful."

—JOHN F. BARNES, P.T., MYOFASCIAL RELEASE TREATMENT CENTERS AND SEMINARS

"I'm impressed. In this time when health-care consumers are rediscovering the value of 'hands-on' bodywork, a book such as this, which accurately describes for the consumer the majority of bodywork approaches and techniques, is of inestimable value. There is no 'high-tech' language here."
—JOHN E. UPLEDGER, D.O., O.M.M.,
MEDICAL DIRECTOR, THE UPLEDGER INSTITUTE

"A complete guide to assessing a wide range of therapeutic practices . . . unique and user-friendly . . . deserves a place on the shelves next to guides on how to choose a lawyer or a physician."
—LIBRARY JOURNAL

"The massage-therapy bible."
—GENTLEMEN'S QUARTERLY

"[This] encyclopedic book . . . is the bible in its field."
—COUNTRY LIVING'S HEALTHYLIVING

"The right touch can do wonders . . . But with all the possibilities . . . how do you choose? . . . Mr. Claire . . . makes a fine guide . . . precise and complete . . . his views from the table are both enlightening and entertaining."
—THE DALLAS MORNING NEWS

"Thomas Claire's *Bodywork* fills the need for a book that describes the many forms of bodywork and massage currently being practiced. Subtitled *What Type of Massage to Get—and How to Make the Most of It,* it delivers that information in an enjoyable and easy-to-use format . . . By giving the reader both theoretical information and an experiential sense of each modality . . . Claire succeeds in conveying a more complete understanding of each modality than any other source I know of."
—MASSAGE MAGAZINE

"Thomas Claire . . . has written a book on massage and bodywork that offers its readers a distinctive feature, that goes further than so many other competent, useful books on the subject. *Bodywork: What Type of Massage to Get—and How to Make the Most of It* is intended to 'convey what each approach actually feels like' . . . an intimate, personal, friendly—and therefore truly helpful—kind of 'hands-on' guide . . . I found most valuable the strongly affirmative human 'spin' Claire brings to a vital subject that has nevertheless too often been presented so objectively and dispassionately."

—MASSAGE THERAPY JOURNAL

"We had the 'baby boom.' Now, we are witnessing the 'body boom.' *Bodywork: What Type of Massage to Get—and How to Make the Most of It* is a . . . much-needed book that answers the multitude of questions repeatedly asked by people who are searching for a clear description of various bodyworks and types of practitioners."

—ILANA RUBENFELD, CREATOR OF THE RUBENFELD SYNERGY METHOD AND FOUNDER OF THE RUBENFELD TRAINING PROGRAM

"Thomas Claire has done a magnificent job of defining and describing virtually every type of bodywork therapy from a firsthand perspective. I believe bodywork is one of the most powerful medicines available. With so many effective techniques to choose from it is often overwhelming. In *Bodywork,* the reader is guided to the best technique for them and their body."

—MICHAEL MURRAY, N.D., AUTHOR OF *NATURAL ALTERNATIVES*

"In *Bodywork* Thomas Claire has illuminated with integrity, compassion and eloquence the interconnective web of holistic bodywork. Each modality explored reveals itself as a valuable strand in this diverse yet unified web that serves to honor the developing field of therapeutic bodywork and its contribution for healing and wholeness. It is a true gift to potential client and professional practitioner alike."

—LAURA NORMAN, REFLEXOLOGIST,
AUTHOR OF *FEET FIRST: A GUIDE TO FOOT REFLEXOLOGY*

BODY WORK

What Type of Massage to Get—and How to Make the Most of It

THOMAS CLAIRE

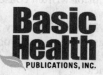

Basic Health
PUBLICATIONS, INC.

The information in this book is intended to increase your knowledge about massage and body-work therapies and by no means is intended to diagnose or treat an individual's health problems or ailments. The information given is not medical advice, nor is it presented as a course of per-sonalized treatment. There may be risks involved in connection with some of the practices sug-gested in this book, just as there may be risks involved in connection with any type of physical activity or therapy. Therefore, before starting any type of massage or bodywork therapy, or before discontinuing any course of medical treatment you may now be undergoing, you should consult your own healthcare practitioner.

The publisher does not advocate the use of any particular healthcare protocol but believes the information in this book should be available to the public. The publisher and author are not responsible for any adverse effects or consequences resulting from the use of the suggestions, preparations, or procedures discussed in this book.

The following trademarks, registered marks, and service marks are used throughout this book: The American Center for the Alexander Technique, Inc., American Massage Therapy Association, AMTA, American Organization for Bodywork Therapies of Asia, AOBTA, Aston-Patterning, Bonnie Prudden Myotherapy, Esalen, Feldenkrais, Feldenkrais Method, Awareness Through Movement, Functional Integration, Feldenkrais Guild, Hellerwork, Holotropic Breathwork, International Association of Infant Massage, IAIM, International Institute of Reflexology, Ing-ham Method, International SPA Association, ISPA, Jin Shin Do, Bodymind Acupressure, Jin Shin Jyutsu, KURED, LooyenWork, MLD, NAVALT, Ohashiatsu, Ortho-Bionomy, Society of Ortho-Bionomy International, Pfrimmer Deep Muscle Therapy, The Radiance Technique, Rolf Institute, Rolfer, Rolfing, Rosen Method, Rubenfeld Synergy Method, Rubenfeld Synergist, Therapeutic Touch, Touch for Health, Trager, Mentastics, Transcendental Meditation, TTouch, The Upledger Insititute, Inc., The Upledger Insititute, Inc. HealthPlex Cliniclal Services, Somato-Emotional Release, and Zero Balancing.

Basic Health Publications, Inc.
28812 Top of the World Drive • Laguna Beach, CA 92651 • 949-715-7327

Library of Congress Cataloging-in-Publication Data

Claire, Thomas.
    Bodywork : what type of massage to get and how to make the most of it/
Thomas Claire.—2nd ed.
    p. cm.
    ISBN-13: 978-1-59120-165-6
    ISBN-10: 1-59120-165-9
  1. Massage. 2. Touch—Therapeutic use. 3. Mind and body therapies. I. Title.

    RA780.5.C57   2006
    615.8'22—dc22
                                        2006002150

In-house editor: Carol Rosenberg • Typesetting: Gary A. Rosenberg
Cover design: Mike Stromberg • Based on original book design by Jessica Shatan

Printed in the United States of America

10 9 8 7 6 5 4 3 2 1

This book is gratefully dedicated to my mother,
for giving birth to the dream; my friend and
colleague Alice Pisciotto, for nuturing it;
my agent, Jeanne Fredericks, for sharing it;
my editor, Will Schwalbe, for giving it a body;
and all other healers, wherever you may be.

CONTENTS

PART III   OTHER CONTEMPORARY WESTERN BODYWORK PRACTICES

PART VI   SUPPLEMENTAL INFORMATION: SIMPLE TOOLS

PREFACE
TO THE REVISED EDITION

Ten years have passed since the first edition of *Bodywork* was released. During that time, massage and bodywork, along with other alternative health practices, have continued to grow in popularity and have entered the mainstream of contemporary life. Indeed, the term alternative medicine is being replaced with increasing regularity by the terms integrative medicine and complementary medicine, further indicating the widespread acceptance of these practices as partners in healing with contemporary Western medicine.

In line with this trend, massage and bodywork practitioners have seen their work embraced by a growing public. When *Bodywork* was first written, nineteen states regulated the practice of massage at the state level. Today, thirty-three states regulate massage at the state level, and the number is growing. Associations of bodywork practitioners, such as the American Massage Therapy Association (AMTA) and Associated Bodywork & Massage Professionals (ABMP) have seen their memberships double and nearly triple in number. The National Certification Board for Therapeutic Massage and Bodywork (NCBTMB), a fledgling organization in 1995, has become an increasingly important and growing factor in massage and bodywork. And massage training has entered mainstream education with traditional educational institutions offering undergraduate degree programs in massage.

Even with all of these changes, the basic approaches to massage remain true to their origins. This revised and updated edition of *Bodywork* retains the strength of the first edition in its presentation of the major approaches to bodywork, while updating the information regarding these approaches to reflect current levels of training, practice, and professional resources. When the first edition of *Bodywork* appeared, the Internet was virtually unknown. This new edition of *Bodywork* not only updates contact information for helpful resources on massage and bodywork, but also includes information on Internet and e-mail addresses for many of the most important bodywork organizations and associations. The resources that are presented in this book have been selected from among the most reliable available. While the Internet has made much useful information accessible to a large population, it has also made each individual an author, capable of posting information on the Web. The reliability of such information is not always of a high order. The Internet resource information that you will find included in this edition of *Bodywork* refers readers to professional organizations dedicated to promoting high standards in massage and bodywork.

As in the first edition of *Bodywork,* I encourage you to experience massage and bodywork for yourself. May this updated resource be a helpful guide to you on your own unfolding journey.

PREFACE
TO THE FIRST EDITION

You might ask what special credentials I bring to writing *Bodywork*. Like you, I'm an ordinary person trying to make sense of a fragmented world, exploring all the amazing potential and beauty it has to offer.

I did distinguish myself academically, where I graduated from some of the country's leading universities with numerous honors, including National Merit and Fulbright scholarships. And I succeeded in the eyes of the business world, where I was a whiz with numbers and financial analysis, so much so that at an early age I became U.S. treasurer of the world's largest and most prestigious luxury goods company.

But I am also, and always have been, a seeker of wholeness and completion. In my late thirties, the mid-point of life, I began to feel a transformation taking place inside myself, almost as though some timed-release capsule had kicked in. I began to know there must be treasures more precious than money, luxuries deeper than skin-care treatments, and more certainties to life than death and taxes. That realization led me on my own journey to examine numerous metaphysical traditions and ways of understanding my own being. The quest ultimately led me to experiment with various bodywork practices, which allowed me to make the shift from head to heart in a gentle, gradual, and undeniably powerful way. Through personal experience, I have learned that we each have teachers who are patiently waiting to guide us when we are ready to begin our journey. My preparation for writing this book has led me to my greatest teachers. The idea for this project was born when I looked for a book that could guide me in the many-faceted world of massage and bodywork. I was unable to find a book that was comprehensive yet individual enough to convey what each approach actually feels like.

I undertook my education in bodywork on my own, beginning tentatively, with a few small steps. I took an introductory workshop and experienced a bodywork treatment here and there. Eventually, though, I left my secure position in the financial world and committed myself to the profession of body-work and to writing this book. I totally immersed myself in this exciting field. I studied countless hours over a course of years to master a variety of techniques as a licensed massage therapist. I attended and graduated from the Swedish Institute School of Massage Therapy and Allied Health Sciences, in addition to completing the Ohashi Institute's advanced program of Ohashiatsu. I am also a practitioner of Therapeutic Touch and a Reiki Master. I've studied CranioSacral Therapy, Myofascial Release, reflexology, and a variety of energetic healing modalities. I progressed to the role of teacher, presenting workshops and lectures on a variety of bodywork practices. I've explored every approach presented in *Bodywork* and have been fortunate to receive treatments from some of the most gifted practitioners of the healing arts. I have read hundreds of books and thousands of articles to synthesize and crystallize the information presented in this book. All of these experiences have served as potent learning tools.

Most important, though, I have been privileged to work with a wide variety of exceptional individuals. It is they who have been my greatest teachers. In Ohashiatsu, we practitioners call ourselves "givers" and those with whom we work "receivers." We quickly learn, however, that the terms are interchangeable for it is my receivers who have given me my greatest understanding of the art of bodywork. It is with deepest appreciation to them that I offer you the fruits of my exploration.

I would also like to thank those of you who are reading this book. It is my goal to make *Bodywork* as useful as possible. I welcome your comments as well as inquiries about my workshops, lectures, consultations, and referral services. Please, write to me:

Thomas Claire
Clairefontaine, Inc.
P.O. Box 1040
Grand Central Station
New York, NY 10163-1040

AUTHOR'S NOTE

The profession of massage and bodywork therapy is an evolving one, with practitioners engaged in discussion as to the best word to use to define their work. I have opted to use the word "bodywork" to include all of the practices presented in this book as it is the most comprehensive term available. "Massage," which is generally used by professionals to refer more specifically to Swedish massage and its variations, is the term that many laypersons have come to equate with any kind of touch therapy. The use of the word "massage" in this book's subtitle is meant to signal to the general reader that this book is about sensitive, skilled touch. However, some practitioners of disciplines presented in this book would not consider their work to fall under the traditional classification of massage. The author respectfully acknowledges that their work is appropriately meant to be considered within the broader context of bodywork.

ACKNOWLEDGMENTS

I wish to express my gratitude to all the teachers, practitioners, receivers, students, friends, and family members who offered support and assistance in completing this project. In particular, I wish to thank the following individuals:

My teachers, who inspired me to pursue a career in healing; Stanislav Grof, M.D.; Brugh Joy, M.D.; Dolores Krieger, Ph.D., R.N.; Ohashi and the staff of the Ohashi Institute; Oh Shinnáh, my Native American medicine woman; Reiki Masters Caroline Boddie, Penny Gnesin, Arthur Robertson, Léonie Rosenstiel, Ph.D., and Elaine Seissler; the faculty of the Swedish Institute, especially Russ Beasley, Lucy Liben, and Jill Thompson; and the faculty and staff of the Upledger Institute, particularly Gayle Breman, Robert Harris, and John E. Upledger, D.C., O.M.M.

Tiffany Field, Ph.D., and her dedicated staff at Touch Research Institute.

The gifted practitioners who shared their time, experience, and enthusiasm for bodywork as they collaborated on the experiential portions of this book: Rob Bauer, Heather Brown, Vicki Calpena-Eklund, Deborah Caplan, Ken Frey, David Frome, Bruria Ginton, Greta, Janet Macrae, Laura Norman, Roger Tolle, Lisa Wiener, and Reese Williams. Without them, this book would be merely words.

Karen Anderson and Richard Kaplan for sharing their experiences of shiatsu and Reiki, respectively.

The following individuals, who, along with those already cited, generously commented on portions of the manuscript of this book so that it might embody the power of their collective wisdom and experience: Judith Aston; John Barnes, P.T.; John Beaulieu, N.D.; Sue Brenner; David Burmeister; Bernard Burt; Dwight Byers; Howard Douglass; Bob Edwards; Cindy Gaydos; Chris Griscom; James Hackett; Brian Ingraham; Arnie Kolodner; Marcy Lindheimer; Kenneth Lubowich, O.M.D.; Keith Miller; David Palmer; Maxine Pannetier;

Ilana Rubenfeld; Iona Marsaa Teeguarden; William Walsh, D.C.; and Zhenya Kurashova Wine.

Christina Newburgh of Spa'Deus in Chianciano Terme, Tuscany, Italy, for her gracious hospitality.

The many professional and helpful people at the many national bodywork organizations I contacted. You are too numerous to cite individually, but you know who you are.

My sister, Dorothy Mraz; my writer colleague Bingo Weyer; and my good friend Ron Mencz, for encouraging me to complete this project.

Victoria Klose and Carol Rosenberg for their thoughtful and careful copy-editing of the manuscript.

I have said that the soul is not more than the body,
And I have said that the body is not more than the soul . . .

—Walt Whitman, "Song of Myself"

GETTING STARTED:
HOW TO USE THIS BOOK

Few things are so endlessly fascinating as the human body.[1]

—*THE NEW YORK TIMES*

Bodywork is intended to answer the questions of everyone who has any interest in the exciting field of bodywork. This includes the one in five adult Americans who receives a massage each year, anyone who has ever experienced aches and pains, anyone who wants to learn more about his or her body, anyone who is curious about all the treatments advertised in the local health club newsletter or favorite spa, anyone considering or embarking on a career in bodywork, anyone involved in the healthcare field, and anyone who has never even thought about bodywork—until now.

This book is designed to be as complete and as user-friendly as possible. You'll find detailed information on a broad spectrum of massage and bodywork practices selected for their popularity, availability, and diversity of approach.

While this book can be read as a whole from start to finish, each chapter can also be read on its own. The key features of each practice are highlighted in a brief "At-a-Glance" section that introduces each chapter. A glossary at the end of the book briefly defines all the bodywork practices profiled, plus many other exciting approaches that have gained popularity.

Bodywork is first and foremost touch communication. The principal challenge in writing about bodywork is how to convey what it feels like. Language tends to reflect the left brain's linear and analytic approach to intellectual understanding while the experience of bodywork is registered in the intuitive and free-flowing right hemisphere of the brain. During a session, an individual might experience concentric spirals of thoughts, emotions, spiritual insights, and physical releases. These sensations can occur all at once in a multidimensional dance that may feel like an instant or an eternity.

The feeling component that emerges during the experience of bodywork cannot be overemphasized. The Western tradition has created duality between thinking and feeling and has clearly given priority to thinking. Ever so subtly, we've lost touch with our feelings, and we wonder where the all-pervading sense of loss that characterizes our way of life comes from.

Bodywork therapies allow us to explore the hidden places of the soul, to own what is there without shame or judgment. They permit us to reestablish a direct link with our feeling selves, including our unconscious desires and fears. In order for us to realize our full human potential, it is essential that we make the shift from thinking to feeling and experiencing. Bodywork is the most effective means I know of arriving at a place of inner certitude and peace.

Bodywork answers the question "What does it feel like?" through a first-hand narrative description of each type of work. These experiential accounts form the heart and soul of this book. Other books on bodywork take a how-to approach that emphasizes photos of strokes and techniques. Pictures are two dimensional and static; they can't capture the dynamic ever-changing feel of a session. They are like listening to a monaural recording versus sense-surround sound.

Bodywork adopts a holistic perspective. The word "heal" literally means "to make whole." Massage and bodywork therapies are holistic practices that aim to help you achieve greater wholeness. Relief of physical symptoms may accompany attainment of this goal. However, practitioners do not set out to fix a broken part, and they are not licensed to diagnose physical illness. To the extent that many illnesses are the direct result of stress or lifestyle habits, these practices can play an important role in promoting health and well-being. *Bodywork* is not a how-to book. It is based on the belief that treatment is best administered by a trained professional and presents the basic facts about each bodywork approach so you can decide which is best for you.

Bodywork methods that share common elements are grouped together in sections. Many professionals agree that bodywork practices are arrayed along a body/mind continuum. Therapeutic practices at the beginning of the spectrum emphasize physical manipulation of the body for the purposes of relaxation and physical rehabilitation. They often employ deep pressure techniques; the client is primarily a passive recipient of the practitioner's active strokes; and the client disrobes to provide full access to the body. As practices proceed along the continuum, they increasingly emphasize the role of the mind and spirit in healing. At the furthest end of the spectrum, practices often involve gentle touch; they are geared toward balancing the mind, emotions, and spirit as well as the body; clients are frequently viewed as equal copartners in their own heal-ing; and they usually remain clad during treatment. Since our culture is tending toward greater inner exploration and integration of body and mind, these lat-ter practices represent exciting areas of development.

This paradigm is by nature somewhat artificial. The inclusion of a bodywork practice in any particular group within the paradigm in no way indicates that it is superior or inferior to any other. This model is used only because it is helpful in underscoring some of the basic differences among approaches. Because a human being is a unified whole, any form of therapy that includes physical touch has the capacity to affect body, mind, and spirit. Our everyday use of the word "touch" to connote both a physical gesture as well as that which emo-tionally moves us illustrates how we take this principle for granted. Addition-ally, many practitioners are conversant with more than one bodywork practice and weave sessions incorporating a variety of techniques.

HELPFUL HINTS

In preparing to receive any type of massage or bodywork, it's helpful to be psy-chologically ready. Often, people feel vulnerable at the prospect of exposing their bodies to a stranger. They also may feel they aren't worth the time or money they spend for a massage or find it easier to give than receive. These fears are often exaggerated and related to issues of self-esteem. Receiving a massage challenges us to grow in our self-confidence, to accept ourselves as we are, including the fact that we are worth every penny and every minute of the massage experience.

Bodywork hopes to take much of the fear out of bodywork by demystifying it. By walking you through a typical session of each type of bodywork, this book will help you understand exactly what to expect. It will empower you to enjoy the nurturing touch that is your birthright.

HOW TO MAKE THE MOST OF YOUR MASSAGE

Here are some tips to help you make the most of your visit to a massage therapist:

- **Do not eat an hour before or after your session.** Digestion diverts circulation to the internal organs and can draw energy and attention away from the massage.

- **Be as relaxed and comfortable as possible.** If the bodywork practice requires you to disrobe, the therapist will drape you with a sheet and uncover only the body part being worked on. While a professional massage may feel pleas-urably sensuous, it is not intended to be a sexual experience.

- **Remove any jewelry and contact lenses.** They may obstruct the therapist's access to your body and cause discomfort to you if pressure is exerted over them.

- **Whether you talk or not during the massage is up to you.** If you prefer quiet and your massage therapist chatters on about the details of a horrific day, let her know you want silence. Keeping talk to a minimum can help you focus your full awareness on the bodywork experience.

- **Be aware of your body.** If something feels uncomfortable or painful, if you prefer unscented oil, or wish to keep part of your clothing on, let your therapist know.

- **Tell your massage therapist about any medical conditions or trouble spots.** Massage therapists will often fill out a short intake form during your first visit.

- **You may find yourself experiencing emotional releases during a session.** This is a normal response, and you shouldn't feel embarrassed. Depending upon the issues that surface, you may wish to seek qualified counseling.

- **You may find your body temperature going down during a massage treatment.** If you get cold, ask for additional covers.

- **Most important: Enjoy yourself.** Massage should be a relaxing experience. After the massage, take a few minutes to revel in the peace and calm of its afterglow. You may feel slightly disoriented because you are so relaxed. Move slowly at first so you can get your bearings.

HOW TO CHOOSE A PRACTITIONER

It's important to choose a massage therapist who is properly trained and skilled and whom you feel you can trust, no matter what type of bodywork you try. Here are some hints on selecting a practitioner:

- **Bodywork is both an art and a science.** As in any healing art, extent of formal training, years of experience, and natural gifts are all important criteria in selecting a practitioner.

- **Check the therapist's background.** Inquire whether the practitioner is licensed or certified and what that entails in your area. Backgrounds vary widely: Some practitioners may have only one or two days of formal training while others may have attended school for years.

- **Ask for personal recommendations from friends or healthcare providers.** Try to pinpoint what they like about the practitioner—what they value may be different from what you do.

- **Check for professional affiliations.** For instance, membership in a professional organization such as the American Massage Therapy Association (AMTA) means that a therapist has completed at least five hundred hours of study in such diverse areas as anatomy and physiology, pathology, hands-on practical work, and supplementary courses such as cardiopulmonary resuscitation (CPR), first aid, and business practices.

- **Look for an affiliation with a professional office.** Some doctors and chiropractors employ massage therapists on staff. Additionally, whatever practitioner you choose should be willing to work with your other healthcare providers.

- **Note the attitude of the practitioner and the environment in which he or she works.** Is he professional? Respectful? Most important, do you feel a rapport? A practitioner must inspire your confidence and trust.

- **Check with your local massage school.** It may provide a list of graduates or operate an on-site clinic.

- **If consulting the Yellow Pages, look for practitioners under the listings "Licensed Massage Therapist" or "Therapeutic Massage."** Be wary of listings for "Massage" and "Massage Parlors" as these are sometimes euphemisms for sex parlors.

- **Be wary of any massage therapist who claims he or she can "cure" you of an illness.** Massage therapists are not permitted to diagnose illness. Most agree their work is geared toward relaxation, which enables the body to rally its own recuperative powers.

- **Fees should be within the prevailing range for your geographic area and background of the practitioner.** Expect to pay $30 to $150 per hour for most types of work.

- **You may want to discuss a typical program of treatment in advance.** For instance, Rolfing typically involves a series of ten sessions; lessons in the Alexander Technique can entail twenty to thirty lessons; while a relaxing Swedish massage can be enjoyed as often as you choose.

- **If you need insurance reimbursement, check beforehand.** When prescribed by a doctor, massage therapy is sometimes reimbursed by insurance plans. You should check with your insurance carrier prior to treatment to determine its policy. Physicians sometimes need to be reminded that they can prescribe massage therapy as an indicated method of treatment.

A NOTE ON GENDER

In order to avoid use of the clumsy s/he construction, this book alternates chapter by chapter the use of *she* and *he* in referring to practitioners and clients. This underscores the fact that practitioners of both sexes provide nurturing, professional treatments.

INTRODUCTION

Massage is the new health treatment in town. Athletes use it. Doctors prescribe it. Lawyers, social workers, artists, computer programmers, stock analysts, plumbers and your neighbor all benefit from it.[1]

—HEALTH MAGAZINE

WHAT IS MASSAGE?

The field of massage and bodywork is rich and varied. While many people associate massage with relaxing touch, a landmark survey in *The New England Journal of Medicine* found no fewer than one hundred varieties of massage in use. Most people's notion of massage—lying on a table in a health spa or resort while a massage therapist plies an oil-soaked body with soothing strokes—is what is called Swedish massage. Sometimes referred to as traditional or Western massage, Swedish massage has historically formed the basis for massage in the United States.

Massage is traditionally defined as the manipulation of the soft tissues of the body for therapeutic purposes, using a system of strokes that include gliding, kneading, friction pressure, tapping, and vibrating. Additionally, massage therapists may engage in active and passive movement of the joints, use auxiliary mechanical devices, apply heat and cold in various forms, and instruct clients on exercises to achieve improved muscle tone, circulation, and range of motion.

The term "bodywork," which until recently meant only "auto repair" to most people, is more encompassing: It includes both traditional massage as well as other approaches to working with the body. Nearly all bodywork practices are united in their common goals of relaxation, pain relief, improved physical functioning, heightened vitality and well-being, and increased awareness.

1

The essence of bodywork is touch communication between a qualified giver and an open receiver. Body/mind modalities, where the recipient does most of the work herself without focused touch from another, such as visualization, biofeedback, hypnosis, and yoga, are not included in this book. Also excluded are other nontraditional therapies that act mainly by introducing external agents into the body, such as homeopathy or Chinese herbal medicine.

BODYWORK IS NOT A SUBSTITUTE FOR MEDICAL TREATMENT

Bodywork practices do not include the diagnosis or treatment of illness or disease, nor any service for which a separate license to practice is required by law, such as medicine, chiropractic, physical therapy, occupational therapy, acupuncture, or podiatry. Anyone who is suffering from a medical problem should seek appropriate attention from a qualified medical practitioner.

A BRIEF OVERVIEW OF THE HISTORY OF BODYWORK

Touch is as ancient as life itself, and it is the sense that is the earliest to develop in the human embryo. The first massage probably occurred spontaneously when the first human instinctively rubbed a hurt.

As long ago as 15,000 B.C., cave paintings in the Pyrénées depicted the therapeutic use of touch. In 8000 B.C., practitioners of yoga in India used breathing exercises to promote healing. More than two thousand years ago the ancient Chinese practice of manipulating pressure points provided the first written reference to bodywork. An ancient Egyptian papyrus from 1700 B.C. provides detailed knowledge of adjusting the spinal column by means of massage.

The ancient Greeks and Romans prized massage for its medical benefits. Hippocrates (c. 460–c. 377 B.C.), considered the father of Western medicine, and the physicians Galen (A.D. 129–c. 199) and Asclepiades of Bithynia (c. 124–40 B.C.) endorsed its therapeutic use. Julius Caesar was massaged daily for his epilepsy. Early Christians and medieval royalty practiced the laying on of hands. In the sixteenth century, Ambroise Paré (1517–1590), a French surgeon, introduced massage for stiff joints and wound healing following surgery. Experimentation with manipulation of bones and soft tissue by "bonesetters" continued during the Renaissance and Industrial Revolution. In the early nineteenth century, the modern Western practice of massage was systematized by Per Heinrik Ling (1776–1839).

Ashley Montagu, anthropologist and author of the acclaimed text *Touching*, has shown that soothing, nurturing touch is essential to life. Newborn animals must be licked by their mothers if they are to survive; rats that are petted grow and learn faster and develop greater immunity to disease than those that are not.[2] Touch deprivation can be devastating. Victorian mothers, schooled in the emerging science of hygiene, maintained a respectful distance from their off-spring with horrifying consequences: In the nineteenth century, more than half of all infants died within the first year of life from what was simply and tragically called "wasting away."[3]

THE ROLE OF MASSAGE AND BODYWORK IN HEALTH CARE IN THE UNITED STATES

As early as 1815, some physicians in America began to incorporate massage into their treatment programs. A well-known proponent and author on the subject of massage was Dr. John Harvey Kellogg, M.D. (1852–1943), who with his brother, Will (1860–1951), developed and established the breakfast cereal company that bears their name. Massage was practiced in hospitals in the United States and included physical therapy until the 1940s and 1950s, as the latter evolved into a separate discipline. As advances were made in the use of antibiotics and surgery, people began to believe that modern medicine could conquer any illness. Massage, as a therapeutic modality, declined.

In the 1970s, the growth of the human potential movement rekindled interest in massage, and many non-Swedish practices were introduced during this time. Interest in massage has continued to grow steadily into the twenty-first century.

With healthcare costs consuming a significant proportion of gross national product and increasing rapidly and no cure for many cancers or AIDS, many people have become disillusioned with orthodox medicine. "Traditional medicine is failing its patients," pronounced a lead-in to a revealing article in *The New York Times*.[4] We are increasingly using complementary and preventive approaches to health treatment. The success of such popular television series as Bill Moyers's *Healing and the Mind* underscores the widespread nature of this concern.

From CNN to *Time*, polls reinforce the same statistic: At least one-third of Americans are turning to alternative health care. *The New England Journal of Medicine* in a landmark 1993 study reported the provocative results of a survey that revealed Americans pay more visits to alternative healthcare providers than to orthodox medical practitioners. These Americans spent $10.3 billion out of pocket on such visits versus $12.8 billion out of pocket for all hospitalization costs. Significantly, this study reported that massage therapy was the third most popular of all alternative therapies.[5]

Responding to the urgency of this message, in late 1992 the Senate Appropriations Committee mandated the National Institutes of Health (NIH) to establish the Office of Alternative Medicine to evaluate complementary healthcare practices. In its first year of issuing research grants, this department awarded the greatest number to projects in the field of bodywork. This department is now known as the National Center for Complementary and Alternative Medicine (for updates on its activities, visit www.nccam.nih.gov).

Bodywork is empowering. It is at the forefront of complementary health practices that will guide us well in the twenty-first century. Up to 90 percent of all visits to medical doctors are prompted by conditions that result from stress and lifestyle choices, such as diet, exercise, and smoking. These are all conditions over which each of us has some control. The practices presented in this book can help you become more aware of your state of health so as to prevent the onset of illness.

THE COMMON FOUNDATIONS OF BODYWORK

While bodywork methods can vary greatly, there are recurrent themes that underlie many of the practices included in *Bodywork:*

- **Nearly all practices were developed by people seeking to cure their own illnesses first and foremost.** The formulation of techniques to teach their successful approaches followed.

- **Movement is life; stagnation is death.** Pain and disease arise from stagnation. ("Disease" literally signals dis-ease, or lack of ease.)

- **The human being is an organized, patterned whole.** Bodywork practices aim to restore balance and wholeness.

- **The self is the healer.** The practitioner, who only encourages the client's innate abilities to self-correct, might better be called a teacher (the literal meaning of "doctor"), facilitator, guide, coach, or midwife.

- **Change is possible.** No matter how chronic a problem may be, some relief is possible.

- **A practitioner's greatest tools are compassion and the intention to help and to heal.** The more our society becomes high tech, the more we crave high touch.

TOUCH RESEARCH INSTITUTE: THE SCIENTIFIC EVIDENCE

As one sign of the growing trend toward evaluating the therapeutic benefits of touch, the University of Miami Medical School established its Touch Research Institute (TRI) in September 1991. Billed as the first center in the world for research on the sense of touch, it provides a home base for a multidisciplinary staff of scientists, including Ph.D.s and M.D.s. Its founder and director, Dr. Tiffany Field, Ph.D., has been studying the effect of massage for many years. She is an unflaggingly eloquent spokesperson for the value of human touch.

Among Dr. Field's earliest findings was that premature infants who received massage treatments for three fifteen-minute periods per day for ten days gained 47 percent more body weight than infants treated with standard therapy.[6] Later studies showed that massage stimulates the release of food absorption hormones.[7] This translates into cost savings: Massaged infants were hospitalized six days less than unmassaged infants, for cost savings of three thousand dollars per infant. With premature births accounting for eighteen hundred or 10 percent of total new births in the University of Miami Hospital, the potential for cost savings is substantial. Significantly, the massaged infants in this study maintained their weight advantage eight months after discharge and exhibited greater motor and mental skills than their nonmassaged counterparts.[8] Other studies conducted by the Touch Research Institute suggest that massage can improve the functioning of the immune system in men infected with the AIDS virus, reduce stress and depression in adolescents, and boost workers' performance on the job.[9]

THE EVOLVING ROLE OF THE MASSAGE THERAPIST

Concurrently with the increasing emphasis on the role of complementary health practices, the profession of bodywork has been developing more professional and organized standards. Spurred on largely by efforts of the nonprofit American Massage Therapy Association (AMTA), the oldest association of massage professionals, massage practitioners have battled for, and won, the right in many states to use the professional title massage therapist. With support from the AMTA, state legislatures have also responded to the call for more organized recognition of the profession. Thirty-three states and the District of Columbia currently have state boards that regulate the profession through licensing, credentialing, or registration and have minimum education and/or testing requirements. Regulation of massage in the remaining states is overseen at the local level. In the early 1990s, a group of professional massage and bodywork volunteers initiated the development of the National Certification Board for Therapeutic Massage and Bodywork (NCBTMB), an independent, private, nonprofit organization. The mission of the NCBTMB is to foster high standards of ethical professional practice in the delivery of services through a recognized credible credentialing program that assures the competency of practitioners of therapeutic massage and bodywork. The NCBTMB developed a national certification exam, which was administered for the first time in the summer of 1992. While voluntary, this examination has come to be recognized or utilized by a growing number of states and local communities as a standard for admission to the practice of massage and bodywork.

The number of practicing massage therapists has grown dramatically over the last ten years. From 1994 to 2004, membership in the AMTA increased more than 270 percent to a current membership of more than forty-nine thousand, and schools that belong to the AMTA's Council of Schools now number nearly 400. Associated Bodywork & Massage Professionals (ABMP), a professional networking organization established in 1986, claims a current roster of more than fifty-two thousand members. The NCBTMB has certified more than eighty-five thousand practitioners since offering its first national exam in 1992.

Skilled in the latest knowledge of anatomy, physiology, and pathology, today's bodyworkers are professionally trained to help you maintain your health and support you in your healing process. Espousing a noninvasive approach to health, they offer you the luxury of uninterrupted attention to your body's needs. As Dr. Tiffany Field reminds us, "Before drugs, there was massage therapy."[10] Massage therapists and bodyworkers are schooled to talk and listen with their hands. It is their mission, and their joy, to serve you with the gift of touch communication. I encourage you to experience this gift, often, for yourself.

PART I

TRADITIONAL WESTERN MASSAGE

Behind your thoughts and feelings, my brother, there stands a mighty ruler, an unknown sage—whose name is self. In your body he dwells; he is your body.[1]

—FRIEDRICH NIETZSCHE

The most well-known bodywork method practiced in the West is Swedish massage, also known as traditional massage. Developed in the early 1800s, it has been refined continually since then. Swedish massage therapists apply oil or lotion to the body in a series of strokes designed to induce relaxation, improve circulation, and increase joint mobility.

The techniques of Swedish massage form the foundation for many contemporary Western-based bodywork practices, but many of these practices also incorporate new information gained from advances in the study of anatomy, physiology, neurobiology, and biomechanics. Generally, these practices are more specialized than Swedish massage and often involve advanced techniques and training. A representative cross section of the most widely available of these therapies follows the information on Swedish massage.

BASIC FACTS

- **Swedish massage is a therapeutic approach to healing.** It applies a scientific system of activity to the soft-tissue structure of the human body.
- **It was introduced by Per Heinrik Ling (1776–1839), a Swede (hence its name), in the early 1800s.** Ling integrated emerging knowledge of anatomy, physiology, and circulation of the blood with traditional Eastern healing techniques and his own set of physical exercises.

THEORY

- **Swedish massage works primarily to induce general relaxation while improving circulation and range of movement.**
- Massage induces the relaxation response, which aids recovery from stress and helps prevent the onset of illness and injury.
- Massage improves circulation, which can help reduce swelling from injury and enhance the functioning of the lymphatic system, which controls the immune response. Massage can also flush wastes, such as lactic acid, from tired muscles to relieve aches and pains.
- Massage breaks up adhesions from scar tissue, which restores flexibility and range of motion.

TYPICAL SESSION

- **Swedish massage sessions are usually a half hour to one hour in length.** (Treatments are shorter for children, the elderly, and the ill.) Treatment is administered on a firm flat padded table. The client disrobes and is draped with a towel and/or sheet. The therapist exposes only the area being massaged. Oils or lotion are applied to the body.
- **Therapists use the basic strokes of gliding, kneading, friction pressure, tapping, and vibration.** They may also incorporate active or passive physical exercises and heat, cold, or water (hydro) therapy to enhance the effectiveness of the treatment.
- Expect to pay $30 to $120 per hour for treatment.

BENEFITS

- **Massage is used to relieve a variety of complaints.** These include the pain and discomfort associated with chronic muscle tension, stiff joints, some forms of paralysis, sciatica, fractures, sprains, and overworked muscles. Receivers of massage often report a sense of heightened well-being.

- Dancers and athletes routinely use massage to enhance performance and speed recovery of sore muscles.

CONTRAINDICATIONS

- **Individuals suffering from any of the following conditions should refrain from any massage:** fever, vomiting, nausea, and diarrhea; jaundice; cancer; bleeding; and acute phlebitis, thrombosis, or varicose veins.

- **People suffering from the following may receive massage, but certain body parts should be avoided during treatment:** in the case of high blood pressure or heart problems, no massage to the abdomen; in the case of chronic varicose veins, fractures, or bruises, no massage directly over the site. Skin disorders may represent a local contraindication, but you should check with your physician first to make sure the condition is not communicable and cannot be spread within your own system.

- **Pregnant women should seek their doctors' advice before receiving treatment.**

BACKGROUND AND TRAINING OF PRACTITIONERS

- **The training of practitioners varies widely.** Thirty-three states and the District of Columbia currently have state boards that regulate the profession through licensing, credentialing, or registration, and have minimum education and/or testing requirements. Their requirements range from three hundred to one thousand hours of formal training. In the remaining seventeen states, massage is generally regulated at the local (city or county) level.

- **It is impossible to estimate precisely the number of practitioners.** Some industry experts place the number of massage therapists in the United States at between two and three hundred thousand. The AMTA, the oldest association of massage professionals in the country, boasts more than forty-nine thousand members who have completed massage school programs with a minimum of five hundred hours of formal training. Professional active members are required to complete forty-eight hours of continuing education every four years. ABMP claims more than fifty-two thousand members, and the NCBTMB has certified more than eighty-five thousand practitioners.

CHAPTER 1

SWEDISH MASSAGE
AND ITS VARIATIONS

The physician must be experienced in many things, but assuredly also in rubbing. . . . For rubbing can bind a joint which is too loose and loosen a joint that is too hard.[1]

—HIPPOCRATES

WHAT IS SWEDISH MASSAGE?

It is appropriate to begin our journey into the rich field of bodywork with Swedish massage as it serves as the foundation for traditional Western approaches to massage and is arguably the most well-known and commonly practiced form of bodywork today.

Swedish massage is a therapeutic approach to healing that applies a scientific system of activity to the soft-tissue structure of the human body by means of a variety of strokes, chief among which are effleurage, pétrissage, friction, tapotement, and vibration. Strokes are generally applied by hand with oil used to lessen friction; however, mechanical devices, such as vibrators, may also be used. In addition to stroking, some practitioners apply hot and cold packs, instruct in remedial exercises, and incorporate hydrotherapy in their treatments. Swedish massage can help the body remove toxins, deliver nutrients to tissues and cells more efficiently, and recover from strains and trauma more quickly.

THE ORIGINS OF SWEDISH MASSAGE

Swedish massage is called Swedish because the principles upon which it is based were most clearly formulated and promoted by a Swede, Per Heinrik Ling (1776–1839), in the early 1800s. Ling's system represents an eclectic synthesis of various healing approaches. He drew on knowledge gained from the emerging science of physiology and circulation of the blood (demonstrated by Harvey). He complemented this with his experience of body manipulations drawn from Eastern traditions and his own system of medical gymnastic rehabilitative exercises.

Ling's life story is a fascinating one with an almost New-Age quality to it. Ahead of his time, Ling might feel at home today teaching at the holistic explorational center Esalen or visiting an ashram in the Berkshires. He was the son of a church minister and earned a degree in divinity at the age of twenty-one. He then took off to see the world. Like many great healers, Ling developed his method in response to the challenge of an illness. He suffered from a debilitating case of rheumatoid arthritis and traveled through France and Germany seeking a cure. Penniless but incorrigibly curious, according to some accounts he went to China, where he studied Eastern principles of manipulation and kung fu with Taoist priests.

Ling was able to cure his rheumatism through the system of massage that he perfected. He introduced this system to the public in 1813, when he founded his school, The Royal Gymnastics Central Institute, in Stockholm. The system he created came to be known as the Ling treatment or the Swedish movement treatment.

Life was an uphill battle for Ling because at first the orthodox medical establishment rejected the claims of his work. By the time of his death, however, his method was widely accepted. In addition to introducing Swedish massage, he completed all the requirements of his day for medical study and bequeathed an impressive corpus of lyric poems, historical dramas, and national epics.

THE THEORY UNDERLYING SWEDISH MASSAGE

Swedish massage has many therapeutic benefits, including physical, mental, and emotional ones. It encourages well-being and optimum functioning by promoting relaxation, improved circulation, and mobility of joints.

Swedish massage promotes relaxation through the release of endorphins and enkephalins. These neurochemicals are dubbed "the body's natural opiates," or painkillers, due to their ability to induce relaxation and reduce pain. (Endorphins, like opiates, are habit forming, so don't be surprised if you become pleasurably addicted to massage.) Massage also promotes what Herbert Benson, M.D., coined "the relaxation response" in his best-selling book of the same title.[2] The relaxation response is an antidote to the fight-or-flight response, which is an excited way in which many of us react to situations of stress. The pressures of modern life are sending us increasingly into this mode.

Massage induces the relaxation response, enabling us to keep stress within a manageable range. Experts underscore how crucial this is to maintaining good health. Stress has been shown to impair the functioning of the immune system, which makes us more susceptible to disease. It also inhibits the restorative process of healing and recuperation and accelerates the aging process.[3] In fact, many illnesses today are psychosomatic, and many experts claim that as much as 80 percent of all illness is caused by stress.

Massage also improves both blood and lymph circulation. They are increased due to the mechanical hand movements applied during massage. In addition to helping nutrients reach their target cells in the body, increased circulation helps the body remove toxins more efficiently. For instance, after physical exercise, we frequently suffer from a buildup of lactic acid, or a lack of oxygen, in fatigued muscles. This results in all too familiar soreness and stiffness. Massage helps to flush out lactic acid, which accounts for massage's ability to remove the achiness caused by overexertion. The lymph system is our key defense in finding and fighting infection in the body. By promoting better circulation of lymph, massage also helps us to strengthen our immune system and protect us from illness. Dr. Field's studies on HIV-infected men indicated that massage—in addition to leading to reduced levels of stress—tended to increase the number of natural killer cells, one of the body's key weapons in the battle against the life-challenging AIDS virus.[4]

Massage improves range of motion in the joints as well as overall mobility. Friction strokes are extremely effective in breaking down adhesions that form around joints, particularly following sprains, fractures, or other injuries where scar tissue forms. Massage can help cut the healing time of minor sprains by as much as one-half.

To accomplish its goals, Swedish massage draws on a repertoire of five basic strokes. Like the techniques of many other great arts, including cooking, skiing, and horsemanship, these strokes have French names. This fact reflects Ling's indebtedness to the French, who first translated an ancient Chinese text, *The Cong-Fou of the Tao-Tse,* which most likely served as the basis for his system of strokes.[5]

Effleurage ("touching lightly") is a smooth, gliding stroke that generally initiates a Swedish massage treatment. It is often performed with the broad palm surface of both hands, but can also use the thumbs, fingers, or knuckles. It is used to relax soft tissue (muscles, ligaments, tendons, and connective tissue) for deeper work as well as being an exploratory stroke, which enables the massage therapist to examine the texture and quality of the tissues on which she will work. Effleurage has the beneficial effect of increasing the circulation of blood and lymph in the body. Effleurage, like all strokes, is generally applied in the direction of the heart in order to encourage the return of blood from the veins.

Pétrissage ("kneading") consists of wringing, squeezing, rolling, and kneading (like kneading bread dough) the muscles, using one or two hands, the thumbs, or the fingers. Pétrissage often follows effleurage. It encourages circulation in the deeper veins and lymph vessels of the body. This increase in circulation has the benefit of bringing nutrients—digested food particles and oxygen—to cells to help them grow and repair. It also helps remove waste products that are released by the cells into the blood.

Friction ("rubbing") is the deepest of all the strokes. It consists of deep circular or transverse movements with the pads of the thumbs or fingers to soft tissue so that the underlying layers of tissue actually rub against one another. This stroke is a powerful tool in breaking down adhesions that form in the body from such processes as formation of scar tissue. Additionally, friction causes an increase in blood flow (local hyperemia) to the massaged area, which aids circulation to provide increased nutrition. A therapist must first warm up a body part with effleurage and/or pétrissage in order to perform the deeper friction strokes.

Tapotement ("tapping"), sometimes also known as percussion or pounding, is performed with cupped hands, fingers, or the edge of the hand. The massage therapist rapidly strikes the client's body with short, alternating blows. (This is the stroke the caricatured, powerful Scandinavian woman uses to pummel a client's back.) Tapotement also increases circulation to the area being treated. When performed for a short period of time (fewer than ten seconds), it helps stimulate circulation to an area of atrophy, for instance. When executed for a longer period of time (up to sixty seconds), its effect is relaxing. When used beyond sixty seconds, it exhausts the body part being worked on. This could be effective in providing relief from complaints such as muscle spasms.

Vibration ("shaking") is performed by placing the hand or fingers on the body and rapidly shaking them as the hand moves over an area. This stroke is particularly effective in working on the nerves. As with tapotement, short-term work is stimulating while longer-term vibration is relaxing.

THE TYPICAL FORMAT OF A SWEDISH MASSAGE SESSION

A typical Swedish massage lasts thirty minutes to an hour, with the longer session allowing for more extensive treatment. (Sessions are generally shorter for children, the elderly, and the ill.) For treatment, the client disrobes, either completely or down to his underwear or other comfortable level of clothing. He lies on a firm, flat, padded massage table, which is covered with a sheet. The massage therapist places a towel, sheet, or blanket over the client's body to ensure modesty. Professional draping also provides additional warmth as well as privacy. The massage therapist uncovers only the particular body part she is working on at any given time.

The massage therapist applies oil to the client's skin. Oil is used to make the massage strokes more smooth and flowing. Because oils are sometimes scented, you should let the therapist know if you are allergic to any aromas or find any scents offensive. The practitioner should be able to work with unscented oils, lotion, talc, or no lubricant if you prefer.

During a Swedish massage, the therapist weaves the five strokes of Swedish massage into a finely orchestrated treatment, like a choreographer constructing a ballet. Her treatment plan is designed to provide the greatest therapeutic benefit. The practitioner may also incorporate active and passive exercises, some with resistance, to help strengthen and tone muscles and increase range of motion in joints. Some practitioners use heat, cold, or hydro (water) therapy in their treatments.

Most Swedish massage sessions are full-body sessions, where the therapist massages the entire body. It is possible, however, to arrange more specialized sessions focusing on particular problem areas.

THE EXPERIENCE: I GET RUBBED THE RIGHT WAY

I arrive at the office of Bruria Ginton, a licensed massage therapist and founder and manager of Associated Massage Therapists, a cooperative association of licensed professionals. She is a past president of the New York State chapter of the American Massage Therapy Association. I've come to receive a session of Swedish massage with Bruria, who has been in private practice for more than fifteen years, on the advice of a friend who recommended Bruria's nurturing touch. Bruria's office is part of QWL Services, which is composed of a variety of healthcare professionals (a psychotherapist, a chiropractor, other bodyworkers, and an acupuncturist) who share a suite of offices on Manhattan's Upper West Side.

As I enter, Bruria warmly greets me at the reception area, which resembles that of a doctor's or any other professional's office. The spacious collection of offices and treatment rooms is painted clean white and decorated with plants and prints. A subtle, pleasing aroma lingers in the air; it smells like a combination of fragrant oils and freshly laundered linen.

Bruria is a short, fair-skinned woman; her long dark hair frames her smiling face. Her eyes shine as she welcomes me into her healing space and hands me a brief questionnaire to complete. In addition to requesting basic information such as name, address, and phone number, it has some questions regarding my medical history, including conditions such as infections, fever, surgery, heart problems, medications, and any skin conditions, as well as a few lifestyle questions regarding exercise and diet.

Once the questionnaire is complete, Bruria shows me to the treatment area, a small studio room. The golden light of a late-October morning streams through the window. A padded massage table is positioned in the center of the room; a white sheet covers it. There is a desk with a stool in front of it and opposite that is a straight-backed chair. Bruria asks me to be seated in the chair while she sits at the stool at her desk.

"I'll just take a few minutes to discuss the work we'll be doing and to get to know one another," she explains.

After asking me about any medical conditions I might have about which she should know, Bruria describes her practice. "Seventy percent of my clients come to me for sports-related treatments. Many of these clients are active in marathon and triathlon activities; some in world-class competition," she explains. (Somewhat modestly, I think later, when I notice photographs of Grete Waitz and Allison Roe, world-famous marathoners, as well as testimonials from other celebrities she has counted among her clients, including figure skater Judy Blumberg and Olympic runner Matt Centrowitz, all of whom have considered massage an important component in their training programs.) "The rest of my clients are stressed-out people, often executives, who want to improve their performance, too.

"I try to approach each client as an individual and design a treatment geared for his or her particular needs. I consider myself client-centered, not technique-oriented. I believe it's important to learn proper technique; however, every practitioner is different, so that no two people even do the same technique the same way.

"Of course, Swedish massage forms the basis of my treatments. Swedish is terribly important, because it improves the circulation, and that is the basis of life. The circulatory system is both the hospital and sewer system of the body. It fosters the functioning of the immune system by improving the flow of lymph; it takes nutrients to where they're needed via the blood system, and then helps to remove toxic buildups through the circulatory system as well. Effleurage, the basic stroke of Swedish massage, is the most important stroke because it is a tremendous aid to circulation.

"It's also important to recognize the role of the mind in healing, too. I have a degree in organizational psychology as well as sports psychology. Both disciplines have a lot in common—they're both about maximizing performance.

Sports psychology uses a lot of visualizations and guided imagery to achieve this. I think that can be helpful in massage also. I've studied hypnotherapy and sometimes I'll incorporate it in my work if it's appropriate—it's important to work with the mind, too. You have to remember that the mind is a fifty percent partner with the body in the healing process.

"The emotional aspect of healing is also important. In our society, we don't have enough touch. Massage fulfills an important need. All of these elements are important, not one more than the other."

Bruria views massage therapy as being therapeutic and educational. It is a valuable adjunct to orthodox health care; both complement one another nicely. She is pleased that massage has gained this status, although she has been practicing long enough to have experienced firsthand its growing pains.

"I remember when I was studying psychology in college years ago. Our professor once said, 'You should be especially nice to Bruria. She gives massages, you know,' punctuating his remarks with a wink. It was frustrating to see a well-educated man equate massage with sex. Fortunately, the profession has come a long way."

Having shared her philosophy and outlook, Bruria explains that she'll leave the room so that I can disrobe, down to my underwear, in privacy. After undressing, I should lie flat on my back on the table and cover myself with the long cotton towel that she points out to me. My face will be pointing toward the ceiling. She suggests that I may want to center myself in quiet meditation for a few minutes in preparation for the massage.

Before she leaves the room, Bruria asks if I like classical music. (I wonder how she knew I once dreamed of a career as a concert pianist.) I tell her I love classical music. Soon the strains of a Beethoven violin sinfonietta begin to relax me as I prepare for a session with her.

I'm all settled when Bruria returns to the treatment room. She asks me if there are any particular areas where I tend to carry tension or to which I would like to direct her attention. I tell her I carry chronic tension in my back. She begins her treatment by sliding her fingers under my shoulder blades, feeling for pockets of tension in the muscle and tissue there, then feels along the side of my spine.

"Not too bad," she says. "There's a little tension, but not too bad."

She then moves on to my shoulders and neck.

Ouch! Are those tight cable wires masquerading as flesh? I wonder, as her fingers slide across the tough muscles that run down my neck from my jaw to my shoulders. I'm not in pain. Bruria's touch feels firm and deep, not invasive. The sensation is more of tenderness, of an area that is tense and wants to be touched so it can release.

"You're a little more tense here," she reports in her understated way.

I sure am and didn't even realize it.

Bruria encourages me to relax as she continues to glide her fingers across my neck muscles. "This time is for you, to take time out of your busy day and just relax." Her hypnotic voice is inducing the same powerful relaxation in my mind as her hands are doing to my neck. She rolls my head from side to side, stretching and releasing my neck as she does so.

Having begun with this preliminary relaxing work performed without oil, Bruria prepares me for the rest of the treatment. She positions a soft cylindrical roll, a pillow that feels as though it's filled with form-fitting sand, beneath the hollow of my neck, which feels firmly and comfortably supported. She has heated the neck roll first, so that it radiates a delightfully soothing heat that further relaxes my recently released muscles. She places a large round bolster under my knees. This allows my low back to sink into the massage table and I feel even more at ease. She wraps a light blanket around my entire body; I feel safe and toasty warm.

"Please let me know if anything is uncomfortable to you as we work," Bruria encourages me. "If my pressure is too deep or too light, please let me know. Also let me know if you feel too hot or too cold or are uncomfortable in any way. I assure you I won't take it personally. I know that no one is perfect and I have a lot to learn." She is a master at making me feel at ease about expressing my personal preferences.

Bruria begins by working on my right arm. She strokes my fingers, wrist, and forearm. She kneads my upper arm and its biceps and triceps as though it was unbaked baguette dough. At times, she applies pressure from her thumb in a deeper friction stroke directly into the tissue. She briskly taps and hacks her fingers along the large surfaces of my arm. She repeats the sequence on my left arm. As she massages, I am aware by the presence of her touch of areas of tenderness I hadn't noticed before. I feel them there, in my forearms, and especially in my triceps, the large muscle at the back of the upper arm. This tenderness signifies places where I'm holding tension.

"Your triceps are very tight, especially the right one," Bruria shares. "Do you work out a lot?" Yes, I do, and I realize that along with my dedication to building my muscles and keeping in shape, I may be working out too much. "When muscles get tight, they block off the flow of circulation. When you work out, you're contracting your muscles. It's important to stretch before and after working out to help the muscles return to their normal resting position," Bruria reminds me. "Also, you can do a little self-massage before and after working out and before you go to bed." As she demonstrates some basic kneading and friction strokes I can do on myself, she adds: "I think it's important for people to learn what they can do to take care of themselves. I see part of my job as educating clients to better maintain their health."

Bruria moves on to massage my abdomen. She lowers the blanket that had covered my chest, moving it to the bottom of my belly, then applies a light coating of oil. The palms of her hands move in a circle around my stomach, first lightly, then more deeply. Gradually she increases the pressure so that her palms are compressing in a clockwise direction around my solar plexus. She asks me to take a deep breath as she compresses further. The pressure is firm, but not painful. I feel as though all my vital organs are being massaged. She further massages the area as she passes her hands back and forth in a crisscrossing motion across my abdomen.

"I think of the solar plexus as the center of our internal environment," she explains. "Not only does it contain the digestive tract, but it also houses the liver, which detoxifies the body; the adrenals and kidneys are behind it; and the stomach is located there, too. This gives a good massage to stimulate the whole internal environment."

Bruria draws the blanket back up over my chest and arms and exposes my right leg. Her hands glide gently up my leg as she applies oil in a long, flowing effleurage stroke that begins at the tip of my toes and progresses to the top of my thigh. She gradually increases the pressure of the strokes as she moves from my lower leg to my thigh. She applies deep pressure strokes with her thumb running up through the midline of my thigh. It feels sensitive, borderline painful, but a good kind of pain. On a scale of 1 to 10, it's an 8.

"Does this feel tender?" Bruria asks. "It seems a little tight."

Are there no secrets I can keep from her?

As she continues her muscle-stripping friction strokes, I continue to feel a combination of pain and release. Ah, yes, it hurts so good!

Bruria finishes with my right leg, drapes it again, then repeats the sequence on my left leg.

She then removes the blanket and, while holding the edge of the towel that covers me, asks me to turn over, so that I'm lying on my stomach. I roll over while maintaining my sense of privacy, my body shielded by the towel. After again covering me with the blanket, she attaches a padded face cradle to the end of the table. I relax my face into it. She places a high stool under the face cradle to support my arms, encouraging me to rest them on it to make myself more comfortable.

Bruria moves to the foot of the table and places a bolster under my ankles, which relaxes and stretches the muscles of my legs. With this positioning, she can work more deeply in the muscles of my legs because they are not contracted. She begins by applying oil in an effleurage stroke to my right leg. The back of my thigh is particularly sensitive, and she observes, "Your hamstrings are very tight." She applies some deep gliding and friction strokes to this set of muscles, from their insertions below the knee up through their muscle bellies to their origins at what is known colloquially as the "sit" bone. Once again, the strokes are slightly painful but releasing. She finishes working on my leg by pressing her thumb into the belly of my calf muscle, then compressing her knuckles into the soles of my foot. She repeats the same treatment to my left leg, redraping each leg as she finishes with it.

Bruria concludes the session by massaging my back. She removes the blanket but is solicitous to know if I am still warm enough or if I would like additional covers. "I often find my body cools down as I receive a massage," she explains. My body temperature does feel a little cooler to me, but I'm comfortable the way I am.

Bruria applies oil to my back with long effleurage strokes. She palpates the tone and texture of the tissue along my spine and asks me if I feel tender in the area of my midback, which is where I tend to hold my tension. She does some friction strokes there to release adhesions, then begins to knead my upper back. That area is indeed tender, much more so than I had realized. "The upper trapezius muscles, which cover the upper back and shoulder area, are tight in nearly everyone," she says. I suppose she's trying to make me feel better, but I'm still aware of the tension. Her strokes do begin, gradually, to assuage the pain. She moves on to my neck, kneading the deep bands of tissue with firm pressure. She performs some large crisscrossing motions with her two hands all along my back; briskly taps the whole large surface area of my back with the outside edge of her hands (which feels invigorating and stimulating); then completes treatment of my back with a few gentle nerve strokes, where she lightly strokes her fingers along my back. I feel both relaxed *and* energized.

Bruria covers my back with the blanket and slowly rubs the blanket and towel underneath it to remove any excess oil from my body. I am floating on a sea of peaceful bliss.

Bruria announces that the session has nearly come to an end. She asks me to remain restfully in the position I'm in and to take a moment to meditate; with my eyes closed to slowly scan my body; to realize as I do so how much more relaxed I feel than when I entered her office; and to take that feeling with me, let it carry forward with me into the rest of my week. "When you feel tense and stressed out, take a deep breath and remember this feeling of peace."

She explains that she'll be leaving the room. Once she's gone, I should rest; then when I'm ready, get up from the table, dress, and meet her at the reception desk.

I slowly take stock of my body. I feel tremendous relaxation. My muscles feel as though they've undergone a meltdown, like pieces of earthenware going in reverse from baked clay to pliant potter's mud. The small pockets in my body where I still feel a little tension are a kind of barometer to me of how relaxed the rest of my body feels, and even of how much better those areas of my body feel relative to how I felt only a short hour ago.

My body has melded with the table. I take a few minutes to savor the sweet sense of relaxation, peace, and wholeness I feel, as though resting in an oasis, and slowly rise, dress, and bid farewell to Bruria.

As I walk outside, I ask myself: *Is the air really cleaner? My body lighter? My mind clearer? Or do I only feel that way?* No matter the answer, I have Bruria, and the restorative strokes of her Swedish massage, to thank for allowing me to feel the questions in the first place.

THE BENEFITS OF SWEDISH MASSAGE

Anyone who has had a Swedish massage knows that it feels good. Aside from being pleasurable, however, it has many added benefits. Individuals have used massage to obtain relief for a host of complaints, including the discomfort and pain associated with chronic muscle tension, stiff joints, some forms of paralysis, sciatica, fractures, sprains, and overworked muscles.

Dancers, athletes, and performing artists routinely use massage to enhance performance and speed recovery of sore muscles. Dance superstar Rudolf Nureyev regularly received massage; Cloris Leachman has been reported to get massaged before her performances and Luciano Pavarotti to take a massage therapist with him wherever he goes.[6] World-class athletes such as Mary Decker Slaney, Judy Blumberg, Michael Seibert, and the New York Giants football team have all benefited from massage. Seven-time New York Marathon champ Grete Waitz says: "I believe everyone who runs should be massaged. In fact, everyone who lives should be massaged."[7]

Massage can actually help reduce pain. Studies at the University of California at Irvine showed that patients given a combination of Swedish massage and acupressure before receiving chemotherapy experienced less pain and nausea during and after treatment. Additionally, surgery patients who were given massage before their operations required less premedication than those who did not.[8]

Contrary to what some people think (or hope), massage will not dissolve fat or increase muscle mass. However, by improving circulation, massage will help bring the nutrients that are needed for muscle development to where they're needed and will help the body's metabolism function more efficiently. Massage can help prevent or reduce muscle atrophy in people who are forced to be inactive due to injury, illness, or age.

In addition to its physiological effects, massage has the benefit of inducing a relaxed state of alertness, resulting in a calmer mind and clearer thinking. In fact, many people who receive massage liken its effects to meditation. It is no wonder that research studies at the Touch Research Institute (TRI) have shown that medical school staff who got a fifteen-minute massage after lunch twice a week were able to solve complex math problems more quickly and accurately than those who didn't.[9] Often clients report feeling taller or lighter after receiving a massage. And their friends, noticing something different about them, may ask, "Have you lost weight?"

Sometimes you may not be aware of any dramatic change. One client once told me after a massage, "You know, I didn't feel anything in particular after the session, but then I realized I had an experience of deep well-being that lasted several days. The only thing I could attribute it to was the massage."

I often feel energized for several days after a massage. I can jump higher in aerobics class, press more weight at the gym, and ideas flow more freely and creatively when I sit down to write. Many of my clients are artists who find that massage gets their creative juices flowing. You may also find your dreams taking on a new dimension following a massage treatment: You may remember them more clearly, they may be more vivid, or they may contain insight into various problems with which you've been grappling.

Massage also has the emotional benefits of satisfying the need for caring and nurturing, reducing anxiety, and imparting a general sense of well-being and harmony. Research studies have shown that depressed and anxious children and adolescents who received massage showed reduced levels of anxiety, were more cooperative, and slept better than a control group who watched relaxing videos but received no massage.[10] Massage was also effectively used to reduce posttraumatic stress experienced by children in the aftermath of Hurricane Andrew.[11] And teams of massage therapists in New York City provided relief to rescue workers in the aftermath of the events of September 11, 2001.

In another TRI study, elderly subjects who themselves received massage and also gave massage to infants reported fewer medical complaints, less anxiety and stress, and fewer trips to the doctor than those who did not.[12] Significantly, they showed the greatest improvement when giving a massage. As a massage therapist, I can totally understand this. I often feel more centered and calmer after I've given a massage. (In fact, this is one of a massage therapist's best-keep secrets.)

CONTRAINDICATIONS TO SWEDISH MASSAGE

Massage is appropriate to use in nearly any situation. However, like any therapy, there are certain situations that indicate massage should not be given, or its use should be modified because it could prove harmful. Generally speaking, a full-body contraindication (meaning no massage at all) is advised for anyone suffering from any of the following conditions: fever; vomiting, nausea, or diarrhea; pain due to unknown cause; arthritis in one joint; or jaundice (in all of the preceding cases, the possibility of infection is present, and massage could spread the infection); cancer; bleeding; some skin disorders; acute phlebitis, thrombosis, or varicose veins (the last three conditions can result in blood clotting, and massage can transport the blood clot, risking stroke or heart failure).

Local contraindications (meaning massage may be given, but certain areas should be avoided) include the following: No massage should be given to the abdomen in cases of high blood pressure or heart problems; in the case of chronic varicose veins, no massage should be given over the site, but massage above the site can help to improve circulation, which will help the varicosities; and no massage should be given directly over the site of fractures, bruises, or keloid scars. Skin disorders may represent a local contraindication, but you should check first with your physician to make sure the condition is not communicable and cannot be spread within your own system.

Pregnant women should check with their doctors before receiving massage. Some massage practitioners specialize in massaging pregnant women, using customized techniques in a side-lying position. (Massage, by the way, is now being provided in some hospital delivery rooms to speed up the recovery period for both newborns and mothers.)

BACKGROUND AND TRAINING OF PRACTITIONERS

The training of practitioners varies widely. Thirty-three states and the District of Columbia currently have state boards that regulate massage therapists. Their requirements range from 300 to 1,000 hours of formal training. In the remaining seventeen states, massage is generally regulated at the local (city or county) level. In a growing number of these states, large cities and counties often utilize the National Certification Exam for Therapeutic Massage and Bodywork (NCETMB) as a criterion for admission to the practice of massage. The NCETMB is a voluntary examination, first offered in 1992 by the independent, nonprofit National Certification Board for Therapeutic Massage and Bodywork (NCBTMB). More detailed information on the NCBTMB can be found in Chapter 18: Resources for Further Exploration.

The American Massage Therapy Association (AMTA) requires that its members be graduates of a 500 in-class hour entry-level massage therapy program, or have a passing score on the NCETMB, or a license from an appropriate state regulatory board. Beginning with the first full year of active professional membership, a member is required to complete forty-eight clock hours of training every four years for renewal as an active professional member. Practitioner level of membership in Associated Bodywork & Massage Professionals (ABMP) requires a minimum of 100 hours of massage and bodywork education, and is available only in states that have not set credentialing requirements. Professional level of membership requires 500 hours of education or state massage licensure or certification. In addition, ABMP offers a certified level of membership and an esthetician level of membership. Details can be obtained from the ABMP, whose contact information follows in the section "For Further Information" below.

Because there is no standardized regulation and no single national association to which all professionals belong, it is difficult to estimate precisely the number of practitioners. The AMTA boasts more than forty-nine thousand members, a 270 percent increase over its 1994 membership and the ABMP claims more than fifty-two thousand members. The NCBTMB has certified more than eighty-five thousand practitioners. Some industry experts place the total number of massage therapists in the United States at between two and three hundred thousand.

FOR FURTHER INFORMATION

If you're interested in further information on massage or would like to find the name of a practitioner near you, the following are among the largest and most informative professional organizations:

The American Massage Therapy Association
500 Davis Street, Suite 900
Evanston, IL 60201-4695
Tel: (877) 905-2700 or (847) 864-0123
Fax: (847) 864-1178
Website: www.amtamassage.org
E-mail: info@amtamassage.org

Associated Bodywork & Massage Professionals
1271 Sugarbrush Drive
Evergreen, CO 80439
Tel: (800) 458-2267 or (303) 674-8478
Fax: (800) 667-8260
Websites: multiple sites for various issues
  www.abmp.com (ABMP's main site)
  www.massageandbodywork.com (an ABMP magazine)

www.massagetherapy.com (ABMP's consumer-related site)
www.bodysensemagazine.com (an ABMP publication)
E-mail: expectmore@abmp.com

SUGGESTED FURTHER READING

The following books are written by massage professionals:

Frances M. Tappan and Patricia J. Benjamin, *Tappan's Healing Massage Techniques: Holistic and Emerging Methods,* 4th Edition (Upper Saddle River, NJ: Pearson Education, 2005). This book details the techniques of Swedish massage while presenting descriptions of other holistic and emerging bodywork techniques.

Elizabeth C. Wood, and Paul D. Becker, *Beard's Massage* (Philadelphia, PA: W. B. Saunders, 1981). This book provides a detailed history of Swedish massage techniques, with black-and-white photos of various strokes.

FOR DO-IT-YOURSELFERS

Fiona Harrold, *The Complete Body Massage: A Hands-On Manual* (New York: Sterling Publishing Company, Inc., 1992). This is a handsomely photographed book by the director of the London College of Massage.

Clare Maxwell-Hudson, *The Complete Book of Massage* (New York: Random House, 1988). A lavishly illustrated and well-written step-by-step guide to giving a massage.

VIDEOS

Esalen Massage (Riverside, CT: At Peace Media, 1997). This hands-on instructional video presents a complete full-body massage session in the style developed and practiced at the celebrated Esalen Institute in Big Sur, California.

Massage for Health (Santa Monica, CA: Healing Arts Home Video, 1988). This is an excellent videotape that demonstrates how to perform a simple, pleasurable, and therapeutic massage, featuring Shari Belafonte-Harper; written and performed by Mirka Knaster and James Heartland, two massage pros.

Massage Your Mate (New York: V.I.E.W. Video Inc., 1987). An excellent videotape for the professional as well as layman, this features New York State–licensed massage therapist Rebecca Klinger demonstrating Swedish massage and acupressure.

VARIATIONS ON SWEDISH MASSAGE

The techniques of Swedish massage form the foundation of many contemporary Western-based bodywork practices. In addition to using the strokes and principles of Swedish massage, many of these practices incorporate new information gained from advances in sciences like neurobiology and biomechanics. Generally, these practices are more specialized than Swedish massage and often involve advanced techniques and training. Many share the common goals of physical relaxation and rehabilitation. The benefits and contraindications of these approaches as well as the fees are also similar to those of Swedish massage.

Medical Massage: Working from a Doctor's Rx

Medical massage has developed specific techniques for treating injuries and a wide variety of illnesses as well as aiding in physical rehabilitation. Massage therapists who practice medical massage work under a prescription provided by a physician or chiropractor directing them in their course of treatment. Medical massage applies the basic strokes of Swedish massage in specialized techniques that are geared toward achieving precise physiological results. Because therapists work under a doctor's prescription, your chances of having massage treatment covered by an insurance plan are generally greater with medical massage than with other types of massage.

Some massage schools, such as the Swedish Institute in New York City, provide extensive training, including hands-on experience treating a variety of medical problems in a supervised clinic, as part of their core curriculum. Other schools, such as the New Mexico Academy of Healing Arts in Santa Fe, have offered medical massage both as part of a core curriculum and as a part-time specialized course of study for those with previous bodywork training or experience.

Massage therapists trained in medical massage are prepared to treat a variety of common pathological conditions. Chief among these are spinal deformities, such as lordosis (an exaggerated anterior tilt to the lower portion of the spine, sometimes also called saddleback or hollow back), kyphosis (hunchback), and scoliosis (lateral curvature of the spine); brachial neuralgia (a pinching of the nerves around the shoulder, causing pain, especially upon raising the arm); different forms of tendinitis (such as tennis elbow); chondromalacia patellae (wearing away or softening of the back surface of the kneecap, which can lead to pain in the knee); bursitis (pain to joint areas caused by pressure on the bursae, or padlike sacs, that surround them); sciatica (inflammation of the sciatic nerve, often accompanying pinched disks in the low back); repetitive stress disorders; fractured bones; and sprained ankles. Medical massage can also be helpful for temporomanidubular joint (TMJ) disorder, a dysfunction that often results in chronic tension and pain in the jaw along with grinding of the teeth. If this sounds familiar, it's no wonder—nearly 50 million Americans are estimated to suffer from TMJ disorder and many other people experience related headaches and stress in the eyes, shoulders, and back.

A medical massage treatment typically differs from a full-body Swedish massage in length of treatment—it's generally shorter—and focus. Medical massage concentrates on a particular medical condition, and while strokes are focused on the problem area, treatment is often applied to adjoining areas to promote circulation to and from the affected part. The corresponding body part on the other side of the body is also often massaged because it may be compensating for the weakness on the problem side. For instance, if a client reported pain from tennis elbow in the right arm, the focus of a medical massage would be to the right arm and elbow in particular. The adjoining areas of the wrist and shoulder would also be massaged. The left arm would be treated, too, which would help the client feel more balanced. In addition, the massage therapist might provide some large, general strokes to the entire body to promote over-all relaxation.

Massage therapists who practice medical massage must be particularly well informed about contraindications to massage as well as about the course of disease processes. They must be familiar with any other medical treatments, including medications, a client may be undergoing so as to be aware of possible side effects. Medical massage therapists are trained to work in concert with an individual's primary healthcare practitioner to administer optimum treatment. This may also include the application of heat and cold therapy to specific areas of the body as well as suggesting physical exercises to benefit a given medical condition.

The Swedish Institute was the first school of massage to operate a full-time medical massage clinic, the P. H. Ling Clinic, and patients there must be referred for treatment by a doctor. Russ Beasley, an administrator of the clinic, says common complaints referred for treatment include rheumatoid arthritis and osteoarthritis, multiple sclerosis, low back pain, osteoporosis, psoriasis, myofascitis and fibromyalgia (generalized muscle and soft tissue irritation and pain), sciatica, whiplash, spinal deformities, brachial neuralgia, HIV-related conditions, and soft tissue joint disorders. Jill Thompson, L.M.T., M.Div., instructor of pathology at the Swedish Institute for more than twenty-five years and former supervisor of its Ling Clinic, is a firm believer in the medical value of massage: "Massage *really, really* helps," she intones with a hint of the fervor of an evangelical minister suffusing her voice. "In the case of a minor sprain to the ankle, massage can help the ankle recover in one third the normal time. In more serious instances, like muscular dystrophy and various forms of spastic and flaccid paralysis, massage can improve circulation to the affected areas. In addition, the therapist can direct exercise movements, thus helping retard muscle atrophy. And even in cases where massage may not offer a physiological 'cure,' like AIDS, it can provide the intangible but valuable benefits of caring human contact and support."

Sports Massage: Maximizing Peak Performance

Sports massage is a specialty area of traditional massage that assists the body to achieve maximum physical results. Administered before physical activity, it can help protect against pain and injuries while boosting performance. Following physical exertion, it helps remove lactic acid and restore normal muscle tone and range of motion. Sports massage is a powerful aid to anyone who wants to use his body at maximum efficiency: not only professional but also weekend athletes; dancers, actors, musicians, and other performing artists; as well as people whose occupations require physical exertion, like painters, construction workers, and busy homemakers. In short, sports massage can help nearly everyone.

Massage has traditionally been used to relieve muscle pains following physical exertion. Ling's original Swedish massage techniques were used by Swedish cavalry officers as a restorative measure in the nineteenth century. In recent times, the dancer Rudolf Nureyev relied on massage to relieve the nearly constant pain he suffered from chronically recurring dance injuries, pain so debilitating he had to measure his steps to the bathroom for fear of aggravating it.[13]

Massage has been used for many years in Europe, especially in the former Eastern bloc countries, not only as a restorative but also as a boost to athletic performance. Jack Meagher, the physical therapist who is credited with introducing sports massage to this country, became interested in it when a German POW at his military base in France during World War II gave him pregame massages to better his performance in camp football games. Meagher's interest in pursuing sports massage was solidified when his career as a professional baseball pitcher was cut short by an old war injury to his shoulder. Appropriate massage to the area provided so much relief that Meagher was able to work semipro. It was not until the 1980s that the medical community in this country began to appreciate the benefits that sports massage can bring. Since that time, sports massage has represented one of the fastest-growing segments of the massage field, becoming a valued adjunct to any situation where peak physical performance is essential. In fact, Jack Meagher claims that sports massage can increase physical performance by 20 percent.

In 1985, the American Massage Therapy Association established a National Sports Massage Certification Program, followed shortly thereafter by the AMTA National Sports Massage Team. More than three hundred massage therapists from this group traveled with groups like the U.S. Olympic teams, among others, to make massage available to every athlete at the Games. While this program has currently been discontinued at the national level, some state chapters of the AMTA have their own sports massage teams. Soviet athletic teams travel with their massage therapists, and the New York Giants started winning around the time they began to receive massage. Local chapters of volunteer massage therapists attend to the pre- and postevent needs of marathoners throughout the country. New York City Marathon champion Grete Waitz has been reported to have received massage as many as four times a week.

What sets sports massage apart is its emphasis on prevention of injury. As Meagher explains, "Always, *maximum effort is bodily abuse* [emphasis in the original]."[14] Muscles that are constantly used become constantly contracted, which makes them less efficient as well as more exhausted and susceptible to injury. Sports massage helps relax these tight, sometimes spasmodic muscles by spreading constricted muscle fibers while also increasing circulation to restricted areas. This allows muscles to operate more efficiently, prevents against injury, and aids in recuperation. It helps to maintain good health, reduce stress, and enhance range of motion. It can help athletes break through plateaulike barriers where they had become stymied because fatigued, contracted muscles had become inefficient. Sports massage can also help extend the working life of a career athlete.

Sports massage uses the basic techniques and strokes of Swedish massage, applied very specifically to contracted muscle areas, to eliminate muscle tightness. This has the added benefit of creating a condition of hyperemia, or increased blood flow. This improves circulation to the area, thereby bringing in nutrients that are needed to fuel physical activity and removing resultant waste byproducts.

The two key strokes sports massage uses to accomplish these goals are compression and direct pressure. In compression strokes, the practitioner uses the palm or heel of her hand to bear down upon muscles, compressing them against the bone beneath in order to separate and relax muscles. Compression is performed only on hard, bony surfaces, such as the legs, arms, and back, and not on soft areas like the abdomen. Direct pressure involves finger or thumb pressure directly on the site of a spasmodic muscle, which is easily identified because it is the area where the client reports pain. Friction strokes are used to separate layers of tissues in these areas, either in round, circular motions (circular friction) or in straight lines perpendicular to the line of the muscle (cross-fiber, or transverse, friction). According to Meagher, these two strokes account for 90 percent of all work done in sports massage. The other strokes of Swedish massage—effleurage and kneading—are also used, but only briefly to warm up the area. Percussion and tapotement are rarely used because they tend to stimulate muscles, and the purpose of sports massage is to relax the muscles.

A sports massage session is usually administered like a Swedish massage session, with the client undressed and covered with a sheet on a massage table, the skin lubricated with oil. It can also be done through thick clothing or tights, however, in the case of athletes or dancers who need quick work before, during, or immediately after an event. A typical sports massage session lasts thirty to sixty minutes. The longer treatment is recommended because it allows thorough preparation, but the shorter session might be used if an athlete is going to perform immediately or if the activity is of short duration. Because sports massage uses the techniques of basic massage, a well-trained massage therapist may also be able to administer a sports massage treatment.

FOR FURTHER INFORMATION

The following text served as the basis for the material on sports massage:

Jack Meagher with Pat Boughton, *Sportsmassage: A Complete Program for Increasing Performance and Endurance in 15 Popular Sports* (Barrytown, NY: Station Hill Press, 1990). This is a classic reference in the field. In addition to providing a general introduction to sports massage, it also gives specific tips relating to a variety of sports ranging from golf to football as well as a description of the stress points most often associated with each type of sport and how you might massage them yourself.

Trigger Point Therapies: Releasing the Pressure Points

Some of you may remember black-and-white photographs from the early 1950s showing a young Senator Jack Kennedy, plagued by pain from injuries incurred during World War II, shoulders crunched over crutches as he hobbled to and from the Senate chambers. A disk operation and spinal fusion failed to provide relief. Contrast that with the image of glowing vitality that a still young and dynamic President John F. Kennedy embodied—a beacon of strength and energy to a nation in need of hope. Kennedy's transformation from a victim of debilitating pain to one of the most admired leaders of his day was due largely to the ministrations of Janet Travell, M.D., pioneer in trigger point therapy. Travell's success was clearly recognized when she was appointed White House physician to both Presidents Kennedy and Johnson, becoming the first woman ever to be so. Travell's work, though, was nonpartisan: Her praises were sung by Senator Barry Goldwater, who claimed Kennedy's greatest gift to the American people was bringing Travell to the attention of the public![15]

The approach to healing researched and developed by Travell seeks out those overly sensitive, irritated points and bands of pain deep in the muscles known as trigger points and applies specific techniques to release their hold. The work she pioneered has been further refined and adapted by other practitioners who have developed methods to work with trigger points. These additional approaches include myotherapy and neuromuscular therapy.

Trigger points are tender areas usually found in tight muscles. They may radiate, or refer, pain to other areas of the body. They can also cause muscle weakness and restricted range of motion. Trigger points can result from a number of causes: direct trauma to the body (such as a blow or a car accident); exposure to cold (such as the draft of an air conditioner or an open window); and overload, caused by overuse of a muscle or chronic postural imbalances. These factors can cause a muscle to contract. As the contraction is held over time, the muscle becomes fixed in an involuntary holding pattern that can become the source of chronic nagging pain. An active trigger point is one in which an individual can feel the pain; a latent trigger point is an area of heightened sensitivity in which one feels pain only when pressure is applied to it. Both types can cause a referral of pain to other muscles and even to the organs of the body, often remote from the original trigger point, resulting frequently in such complaints as headaches, indigestion, and upset stomachs.

There are certain common areas of the body that are more susceptible to the development of trigger points and pain because they are located at sites of greater biomechanical stress. One common site for trigger points to develop is in the trapezius muscle of the shoulder, the thick, massive muscle that lies between the shoulder blade and the neck. Trigger points in this area are often associated with pain in the back of the neck and around the eyes and ears, which is why you might experience a tension headache when your shoulders feel sore. Interestingly enough, Travell has observed that nearly 75 percent of trigger points are identical with the points used in acupuncture and acupressure.

The goal of trigger point therapy is to apply sufficient pressure to trigger points to release their chronic contraction. Following release, muscles containing and surrounding the trigger point are stretched to help prevent a recurrence of the trigger point. To the extent that such structural factors as leg length discrepancies or habitual factors such as diet, poor posture, and lack of exercise contribute to the formation of trigger points, the client may be counseled on other measures to take to prevent recurrence, such as reconfiguring a work station to promote proper body position while performing routine tasks. In the case of President Kennedy, Travell ordered an orthopedic lift for the heel of his left shoe to reduce a postural imbalance that contributed to the formation of his trigger points. She also redesigned all of his seats, including those in his helicopter, airplanes, and boats, for proper posture and prescribed an old-fashioned rocking chair for mild exercise.[16]

Dr. Travell's work is based on a technique she terms "spray and stretch," in which a vapocoolant is applied to trigger points in order to anesthetize them and the area is then stretched to release tension. A number of physicians, chiropractors, and dentists have incorporated Travell's techniques into their work.

Today, many massage therapists use manual techniques to release trigger points. Bonnie Prudden, who developed and popularized myotherapy, is a leading proponent of using finger, knuckle, and elbow pressure to release trigger points through her work known as Bonnie Prudden Myotherapy. The success of this method depends on the use of specific corrective exercises for the released muscles. Paul St. John developed a system of working with trigger points known as neuromuscular therapy, whose goal is to relieve soft tissue pain and dysfunction.

Jim Hackett, a leading practitioner and teacher of trigger point therapy, recommends the use of friction strokes (to release the tight bands associated with trigger points) combined with strokes to lengthen muscle and connective tissue, deep sustained pressure, and general relaxing strokes to promote circulation. "Most areas where there are trigger points have been cut off from circulation, and the buildup of metabolic waste in the area results in pain. Bringing in new circulation helps to remove the wastes and provide nutrition for tissue maintenance and repair," he explains. "An important aspect of trigger point therapy is to follow up with appropriate stretching and physical exercise to maintain the area in full function," he adds.

The background of practitioners of various trigger point therapies differs. For instance, certification in Bonnie Prudden Myotherapy requires 1,300 hours of training. Additionally, myotherapists require a physician's referral for treatment. Other forms of trigger point therapy, such as neuromuscular therapy, are taught in a series of weekend workshops. Many massage schools incorporate training in trigger point therapy as part of their core curriculum while others offer training through specialized continuing-education courses.

A trigger point therapy session focuses on treating specific physiological complaints and is performed in much the same setting as a Swedish massage. The client undresses and is draped on a massage table. Oil is used, although more sparingly than in Swedish massage because more friction is desired to release the trigger points. The trigger point therapist must possess a detailed knowledge of muscles and their origins and insertions as well as of the map of trigger point referral areas. A trigger point session typically lasts an hour.

During a trigger point therapy session, the massage therapist will generally warm up an area and relax it with general effleurage and kneading strokes. Friction or compression strokes to the trigger points will follow, with pressure being applied to tender areas for about eight to twelve seconds. While this pressure will most likely be uncomfortable, it should not be overly painful. "This is one area where clients who think 'No pain means no gain' need to be reeducated," Hackett advises. "If the pain is too great, the muscle will contract farther to protect itself, and that will be counterproductive." On a scale of 1 to 10, with 10 being the most painful, a therapist works between a level of 6 and 8 of client tolerance while treating a trigger point.

Trigger point therapy is used to treat a variety of complaints, including low back as well as all types of muscle pain, whiplash, tennis elbow, frozen shoulder, fibrositis, and TMJ disorder. Many clients report significant relief from pain after only a few sessions of trigger point therapy. Trigger point therapy has proven effective in some instances where other forms of therapy, such as physical therapy and painkillers, provided less relief.

Following a trigger point therapy session, an individual may feel sore for a day or two. This is a normal response of the body to the removal of toxins. Drinking lots of fluids and taking a warm shower or soaking in a hot bath may help reduce the feeling of discomfort.

FOR FURTHER INFORMATION

For information on Bonnie Prudden Myotherapy, contact:

Bonnie Prudden Myotherapy
P.O. Box 65240
Tucson, AZ 85728-5240
Tel: (520) 529-3979 or (800) 221-4634
Fax: (520) 529-6679
Website: www.bonnieprudden.com
E-mail: info@bonnieprudden.com

For information on training and certification in St. John Neuromuscular Therapy contact:

St. John Neuromuscular Therapy Seminars
6565 Park Boulevard
Pinellas Park, FL 33781
Tel: (727) 547-5424 or (888) NMT-HEAL (668-4325)
Fax: (727) 547-0962
Website: www.stjohnseminars.com
E-mail: registration@stjohnseminars.com

The following books are recommended:

Bonnie Prudden, *Myotherapy: Bonnie Prudden's Complete Guide to Pain-Free Living* (New York: Ballantine Books, 1985).

_____. *Pain Erasure: The Bonnie Prudden Way* (New York: M. Evans and Company, Inc., 2002).

Janet G. Travell, M.D., and David G. Simons, M.D., *Myofascial Pain and Dysfunction, the Trigger Point Manual,* 2nd Edition (Baltimore: Williams and Wilkins, 1998). The bible of trigger point therapy, this book is detailed and technical and intended for the professional.

On-Site Massage: Chair Massage

"Like a 72-hour vacation in 10 minutes. I learned my trade in China, Japan, India, Egypt, Israel, Lebanon, and Nirvana," modestly proclaims the eye-catching placard next to the padded chair of a purveyor of massage on a crisp autumn day in New York City's well-traveled Central Park. His competitor across the way counters with: "Like 12 hours of sleep . . . a 2-week vacation in Tahiti . . . 5 weeks of rest . . . heaven . . . "

Can't find time to get to the massage therapist? What's the next best thing to a trip to paradise? With on-site, or chair, massage, the massage therapist comes to you—whether it is in your office, the lobby of a bustling airport or shopping mall, an aircraft winging its way across the Atlantic, the park on a beautiful day, or the sidewalk at the corner where you live. On-site massage is one of the hottest, fastest-growing fields for massage therapists.

On-site massage is often referred to as chair massage because the client generally sits comfortably in a chair, often right in front of his desk. Special lightweight portable padded massage chairs have been developed that can be easily folded up and taken anywhere. Generally, these chairs slope forward to provide easy access to the largest, and often most tense, muscles in the body—the large muscles of the back. In a pinch, a massage therapist can use any chair and still provide a relaxing, energizing treatment.

On-site massage is administered with the client clothed. Strokes include friction, compression, tapotement, and range-of-motion stretches. Electric vibrators and mechanical devices may complement manual strokes. Many of the techniques employed are borrowed from shiatsu, which has developed a long tradition of pressure strokes applied through clothing, without the benefit of oil. On-site massage is more like Swedish massage, however, in its goal of relaxation.

On-site massage is generally short, lasting from fifteen to thirty minutes. It aims to relax constricted musculature and improve circulation. While the back is the chief area treated, on-site massage therapists may also minister to the neck and head, scalp, arms, legs, and even the front of the torso. Because massage is provided through clothing, a busy executive need take only a brief time out of a busy schedule to receive an energizing treatment to help put a hectic workday back on track.

In more and more cities and venues as diverse as corporate offices and airport lobbies, chair massage is becoming available to increasingly more people. Practitioners typically provide ten-minute on-site massages for about $10, with additional increments available. Treatments are geared to providing a quick pick-me-up in the middle of a busy day. David Palmer, dubbed the "father of contemporary chair massage," predicts that most on-site massage in the future will be done in retail settings, such as airports and shopping malls, making massage as common and accessible as a haircut.

Many businesses (American Express, AT&T, Lotus Development Corp., Merrill Lynch, and State Farm Insurance, for example) have allowed massage therapists to give on-site massages on their premises to promote employee efficiency and well-being. If you're not so lucky as to work for such a company, keep your eyes open: An on-site massage therapist may be waiting just around the corner.

FOR FURTHER INFORMATION

Check with your local massage school: Many massage schools incorporate some on-site massage training in their programs.

David Palmer has trained more than four thousand bodyworkers in the techniques of chair massage. For information on his programs, contact:

TouchPro Institute
584 Castro Street, #555
San Francisco, CA 94114
Tel: (800) 999-5026 (United States and Canada) or
  (415) 621-6817 (international)
Fax: (415) 621-1260
Website: www.touchpro.com
E-mail: info@touchpro.com

Specialty Practices: Endless Variations

The world of traditional Western massage is extremely rich. The specialized uses to which massage has been adapted are as limitless as the human imagination and need for touch. Here is a sampling of some further possibilities.

Pregnancy massage caters to the special needs of pregnant mothers. At least one enterprising massage team has even designed a tailor-made massage table with a hole in the middle so a pregnant woman can lie on her stomach without discomfort; a sling attached underneath provides gentle support. Enthusiastic mothers-to-be report it feels wonderful to be able to lie on their stomachs. Some massage therapists have obtained special privileges at hospitals to assist during labor, massaging the mother as she gives birth and both mother and newborn following delivery.

Infant massage deals with the special needs of newborns, including prematurely delivered babies. Massage is a wonderful way to help improve circulation in newborns; it also can help relieve some common infant ailments like gas, constipation, and colic. In addition, it promotes the formation of strong nurturing bonds and helps relax both parents and newborn. *Mothermassage: A Handbook for Relieving the Discomfort of Pregnancy* (New York: Delacorte, 1992) by Elaine Stillerman addresses techniques for massaging both the mother-to-be as well as the newborn. For those readers with a particular interest in this aspect of massage, associations such as the International Association of Infant Massage (IAIM) offer information and training in infant massage (www.iaim-us.com).

Some well-known resorts and holistic centers have pioneered their own forms of massage, integrating the techniques of traditional massage with other healing methods. **Esalen massage**, named after the Esalen Institute in Big Sur, California, combines Swedish massage with sensory awareness. **Kripalu bodywork**, named after the Kripalu Center for Yoga and Health in Lenox, Massachusetts, incorporates techniques drawn from Swedish massage, energetic bodywork, and breathing practices.

In case you're concerned about your brethren in the animal kingdom, yes, there are practitioners of **pet massage**, which is geared toward increasing the health and happiness of your favorite pet. Alice Brock, former owner of Alice's Restaurant, has even written a comical book about cat massage (*How to Massage Your Cat*, San Francisco, CA: Chronicle Books, 2003). There is a well-established subspecialty of pet massage for horse lovers, **equine massage**. Jack Meagher, a sports massage expert, also works with the U.S. Equestrian Team. His book *Beating Muscle Injuries for Horses* (Hamilton, MA: Hamilton Horse Associates, 1985) explains how you can help massage your horse to better competitive performance as well as relieve its aches and pains. No, the book proclaims, it "can't make a 'ten' out of a 'six,' but it does allow the athletic, conditioned horse to take advantage of his potential." Of special note, animal trainer and author Linda Tellington-Jones has pioneered a gentle system of bodywork known as TTouch that has been used successfully with horses and other animals, including humans, to reduce stress, enhance healing, and improve self-awareness (www.TellingtonTTouch.com).

PART II

STRUCTURAL/FUNCTIONAL/MOVEMENT INTEGRATION: SOMATIC EDUCATION

One individual may experience his losing fight with gravity as a sharp pain in the back, another as the unflattering contour of his body, another as a constant fatigue, and yet another as an unrelenting threatening environment. Those over forty may call it old age; yet all these signals may be pointing to a single problem so prominent in their own structures that it has been ignored: they are off-balance; they are all at war with gravity.[1]

—IDA P. ROLF, PH.D.

Bodywork practices grouped under this heading are concerned with the most appropriate alignment of the body in space. Practitioners of the disciplines that follow use a wide variety of methods to affect the body. They view themselves as somatic educators, teaching you new ways of integrating body and mind. Proponents of these methods maintain that structure and function are inextricably intertwined: If your body is free of restriction, then you'll be able to function more efficiently. Your movement and behavior will be free, spontaneous, and unrestricted.

THE ROLFING METHOD OF STRUCTURAL INTEGRATION AT A GLANCE

BASIC FACTS

- **Rolfing is a method of manipulating the soft tissue of the body.** It aims to restore flexibility and ease of movement by freeing major segments of the body.

- **Rolfing was developed by Ida P. Rolf, Ph.D. (1896–1979).** Rolf pioneered the approach to bodywork known as Structural Integration.

THEORY

- **The most important factor impacting human structure and function is gravity.** The constant unconscious battle with this force results in physical dysfunction and psychological, mental, and emotional fatigue and stress. Structural Integration restructures the body in optimal alignment with gravity.

- **Rolfing restructures the body through manipulating the body's myofascial system.** The myofascia consists of muscles (Greek *myo*) and the soft connective tissue (fascia) that intertwines the muscles and forms a continuous web throughout the body. The average body has experienced a history of trauma, including poor postural habits, accidents, and emotional stress, which have resulted in tightening and distortion of the myofascia.

- **Structure determines function.** A properly organized body is able to function more efficiently (physically, mentally, and emotionally) in everyday life.

- **Rolfers consider themselves teachers.** Rolfing is not an end in itself, but initiates a series of changes that will continue to unfold.

TYPICAL SESSION

- **Rolfing is conducted in a series of ten sessions.** Sessions last from one to one and a half hours each and are typically spaced about one to two weeks apart.

- **The Rolfee lies on a firmly padded massage table.** Treatment sometimes involves a standing or seated position. The Rolfee disrobes to underwear. No oil is used, in order to intensify the benefit of friction.

- **Rolfers use their fingers, forearms, and elbows to stretch and free the fascia.** These strokes employ deep pressure; the individual being Rolfed may experience occasional fleeting pain and might recall prior emotional trauma.

38

- Expect to pay $75 to $125 per session, depending upon geographic location and background of practitioner.

BENEFITS

- **Rolfing aims to realign the body to function most efficiently.** Its goal is to optimize health, not cure disease. Rolfing is better suited to alleviating chronic rather than acute pain.

- **People who have been Rolfed report feeling greater ease and freedom in body movement.** This is often accompanied by a sense of centeredness and balance, increased energy, and reduced anxiety.

CONTRAINDICATIONS

- **Because Rolfing manipulates deep tissues of the body, the contraindications for Swedish massage should be observed** (see Swedish Massage at a Glance on page 8). Additionally, anyone with acute pain or illness and prolonged or massive addiction should postpone Rolfing.

BACKGROUND AND TRAINING OF PRACTITIONERS

- **Only practitioners trained and certified by the Rolf Institute in Boulder, Colorado, can call themselves Rolfers.** The Rolfing course requires approximately 600 to 700 hours of formal study, including lecture and hands-on work.

- **The Rolf Institute has certified more than thirteen hundred Rolfers** who practice throughout the world.

CHAPTER 2

THE ROLFING METHOD
OF STRUCTURAL INTEGRATION

For it is not structure alone, but the integration of structure that is the key. We seek to create a whole that is greater than the sum of its parts. We are searching for a method to foster the emergence of a man who can enjoy a human use of his human being.[1]

—IDA P. ROLF, PH.D.

WHAT IS ROLFING?

The Rolfing Method of Structural Integration is a technique of manipulating the soft tissue of the body. It aims to restore flexibility and ease of movement by freeing the major segments of the body, which over time become locked in habitual patterns of tension. Rolfing was developed by Ida P. Rolf, Ph.D. (1896–1979), who considered her approach a form of somatic education where a practitioner instructs a client in new ways of organizing the body. Rolfers maintain that the body is a whole; an appropriately structured body will function more efficiently and economically. Rolf summarized her guiding principle in the maxim "All function is an expression of structure."[2]

THE ORIGINS OF THE ROLFING METHOD OF STRUCTURAL INTEGRATION

Structural Integration is a term coined by Rolf and that refers to a type of bodywork that is sometimes called deep tissue massage or bodywork. It tries to release both superficial and deep structures in the body. Over time her students came to call her work simply Rolfing in affectionate tribute. Rolf's influence was so seminal to bodywork that her method forms the foundation for a number of other approaches to structural and movement integration, which are highlighted at the end of this chapter.

Rolf was born in 1896 in the Bronx, New York. She was raised in a comfortable Victorian household ruled with authoritarian firmness by her father, an electrical engineer. Rolf earned her undergraduate degree from Barnard College in 1916, followed by a Ph.D. in biological chemistry from the College of Physicians and Surgeons at Columbia University in 1920. World War I afforded her a position as research scientist at Rockefeller Institute, an opportunity that was unique for a woman of the time.

Rolf traveled widely, complementing her academic background with studies in unorthodox healing modalities, including homeopathy, yoga, osteopathy, chiropractic, and the Alexander Technique. Her divergent interests coalesced in Structural Integration. Like many other healers, Rolf developed this approach to solve her own health problems (she suffered from scoliosis and spinal arthritis and was prediabetic) as well as those of her son and friends. Through trial and error, she combined her knowledge of science and physical manipulation to develop a technique for balancing the human body.

In the 1950s and 1960s, Rolf toured the United States, Canada, and Great Britain, teaching her technique to chiropractors and osteopaths, mainly because they were the only professionals who were interested in it. Rolf was dissatisfied with this situation, though, because her approach was viewed as an adjunct technique to be used among others in fixing a particular complaint. She considered her approach a complete method for integrating the human being.

In the 1960s, Rolf gained greater recognition when she visited Fritz Perls, the founder of Gestalt therapy and director of the Esalen Institute in Big Sur, California. In the sixties, Esalen was the focal point for the new and exciting developments that formed the emerging human potential movement. Rolf established a relation of mutual respect and trust with Perls when she was able to relieve severe attacks of chest pain he was experiencing from a heart problem. Ida Rolf continued to practice and teach at Esalen each summer, feeling that at last she had found a home for her work. In 1972, she and her followers established the Rolf Institute in Boulder, Colorado.

Rolf spent most of her life in relative obscurity. She gained a reputation as a strong-willed, generous, and feisty iconoclast, and someone outspoken in her conviction in the absolute correctness of her approach to the body. Despite the sophistication gained from her studies and travels around the world, she remained Victorian enough in spirit to require her clients to wear underwear when being worked on, yet she was kind and gracious enough to lend them her own in a pinch if they failed to be aware of her decorum.

It was not until Rolf was seventy years old that Esalen gave her the opportunity of sharing her work with a wider audience. Her book *Rolfing*, which presents her teachings, was not published until 1977, when she was in her eighties. Late in her career, she was still convinced that Rolfing would die with her. But by the time of her death, she had trained more than two hundred Rolfers and had personally Rolfed thousands of people around the world, including such celebrities as Cary Grant, Georgia O'Keeffe, Greta Garbo, and Adam Smith. Today, there are more than thirteen hundred certified Rolfers practicing worldwide.

THE THEORY UNDERLYING ROLFING

Rolf maintained that the basic force affecting our organization in space and physical movement is gravity. "Gravity, man's name for the energy of the earth, is the never-sleeping therapist and teacher," she claimed.[3] While most of us are usually unconscious of the powerful force gravity holds over us, life might be described as one long, constant battle with it. And gravity usually wins.

Each individual experiences this defeat in a different way: a slumped-over posture; muscular aches and pains; or emotional, physical, and psychological weariness. Rolf claimed that as gravity shortens tissues in the body, it can lead to psychological changes. "When his physical body gets into difficulties, trouble spreads to the whole man. It affects his consciousness, and he calls it stress."[4]

Rolfing focuses on the myofascial system, which is the soft tissue system of the body. It includes the muscles (Greek *myo*) and the connective tissue known as fascia. Fascia is referred to as the packing material of the body because its fibers surround and intertwine with all the muscles, organs, and bones in the body. It is like a continuous body stocking, or bandage, that ensheathes and binds from head to foot. Many common chronic aches and pains can be traced to imbalances in the myofascial network.

Fascia is composed principally of collagen, which is tough, strong, white, and flexible and has a tendency to form a rope-like consistency in the body. Rolf considered fascia the organ of support because it is what gives shape to the body; it holds the bones and organs in place and allows them to move. When the soft tissue structure of the body gets out of balance, it can pull bones, muscles, and organs out of position and lead to structural misalignment. Rolf compared this with the lining of a coat that has become misshapen.[5] Myofascial imbalance leads to pain and dysfunction.

There are many ways in which soft tissue can become distorted. Early trauma—as far back as physical trauma in the birth canal or early falls and accidents—can set the process in motion. Unconscious patterning of our parents' postural habits when we first hold ourselves erect and begin to walk can cause distorted holding patterns, not to mention emotional trauma. Our mothers scold us and we raise our shoulders to protect ourselves. We become angry and want to strike someone with our fist but are prevented from doing so because that's not a "nice" thing to do, thereby reinforcing a pattern of tension and holding in the hand and arm. (As an experiment, try paying attention to what is happening in your body when you're in a stressful situation, such as asking your boss for a raise or standing alone at a cocktail party. You might be surprised to find you're unconsciously tensing your jaw, shoulder, or neck.) Such unconscious holding patterns can become habitual. Subsequent accidents and physical trauma to the body (such as car accidents, falling on one's tail-bone, or surgery) can further cause shortening and distortion in the body.[6]

Rolfers emphasize that the body is a plastic medium. Under stress or pressure, it can be molded out of its original shape without breaking, yet on release of the stress it can be restored to its original state. Traumatic experiences can cause shortening of muscle and fascia in the body. Under tension, muscles contract. If forced to maintain a contraction for an extended period of time, the shortening becomes permanent. The fascia begins to bind muscle into shortened patterns and, in fact, to become entwined with the muscles. In so doing, it becomes hard, like bone, and supports the body in a deviated position. (It is collagen's ability to form into a hard ropelike substance that makes this possible.) But that's not all. Because the fascia is continuous throughout the body, and because muscles complement and balance one another, a distortion in one part of the body is reflected in a compensating distortion in another part, much as a snag in a sweater can pull the whole garment out of shape.

Such distortions are typical of what Rolf called the chaotic, disorganized, or random body, which is the average body of anyone who has experienced trauma and not had her body reeducated by a Rolfer. These distortions result in problems in any area that is shortened, including poor circulation, feelings of pain and irritation, and a hardening of the affected tissue. The area begins to feel and act like bone. It lacks blood supply and warmth. An individual can feel fatigued as energy is consumed to maintain tensed musculature.

Fortunately, the process of deterioration caused by life's traumas is reversible. Because the body is pliant, it can be manipulated back into shape. Even bones can change: They are like green trees—living, supple, flexible, with some movement and some fluid. The goal of Rolfing is to realign the body so as to unveil its more naturally occurring structure. The Rolfer puts energy into the body through the use of the mechanical pressure of his strokes. This energy produces heat, which softens and releases contracted muscles, leading to greater balance in the body. Once constricted soft tissue is released, an individual has more energy available for other uses, and the body's healing energy can enable the body to heal itself. Rolf said, "This is the gospel of Rolfing: When the body gets working appropriately, the force of gravity can flow through. Then, spontaneously, the body heals itself."[7]

Rolf's background as a research scientist made her extremely interested in mechanics. She looked at the body as an engineer or architect might. She saw the body as a structure that can go awry and needs to be put right. Rolf's criteria for an appropriately aligned body focus on the proper relation of vertical and horizontal planes in the body. A key factor that distinguishes us from other animals is our erect posture. Ever since we evolved from a four-legged animal to a two-legged primate, we have been waging a war with gravity. Part of our evolutionary development is to continue to adapt to gravity. Rolf saw her method as one aid in meeting these evolutionary demands, contributing to the fulfillment of human potential.

In order to be aligned vertically, a plumb line dropped from an individual's head to her feet should form a straight line. This line should pass through the midpoints of five key landmarks: the ears, shoulder joints, hip joints, knees, and ankles. This line is not inflexible but should be capable of movement and resilience, like the supple branch of a willow tree. (The rigidly erect military stance, considered by many to be the model for posture, is deviated posture because it holds the body in an unnatural rigid position.) In appropriate alignment, the elbows, hipbones, kneecaps, and ankles should align at right angles to the vertical plumb line. The pelvis is the keystone to the body. An improperly aligned pelvis can be responsible for distortions throughout the body, all too often including low back pain.

In random, or disorganized, bodies, the vertical and horizontal landmarks are not in appropriate alignment. This situation is depicted schematically in the logo of the Rolf Institute, which compares a random body to a properly aligned body. The role of the Rolfer is to realign the body in such a way that all the major body segments regain their natural alignment. This frees the body of unnatural constrictions, resulting in feelings of enhanced movement, better balance, and increased energy and vitality.

A Rolfer does not deal only with a client's presenting symptom, but also aims to reorder the entire body into a properly structured whole. An analogy to this would be a house that is tilting to one side. One way of approaching the repair of this house might be to jack up one side. Rolfers would see this as a makeshift measure and not really repairing the house in the long run. A Rolfer would look at the house and see that the foundations needed to be repaired and that other adjustments might have to be made throughout the structure to bring it into proper alignment. Rolfers are not concerned with the source of the trauma that originally sent the body into misalignment. So many compensations will have occurred since then that the structure of the whole body must be evaluated.

A TYPICAL ROLFING SERIES

Because Rolfing involves a comprehensive restructuring of an individual's body, it requires a series of sessions that last from one hour to one and a half hours each. The amount of time between each session varies, but is usually one or two weeks.

During treatment, the client disrobes to underwear. No oil is used, in order to increase the amount of friction involved. For the most part, the client lies on her back or stomach on a firmly padded massage table while the Rolfer applies slow, deep gliding strokes to stretch and free the fascia. Some treatment may also be done with the client seated or even standing or moving about. While each session focuses on a particular area of the body, all sessions usually incorporate work on the back, neck, and pelvis so that the individual being Rolfed has a sense of having every part of her body worked on.

The basic Rolfing series consists of ten sessions that progress from superficial to deeper layers of the body and from the extremities of the body to the core. The first three sessions deal with the superficial envelope of the body, which includes the layer of fascia that is just below the skin, plus the extremities of legs and arms. The next four sessions deal with the body core, which is comprised of the deeper layers of fascia and body segments that are closest to the midsection. The first seven sessions deal with specific local areas. The last three sessions focus on reorganizing the relationship of the major segments of the body, integrating all the preceding treatments. Consequently, these sessions are more personalized and address whatever areas of the body require attention.

A Rolfing series follows a systematic scheme that reflects optimal progression for restructuring the body. For instance, in the first session the Rolfer treats the chest to open up breathing and allow for increased oxygenation to support more efficient functioning. In the second session, he manipulates the feet and ankles to provide a secure foothold for the body in the gravitational field. Rolfing is not merely cookbook-like in its approach, however: While Rolfers focus on a specific part of the body in each session, the precise nature of what they do is determined by the needs of the individual client. A Rolfer, therefore, develops a unique treatment plan for each client.

The Rolfer effects change in the body by adding energy through the refined and intelligent use of manipulative strokes. Using fingers, elbows, and forearms, the Rolfer adds energy, which heats the collagen and makes it more fluid. This allows the practitioner to stretch the fascia out of its hardened, restricted position. Once the fibers are properly aligned, the ground substance hardens, returning them to position in the appropriate line of force.

Part of the traditional protocol of being Rolfed is having your photo taken before and after each session in order to chart the progress of change. At the beginning of each session, the Rolfer evaluates a client's body to fine-tune the work plan for that session. During the course of the session, the Rolfer sometimes offers guided visualizations to help release areas of holding. At the end of the session, the Rolfer may ask the client to walk about, observe herself in the mirror, or provide feedback on how she feels. The Rolfer may also recommend exercises to do at home. For instance, after working on the feet and ankles, the Rolfer might suggest a client stand like a tree, blowing in the wind, with movement coming from the ankles as they swing freely and openly like hinges. The Rolfer may then suggest expanding that notion of suppleness into movement: walking as though being pulled from the chest—with the feet just following along from the hinges at the ankles. These exercises help bring the structural changes of Rolfing into conscious awareness.

Practitioners maintain that the changes effected by Rolfing are permanent. In one famous incident, Greta Garbo, who was Rolfed by Ida Rolf, maintained that Rolfing had changed the shape of her face, creating more space in her mouth. She threatened to sue Rolf but changed her mind when the celebrity photographer Cecil Beaton photographed her and convinced her that her looks had improved.[8]

It can take the body a long time—months, and in some cases even years—to assimilate the changes from the initial Rolfing series. For this reason, Rolfers recommend allowing at least six months following the initial series before undertaking any further sessions. After this time, individuals may choose periodically to have one or several tune-up sessions. An Advanced Rolfing Series of five sessions is also available, with the recommendation that individuals wait at least a year before embarking on this program.

In addition to Rolfing sessions, the Rolf Institute offers a program in Rolf Movement Integration to teach clients to move more efficiently with gravity. As senior Rolfing instructor Jeffrey Maitland explains: "Rolfing frees and integrates the body's structure so the client has more movement options, and Rolf Movement teaches the client how to use these possibilities in everyday life."[9] Rolf Movement Integration is taught one on one in a series of eight sessions, which are often integrated into the ten basic Rolfing sessions.

THE EXPERIENCE: I GET ROLFED

I arrive for my first Rolfing session. My Rolfer is David Frome, a physical therapist who specializes in Rolfing. I obtained David's name from a list of referrals of certified Rolfers furnished me by the Rolf Institute. I selected David after interviewing several Rolfers over the phone. David's low-key caring attitude toward his work made me feel we'd be a good match.

I arrive at David's office on a sunny midsummer afternoon. His practice is affiliated with the New York Rolfing Associates, a group of Rolfers united in a professional suite occupying a sprawling apartment on Manhattan's Upper West Side. He also maintains a practice in suburban Montclair, New Jersey, which includes Rolfing for infants and children.

David shows me to the treatment room. It's a bright, sun-filled room with a padded massage table in its center. David asks me to undress down to my underwear. He leaves the room, then reappears after I have disrobed. I stand before him while he appraises me and takes Polaroid photographs of me from front, back, and in profile. These are the before photos.

David asks me what my major complaints are.

"Tension," I reply. "Chronic tension, in my back, in my thoracic area, especially on the right side. Plus my hamstrings, which get tight. And my spine is curved due to a scoliosis, so that my head tilts to the left side. And, oh, yes, most important of all, my posture: My chest is rounded forward so that I feel like it's sunken in. I'd like to stand tall with good posture."

David eyes me like a painter scrutinizing a blank canvas. I can sense his mind working as he evaluates my structure. He agrees with all I've said, then adds: "Plus I'd like to see you lengthen, become taller, relieve some of the compression in your body."

David asks me to lie down on my back on the massage table. He begins to stroke my chest with long, slow, deep strokes. At first there is no discomfort, just a sensation of pressure. But the work seems to go deeper, and soon I feel he is stretching layers well beneath the skin into long strands, like separating tufts of taffy and lengthening them. I experience some pain, but it is a kind of pain that feels good. Part of the pain comes from the fact that no oil is used, which increases the friction and pressure of the strokes. Because my chest is hairy, the pain is accentuated by hairs being pulled.

David's hands are firm, strong. They belie his slim, nonmuscular appearance. As the strokes deepen even more over my pectoral muscles, I feel as though a roller is flattening the asphalt of my tissues. And as I look at David's hands, I notice that his fingers are held closely together, forming a shape like a shovel, and that he's using them to press and stretch the fascia beneath the skin.

I can feel a lengthening taking place. Are those little pockets of bubble wrap I hear popping as his hands glide up my pectoral muscles? At times I feel as though he's coming up against little knots or nodules, like small stones or pieces of gravel, and I ask him what they are. He says a buildup of different things over the course of years. Rolfing will remove them as well as lengthen my fascia.

"Your chest feels like it's been wrapped too tightly in cellophane," he observes. "That's very common."

I can feel my chest starting to lengthen and expand. My breath swells to a volume I had not known before. David explains that he's working to free up the chest to increase my breathing capacity. His goal is to turn my ribs into something like venetian blinds that open and close independently rather than as a single large shutter with no flexibility. He also works on the fascia of the upper abdomen, where it meets the rib cage, and along the side of the body.

"Try to picture your breath as coming all the way from your pubic bone and fanning out laterally to the shoulders, forming a V shape," David coaches me with his verbal imagery.

I follow his subtle suggestion—and my abdomen fills with breath.

"Good. That's good breath," David coaxes and encourages me. He then works on the fascia of my thigh. He asks me to raise my knee to a flexed position in preparation for separating the fascia of the hamstrings and the outer thigh. As he works, I slowly flex and extend my foot.

I can feel the tightness as he remarks that I'm tense there. "Many people are," he adds. I can feel the pressure here, a searing pain, and I ask if he's using his forearm. No, he's pressing his elbow into me, slowly sliding it along, using it to spread fascia masquerading as bone.

David also adds that my abductor muscles, the muscles of the outer thigh, are confused with the quadriceps, the muscles that form the bulge at the middle top of the thigh above the knee. I like his use of the word "confused," because it can be interpreted both physiologically and mentally. I can't help but wonder, if the fascia is confused, can my mind, which is connected to my body, not help but be confused, too?

After working the right side of my body, David asks me to stand up. I feel light-headed, very relaxed, almost groggy. Despite the pressure and mild passing pain I experienced, the work has been very relaxing. (David tells me some of his clients actually fall asleep while being Rolfed.)

David asks me how I feel, what I notice. I report that my right side feels much more open than before, much lighter; my left side, which has not yet been worked on, feels tense and tight.

I return to the table, and David repeats his maneuvers on my left side, which is less constricted than the right. David explains that he usually begins a session working with the tighter side and moves to the less tight side. My right foot has always turned out, and I ask if that is because my right leg is tighter, shorter. David affirms that, yes, the fascia on that side is shortened, tighter, so it pulls on the bone, rotating it into a distorted position. Future sessions will address that problem.

Periodically, David steps back and, even with my eyes closed, I can feel him observing me, like a sculptor eyeing a blank block of marble waiting to be carved. He says, "You may think this strange, but I sometimes feel like I'm making a sculpture." No, I don't find this strange, because Rolfers seem a powerful combination—part scientist, part artist. I can understand how David could stand there and appraise the plastic medium before him to see how he should mold it next. I am reminded of a famous comment attributed to Michelangelo about how he would just look at a cube of marble and see what its final form should be. He felt he was just liberating the form that was already contained inside the marble. And, yes, I feel as though David is looking beyond the constraints of my current physical organization to liberate the structure of the unique and free being within. Ida Rolf herself described beauty as "an intuitive appreciation of normalcy."[10]

David completes this first Rolfing session by having me sit erect on a round, low stool. He has me slowly curl my head and neck and then whole spine, down, until my back is parallel to the ground. He places his elbows in the grooves in the middle of my shoulders. His elbows glide slowly, firmly, deeply down my back, along the length of the ropelike erector spinae muscles that line either side of the spine. This is painful at moments as the bony surfaces of his elbows work their way down the bony surfaces of my back with its tight muscles.

"Your right side is especially tight," David explains, then repeats this maneuver several more times.

As painful as this experience is, it feels good to be stretched to such an extent, to reach positions I could not reach on my own.

David then has me return to the table. He encourages a lengthening in my pelvis by having me tilt it forward and up.

"If I had to reduce our goal in Rolfing to one precept, it would be this: to make the pelvis horizontal and the fifth lumbar vertebra, the last lumbar vertebra, sit properly on the sacrum. "

As David works on my pelvis, I can feel my abdomen opening up even more and the breath filling it more deeply. I have seen pictures in various books of people before and after Rolfing treatments. One in particular caught my attention—that of a middle-aged man who lost his love handles during the course of treatment. I would love that result.

"Can I expect such a result," I ask David, "as you lengthen my spine and my abdomen sits back into my pelvis?"

"I can't say what will happen," David says candidly. "I've only been doing this work for eight years. But often that is the case." David's modesty and lack of expectation impress me as hallmarks of a healer.

David moves to the head of the table and begins to apply traction to my neck, manipulating it from below the prominence of the occipital ridge. He massages this area where the neck begins, and I can feel its effect all the way down to my abdomen, which opens up even more as my breathing becomes deeper.

"Good job," David coaxes me again. "Good breathing." He seems to be aware of the changes taking place in my body as quickly as I, attesting to his keenly honed powers of observation.

An hour has passed. We conclude the session. David has me stand tall in the first position again, toes together, facing forward.

"How do you feel?" he asks.

My left side feels fuller, more open now. The right side had felt that way after he had finished working on it, but now the left side feels fuller.

"That's natural," he says, "because your left side was more open, fuller, to begin with.

"What we are providing here is an opening, and your body will continue to change. Rolfing, even if done for only one session, can have a permanent effect on you. Sometimes people go through a whole series of Rolfing sessions and don't feel or see that much change, and then two years later they experience major changes. The work provides an opportunity for your body to change."

The format for this first session turned out to be typical of the ten in my Rolfing series. We would begin each session with David's evaluating my structure and then proceeding to work on a specific area. During the course of the work, he would often provide visualizations to help me, release tensed areas, would reevaluate me periodically, ask for my feedback on the changes I felt in order to help me own them, offer a homework exercise, and complete the session with a final appraisal of the progress made in that session, which was recorded on a Polaroid photograph.

As my Rolfing treatments progressed, I occasionally asked myself, "Am I really changing?" The world around me said yes. One of my regular massage clients observed after my third session, "What have you done to yourself? You look fifteen years younger." My doorman remarked as I passed through the lobby after my fourth session, "You look different. Did you shave your beard?" I reminded him that I never had a beard. At the gym, the fellows I work out with, the ones whose names I don't know and who know me only by sight and who are therefore in a position to be most objective, remarked after my fifth session on how I'd changed. "Your chest is wider, your torso longer." They added, "You've been working your body hard." I accepted the compliment, but kept the secret to myself: My body is working smarter, not harder. After my sixth session, I went for a walk in Central Park. A middle-aged matron came up to me and said, "You look fantastic; you've got a great body!" Then apologetically remarked, "I'm sorry. I don't know what came over me. I've never said anything like that to anyone before. But it's true. Your body is so long and tall." After my seventh session, my psychotherapist said to me, "I don't care what you say, you're getting taller!" After the tenth session, my "graduation," my yoga partner inquired, "Have you lost weight? You look taller." When I bumped into a friend I hadn't seen in two years, he exclaimed, "I didn't recognize you. You've grown an inch or two!" All of these people were responding to significant, noticeable differences in my physical appearance and structure.

But what is even more revealing is that I noticed the changes myself. And I believe that shows the deepest level of transformation. Throughout my experience of Rolfing, I was acutely aware of the changes that were taking place in the physical structure of my body in myriad subtle and unexpected ways. My T-shirts, which used to fit securely in the waistband of my trousers, began to rise up and expose the bottom of my belly: I must be growing taller. When I looked in the mirror, I saw a new firmness and squareness to my jaw: This must reflect the release of tension and the arrival of a new level of inner confidence. The muscles of my body stood out with greater definition: They must be developing new integrity. When I engaged in aerobic exercise, my lungs seemed to expand more fully: I must be taking in more oxygen. As I walked, I felt my feet planted firmly on the ground, the weight of my upper body transferred all the way down and through my heels: This must be a new relation to gravity. When I stood at the kitchen counter and unscrewed a jar, I realized I didn't need to twist my body, too: I must be developing inner structural clarity.

When I told my friends and colleagues about my Rolfing experience, the most common remark I heard was, "Oh, that must have been painful," reflecting a prevalent notion that Rolfing hurts. This need not be so: In fact, Rolf treated four-month-old infants and ninety-one-year-old women. Rolfers have refined their technique over time so that Rolfing need not be painful to be effective. Ida Rolf acknowledged that this work could be painful, but taught that pain often results from resistance to change, much as an individual in psychotherapy refers to sessions where she resists change as painful. While being Rolfed, I did experience occasional pain; however, it was transitory and not as severe as many people seem to imagine. At times I felt a burning, searing pain that would last for only the few moments or minutes while David was working on an area of my body where I was holding especially hard. I felt this pain had a large emotional component related to my fear of allowing a sensitive area to become vulnerable. The areas where I felt pain when they were worked on were often the very areas of tightness that needed to be opened up. I was able to overcome this fear because I knew I could always tell David if the work felt uncomfortable. After some sessions, I experienced the dull kind of ache one might feel after physical exercise. I would drink lots of fluids after my sessions to help stem this inflammatory response.

Often, Rolfing can facilitate emotional as well as physical releases. Rolfer Kalen Hammann has reported that about one-third of his clients experience emotional releases, with these usually occurring in only one or two of the ten-session series.[11] I found painful memories from my childhood sometimes surfacing as David worked on painful areas of holding. I also found myself letting go of old patterns of behavior. After one particularly releasing session, for example, I found myself spontaneously stopping at a store to purchase some new clothes. This was a new and liberating experience for me: As the fourth-born child of parents raised during the Depression, I'd developed a long-ingrained pattern of not permitting myself to buy new things. It was immensely energizing to be freed of this pattern of behavior.

Am I perfect after my Rolfing experience? As David and I evaluated the before and after photos, we noted that my pelvis is still not completely horizontal. My left hip, which was higher to start with, is still higher but less so. My left shoulder is still higher than my right but not in as pronounced a way. But my neck and torso are much longer. Most important, I *feel* much better.

THE BENEFITS OF ROLFING

Rolfing aims to teach individuals to achieve and maintain optimum health, not cure disease. Consequently, it is not recommended for acute conditions of pain or for relieving any particular physical symptom, such as a sore shoulder or back. However, improved structural integration can result in improved function so that chronic symptoms, such as back pain caused by chronically shortened muscles, may be alleviated. Rolfing can help improve circulation, relay nerve impulses more smoothly, encourage more efficient breathing, and enhance removal of waste products from the body. Additionally, Rolfing may enhance physical performance in professional and daily activities. As a Rolfee's musculature relaxes, she often feels a heightened sense of wholeness and vitality.

Rolfing may cause occasional physical or emotional discomfort. Having a psychological support system in place while undertaking Rolfing can be a valuable adjunct. Rolfing can be a powerful complement to psychotherapy as well as an aid to deepening such practices as meditation, yoga, and martial arts.

Rolf Movement Integration can result in increased grace, ease, and efficiency of movement; an increased sense of balance and centeredness; and the relief of physical stress caused by resistance to gravity.

Ida Rolf claimed not to understand how Rolfing works. "I don't know *why* it works, I only know *that* it works. I invent all these explanatory rationalizations later on," she said [emphasis in the original].[12] Nonetheless, several scientific studies have been performed to evaluate the effects of Rolfing on the body. One of the most ambitious and interesting studies was undertaken by Valerie Hunt, Ph.D., director of the Movement Behavior Laboratory at UCLA. Among the empirical findings of this impressive study, which evaluated subjects both physiologically and energetically, were the following: After Rolfing, Rolfed subjects demonstrated major improvement in muscular efficiency; used energy more efficiently; and showed more spontaneous behavior and a greater propensity for creative thinking. Among the more esoteric of her findings was that Rolfing altered subjects' perception of time so that it seemed to slow down in a state of expanded consciousness while improving their organization of energy toward more refined, equal, and higher frequencies. To the extent that Rolfing counters the body's tendency toward disorganization, this study suggested that Rolfing can mitigate the effects of aging.[13]

Another group of scientists, led by Julian Silverman of the California Department of Mental Hygiene, found that Rolfed subjects demonstrated increased openness and sensitivity to environmental stimulation, which is associated with decreased levels of stress.[14] Studies led by Rolfer John Cottingham indicated that Rolfing may be able to help alleviate many chronic low back problems, which are often caused by misalignment of the pelvis, as well as help reduce levels of stress.[15]

CONTRAINDICATIONS TO ROLFING

Because Rolfing goes into deep layers of tissue and the work can involve a great deal of physical pressure on the body's connective tissue, Ida Rolf recommended that anyone with acute pain or illness as well as anyone with prolonged or massive addiction should defer Rolfing. Additionally, the contraindications for Swedish massage (Chapter 1) should be observed.

BACKGROUND AND TRAINING OF PRACTITIONERS

Rolfing practitioners undergo rigorous training. Prior to admission to Rolfing, applicants must have completed Foundations of Somatic Practices (Unit 1) or the Advanced Unit 1, which includes extensive training in anatomy, physiology, and kinesiology. They must also possess good health, physical stamina, and a strong commitment to Rolfing. Following acceptance into the program, Rolfers undergo 588 to 731 hours of training in Rolfing. Practitioners of Rolf Movement Integration receive an extra three weeks of training. In order to be entitled to use the word "Rolfer," a practitioner must be trained and certified by the Rolf Institute. In becoming a Rolfer, a practitioner agrees in writing to pursue a program of continuing education and to complete training to become an advanced Rolfing practitioner within three to nine years of receiving basic Rolfing training.

There are currently more than thirteen hundred Rolfers throughout the world who have been certified by the Rolf Institute. Rolfing training programs are offered at the Rolf Institute in Boulder, Colorado, as well as at sites overseas, including Brazil, Europe, Australia, and Japan.

FOR FURTHER INFORMATION

The nonprofit Rolf Institute is dedicated to training Rolfing practitioners, sponsoring scientific research on Rolfing, and serving as a clearinghouse of information on Rolfing. For further information on its programs, literature, and video programs, as well as a list of certified Rolfers in your area, contact:

Rolf Institute
5055 Chaparral Court, Suite 103
Boulder, CO 80301
Tel: (800) 530-8875 or (303) 449-5903 (Colorado residents)
Fax: (303) 449-5978
Website: www.rolf.org
E-mail: info@rolf.org

SUGGESTED FURTHER READING

The following books are by Ida Rolf:

Ida P. Rolf, Ph.D., *Rolfing: Reestablishing the Natural Alignment and Structural Integration of the Human Body for Vitality and Well-Being* (Rochester, VT: Healing Arts Press, 1989). This is Ida Rolf's textbook on Rolfing and is geared to the practitioner.

_____. *Rolfing and Physical Reality* (Rochester, VT: Healing Press, 1990). This highly accessible anthology of Rolf's thoughts is edited and introduced by Rosemary Feitis, Rolf's longtime assistant. Highly recommended as an introduction to Rolf's work.

The following books are out of print, but worth looking for in your local library:

Don Johnson, *The Protean Body: A Rolfers View of Human Flexibility* (New York: Harper & Row, 1977). This is an early Rolfer's insightful look at the art of Rolfing.

Will Schutz and Evy Turner, *Evy: An Odyssey into BODYMIND* (New York: Harper & Row, 1976). These are the impressions, in journal form, of a Rolfing client as she is being Rolfed.

OTHER APPROACHES TO STRUCTURAL INTEGRATION

The approach of Structural Integration that Ida Rolf developed has served as the basis for a number of other approaches to structural and movement integration.

Aston-Patterning is a form of movement reeducation developed by Judith Aston. Aston is a former teacher of dance, physical education, and theater movement whose career was stopped short by a car accident. She turned to Rolfing for relief, and found it. Working with Rolf, she developed the system of movement education that later became Rolf Movement Integration. Her own work developed beyond the scope of Rolf Movement Integration to include fitness training, bodywork, ergonomics, and product design. For more information on Aston-Patterning, contact:

Aston Enterprises
P.O. Box 3568
Incline Village, NV 89450
Tel: (775) 831-8228
Fax: (775) 831-8955
Website: www.astonenterprises.com
E-mail: info@astonenterprises.com

In 1990, a number of instructors left the Rolf Institute to form their own association, called the **Guild for Structural Integration**. For information on its programs, contact:

Guild for Structural Integration
P.O. Box 1559
Boulder, CO 80306
Tel: (800) 447-0150 or (303) 447-0122
Fax: (303) 447-0108
Website: www.rolfguild.org
E-mail: gsi@rolfguild.org

Hellerwork is a type of bodywork that combines realignment of the fascia, movement education, and interactive dialogue between practitioner and client. This method was formulated by Joseph Heller, a former aerospace engineer (and no relation to the novelist Joseph Heller). He was one of Rolf's first students and the first president of the Rolf Institute.

A complete Hellerwork series addresses eleven thematic sections of the body. These sections are covered in a series of eleven to twenty sessions, with each session lasting sixty to ninety minutes. For further information on Hellerwork, contact:

Hellerwork International LLC
326 "I" Street, Suite #146
Eureka, CA. 95501
Tel: (800) 392-3900
Fax: (425) 642-8400
Website: www.hellerwork.com
E-mail: info@hellerwork.com

THE ALEXANDER TECHNIQUE AT A GLANCE

BASIC FACTS

- **The Alexander Technique is a system of reeducating the body/mind.** It aims to facilitate appropriate posture, ease of movement, and optimum health.

- **This technique was developed by F. Matthias Alexander (1869–1955) at the turn of the twentieth century.** An Australian actor, Alexander developed this technique to cure his own chronic laryngitis.

THEORY

- **The Alexander Technique teaches proper use of the self.** Through such stresses as improper handling by their parents, emotional and physical trauma, and being forced to sit in uncomfortable chairs at early ages, most people learn to misuse their bodies. Misuse of the body can result in stress that leads to tension, aches, and pains.

- **The most important relationship in the body is the relationship of the head to the neck and torso.** The Alexander Technique aims to promote optimal alignment in which the head releases up and the neck and spine lengthen.

- **Alexander Technique practitioners are called teachers.** Their goal is to teach the client (called a student) how to consciously control responses to stimuli, thereby allowing him the freedom to choose new, less stressful, and more efficient patterns of behavior.

TYPICAL SESSION

- **An Alexander lesson generally lasts forty-five minutes.** The student wears loose, comfortable clothing. He may lie on a firm, padded table, head supported, or sit, stand, or walk.

- The Alexander teacher uses a combination of gentle manual guidance coupled with verbal directions to break up old patterns of holding and movement and to initiate new ways of functioning.

- Alexander lessons are usually taken in a series. Typically, students begin with twenty to thirty lessons, spaced one to two weeks apart.

- A typical Alexander lesson ranges in cost from $45 to $100.

BENEFITS

- **An Alexander lesson is designed to teach better conscious control of the self.**

Learning a better use of the self is often accompanied by improved functioning. In particular, contracted musculature associated with back pain, TMJ disorder, and spinal deformities, such as scoliosis, kyphosis, and lordosis, can be relieved. Individuals who receive Alexander lessons often report reduced levels of stress, a feeling of "lightness" and "tallness" as their spines lengthen, and increased energy and vitality.

- **The Alexander Technique is frequently used by people suffering from back pain,** either following surgery or as a possible preventive measure to avoid surgery.

- **The Alexander Technique is a favorite among performers** as their livelihood depends upon proper awareness and use of their bodies.

CONTRAINDICATIONS

- Because the Alexander Technique involves gentle movements, there are no contraindications.

BACKGROUND AND TRAINING OF PRACTITIONERS

- **The American Society for the Alexander Technique (AmSAT) maintains standards for the training of Alexander teachers.** These standards require 1,600 hours of training over a minimum of three years.

- There are approximately five hundred teachers of the Alexander Technique in the United States and additional practitioners worldwide, including Australia, Israel, South Africa, South America, and Western Europe.

CHAPTER 3

THE ALEXANDER TECHNIQUE: ALIGNING THE SPINE

I discovered that a certain use of the head in relation to the neck, and of the head and neck in relation to the torso and other parts of the organism . . . constituted a primary control of the mechanisms as a *whole* . . . and that when I interfered with the employment of the primary control of my manner of use, this was always associated with a lowering of the standard of my general functioning" [emphasis in the original].[1]

—F. MATTHIAS ALEXANDER

WHAT IS THE ALEXANDER TECHNIQUE?

The Alexander Technique is a system of reeducating your body and mind so you can use your self in a way that facilitates proper posture, ease of movement, and attainment of optimum health. Through gentle manual guidance accompanied by verbal directions, the Alexander teacher coaches a student to become aware of and to inhibit unnecessary movement and to achieve greater ease and efficiency in performing physical tasks. As the body regains more optimum functioning, the student often gains relief from stress and chronic pain. F. Matthias Alexander (1869–1955), the originator of this technique, summarized his subtle goal in the elegantly simple dictum of "developing a better use of the self."

THE ORIGINS OF THE ALEXANDER TECHNIQUE

The Alexander Technique is one of the oldest of the Western mind/body therapies currently in use. It was developed at the turn of the century by Alexander, an Australian actor who was born in Tasmania and who moved to Melbourne as a young man. He embarked upon a career as a Shakespearean reciter, performing dramatic monologues. He constantly lost his voice in the middle of a performance and experienced lowered energy and vitality. Medical doctors offered the standard advice: Get plenty of rest. Unfortunately for Alexander (but fortunately for us), this cure provided only temporary relief and led Alexander on a decade-long quest to heal his physical problem.

From about 1890 to 1900, Alexander carefully observed himself in front of a three-part mirror. He noted, through careful and meticulous empirical observation, that when he lost his voice he was distorting his head and neck in a characteristic way—his head and neck slumped downward. This resulted in compression of his larynx, which caused him to pull in his chest to suck in air. By allowing his head, neck, and torso to achieve a more appropriate alignment, he completely eliminated his hoarseness. Alexander also observed that his misuse of his body did not occur in isolation, but was related to other patterns of stress that sometimes affected his legs, feet, and toes as well. As he corrected the relationship of his head, neck, and spine, he registered improved coordination in his overall physical, mental, and emotional functioning.

From this method of self-exploration, which John Dewey maintained satisfied "the most exacting demands of scientific method," Alexander developed a technique of reeducating the body that became the focus of his life's work.[2] In 1904, he moved from Australia to England so that he could bring his work to a wider audience. When World War I broke out, he toured the United States to promote his work and to train future teachers. Thereafter, Alexander divided his time between the United States and England. His brother, Albert Redden, known as A.R., took up permanent residence in Boston, where he also trained teachers. Alexander's technique was studied and applauded by leading intellectuals and educators of his day, including George Bernard Shaw; William Temple, Archbishop of Canterbury; Aldous Huxley; and John Dewey.

Unfortunately, many of Alexander's students were killed during World War II, and Alexander was afraid his technique would die with him. However, the reputation of the Alexander Technique enjoyed an unexpected boost in the early 1970s. Oxford biologist Nikolaas Tinbergen became intrigued by the Alexander Technique and arranged lessons for himself and his family. Shortly thereafter, he was awarded the Nobel Prize for Physiology or Medicine and gave public support by devoting half his Nobel Prize acceptance speech to praising the Alexander Technique.[3] Alexander's work is now carried on in a number of schools throughout the United States, Europe, Israel, South Africa, and Australia that are devoted to the teaching of his technique.

The use of the Alexander Technique has been particularly embraced by performing artists who recognize the need to keep their instruments (that is, their bodies) in top shape. In his time, Alexander would make daily rounds to visit as many as five theaters per afternoon to help leading men and ladies prepare for their performances. He treated many of the famous stage and film stars of his day, including the legendary figure Lillie Langtry. Today, the Alexander Technique has been incorporated in the drama departments of such prestigious schools as New York University, the San Francisco Conservatory, and the Juilliard School, where it has been a required course since the department's inception in 1968. In England, it has been part of the curriculum of the Royal College of Music and the Royal College of Dramatic Arts. The list of celebrities who have availed themselves of the technique reads like a *Who's Who* of the entertainment world: William Hurt, Kevin Kline, Patti Lupone, Paul Newman, and Irene Worth, to name just a few.

THE THEORY UNDERLYING THE ALEXANDER TECHNIQUE

The Alexander Technique is based on straightforward principles: There are certain ways of using our self that are better than others; most of us have adopted ways that are less than optimal; because of our improper use of our self, we suffer in our way of functioning. Studies performed by Alma Frank, one of the first American practitioners of the Alexander Technique, confirmed that we develop distorted patterns of use early in life. Young children already show signs of miscoordination due to improper stimulation and handling by their parents beginning from the age of two. A particular source of distortion is introduced as young children are required to sit for hours at a stretch in poorly designed chairs when they first start school. By the time most of us are adults, we have established unique patterns of distortion that give us our individual characteristic habits.[4]

Because the Alexander Technique is a system of education, the practitioner is called teacher and the client student. The Alexander teacher instructs the student to exercise greater use of what Alexander termed "primary control," or the proper relationship of head, neck, and torso. The Alexander teacher herself undergoes extensive training in refining her primary control. This empowers her to communicate, through her touch as she applies it to a student, the sense of the right feeling that goes with primary control.

To use the self properly, we actually must progress through what Alexander broke down into three steps.[5] We must: (1) become consciously *aware* of ourselves and our posture, of how we hold ourselves and move; (2) master the ability to *inhibit* conditioned patterns of movement before they occur; and (3) consciously *direct* our responses to break old habits and establish new, better uses of our self.

This may sound simple enough, but as anyone who has taken lessons in the

Alexander Technique knows, it is one thing to understand this process intellectually and quite another to know it at the experiential level. Because the Alexander Technique is based upon the hypothesis that the mind and body are one, all learning must take place both within the mind and within the body. This means we must develop our kinesthetic sense, the internal mechanism that enables us to feel the position of our bodies in space. Most of us have little experience in doing this, with the result that this sense is undeveloped or unreliable: Often we feel that what we do is correct, when we are actually reinforcing a bad habit. We must develop kinesthetic awareness slowly over time.

Learning the Alexander Technique presents us with an additional challenge: In order to allow our bodies to assume an improved alignment, we must inhibit our familiar habitual responses. Unlike the Freudian use of the term, which is associated with suppression, Alexander used the concept of inhibition to describe a conscious decision not to react to a stimulus with a habitual response.[6] This requires us to do nothing, which is hard for most of us because we are used to exerting some effort to achieve a goal. The Alexander Technique involves consciously inhibiting the preconditioned automatic reflex reactions that put us into improper alignment in the first place. The Alexander Technique is, on the deepest level, a process of allowing ourselves to unfold naturally rather than with striving toward a preconceived end. It is easy to see why John Dewey held the Alexander Technique up as a model for what true education should be.

Alexander taught that the key relationship in the body is the relation of the head, neck, and torso, or primary control. When these body segments are properly aligned, the head floats upward, and the neck and spine are lengthened and released. As Frank Pierce Jones, Ph.D., a student of the Alexander brothers and a distinguished researcher into the physiological basis of the technique, explains: "When the primary control is functioning as it should, it is sensed as an integrating force that preserves freedom of movement throughout the system, so that energy can be directed to the place where it is wanted without developing strain either there or elsewhere."[7] In the field of biology, G. E. Coghill supported Alexander's findings by reporting that the proper relation of the head to the neck that Alexander observed as primary control also characterizes movement throughout the animal kingdom. One of Alexander's most important contributions is his discovery that modern civilization interferes with this relationship and his subsequent development of a system of education to restore natural function.

You may appreciate more the prime importance of the neck when you consider that it forms the all-important passageway between the brain, which is our central processing unit, and the rest of the body, whose functions it directs.

Specifically, the neck is the area through which all the nerves that receive sensory input from, and direct motor activity to, nearly the entire body pass. In addition, because all the vertebrae of the spinal column are interconnected through a series of complex joints, pressure or compression on the vertebrae of the neck can cause compression throughout the rest of the vertebral column. This results in pressure on nerve roots as they exit the spinal column, causing aches, pains, and contracted muscles throughout the body.

According to Alexander, most of us misuse our bodies. We tend to throw our heads backward, which causes us to shorten and stiffen our necks. In fact, Dr. Wilfred Barlow, a British physician, Alexander teacher, and founder of the Society of Teachers of the Alexander Technique in London, performed an experiment in which he took measurements of 108 young men between the ages of seventeen and twenty-two: Astonishingly, only one of these subjects did not exhibit a characteristic misuse pattern.[8] In another study undertaken of 112 physical education students, whom you might expect to represent the epitome of physical well-being, Barlow observed that 62 percent exhibited severe postural defects; 11.5 percent slight defects; and 26.5 percent very severe defects.[9]

Alexander taught that this basic misuse pattern is central to all the other deformities that occur in the body. The Alexander Technique therefore mainly deals with reestablishing a proper connection between the head and spinal column. It is no wonder that teachers of the Alexander Technique often present images of attractive balanced posture and flowing poise. People wanting to improve their posture and presence or to achieve relief from back injuries and chronic pain frequently turn to the Alexander Technique for help.

Alexander believed that misuse of the body cannot be corrected just by the desire to do so. In fact, in the first study cited above, the 108 young subjects were asked to correct the alignment of their heads to their necks. No matter how hard they tried, only eleven were able to do so.[10] This is because once we have established a misuse of our bodies, we are unable to recognize a proper use. Our efforts to correct simply put us into another misuse pattern.

You might ask: "If Alexander was able to correct his defects on his own, without the help of a teacher, why can't we do the same?" Alexander's stock response to this question, frequently posed to him during his life, was: "You can do what I do, if you do what I did."[11] Most of us are so oblivious to our own ingrained patterns of misuse that we need the help of an experienced instructor who has been properly trained to awaken our kinesthetic sense and guide us toward proper use of our self.

The Alexander teacher educates the client to consciously sense and control the body through a series of lessons geared to increase self-awareness. During the lessons, the teacher gently guides the student's body in such a fashion as to help it release. The teacher's touch is gentle; she uses her hands more to arrange a student's body in proper alignment than to massage, manipulate, or exercise it. At the same time that she physically adjusts the student's body, the teacher provides verbal directions, or orders, to reinforce the student's awareness of enhanced ease. Alexander believed that the mind and body are inextricably connected and that most therapies fail to provide full relief because they focus either on the body or on the mind to the exclusion of the other. The combination of gentle guidance by touch and verbal instruction is meant to register awareness at the level of the body/mind.

THE TYPICAL FORMAT OF AN ALEXANDER LESSON

A typical Alexander lesson lasts forty-five minutes during which the student remains dressed in loose, comfortable clothing. He may lie on a massage table, head resting on a firm support, or receive instruction in proper use of the body while sitting, getting up from a seated position, standing, walking, or even crawling. In the case of people who want to improve their performance at a particular task, such as a pianist who wishes to improve arm movement at the keyboard or a receptionist who suffers from neck and shoulder problems from holding a phone all day, the teacher may evaluate and instruct better ways of performing specific routine activities.

During a typical session, the teacher's goal is to teach students how to give up habitual patterns of holding and relinquish with awareness any improper control they had been exercising. In effect, the teacher is asking the student to inhibit the normal tendency to contract a given muscle reflexively. In that moment of stopping action, a new pattern of ease is allowed to take over. The teacher shows the student what a new pattern of movement might feel like by guiding the student's body through a motion from beginning to end. The teacher's physical guidance is accompanied by directions that reinforce at the level of conscious mental activity what is happening in the body: For instance, guiding the head upward with a consequent elongation of the neck might be accompanied by the verbal direction, "Head forward and up," offered repeatedly until the student makes the connection between the physical feeling of what is happening and the conscious mental awareness. Some teachers may suggest visual images to reinforce what is taking place physically. These verbal cues also serve as a kind of key that the student can use after the session to remind himself of the feeling/tone of the lesson.

The Alexander Technique is ambitious in the extent of its undertaking. It aims at no less than a total reeducation of the way we use our selves in all of our activities. It involves a process of learning rather than achieving a fixed end goal. While some people seem to be gifted with proper natural use of the self (witness the grace of Fred Astaire or the flexible nimbleness of Muhammad Ali), most of us require a period of time in which to acquire it. Most Alexander teachers recommend a series of twenty to thirty lessons, undertaken once or twice a week, in order to learn the proper use of the self.

The Alexander Technique is very subtle. Its movements are gentle, slow, and painless. It requires a commitment to concentration, awareness, and greater conscious control of activities that previously seemed beyond conscious control. The rewards for this include a greater sense of ease, vitality, and improved functioning. Because of its emphasis on bringing more conscious awareness to bear upon habitual states, the Alexander Technique can be a powerful adjunct to psychotherapy.

THE EXPERIENCE: I ALIGN MY SPINE

I've arrived at the spacious apartment/office of Deborah Caplan, one of the foremost teachers of the Alexander Technique, for a lesson. I'm excited to meet and work with Deborah because she has the distinction of having known Alexander and received lessons from him as a child. Her mother was an Alexander teacher, and Deborah followed in her footsteps, becoming certified as an Alexander teacher before earning a degree in physical therapy from New York University. She is the author of *Back Trouble: A New Approach to Prevention and Recovery*, which provides valuable insights into avoiding and alleviating back pain, based on the principles of the Alexander Technique. Deborah, who was on the faculty of the American Center for the Alexander Technique, was instrumental in establishing the standards of training for Alexander teachers in America.

Deborah is a short, trim, attractive woman with long flowing hair. What strikes me immediately about her, though, is the beauty and ease of her posture, the calmness of her bearing. Deborah has poise and grace, qualities regrettably lacking today. What I have observed in all the Alexander teachers I've encountered is their supple and seemingly effortless carriage. Their torsos appear long and open, flexible, and easy; their faces exude a kind of self-contented radiance. They do practice what they preach. One of my colleagues calls Alexander teachers the "nuns of bodywork," suggesting the deep sense of inner calm and wholeness that is the hallmark of well-organized structural alignment.

We are in Deborah's office, a sunny, spacious room with windows overlooking the Hudson River. Its furnishings include a desk, where Deborah sits when recording intake information. Her "equipment" is a massage table covered with a sheet, a chair, and a stool. Charts of the body's muscular and skeletal systems line the wall, much like in a physician's or chiropractor's office.

She begins our session by taking a short medical history, then instructs me in an introductory lesson. "We'll be doing most of our work in positions of move-ment—standing, sitting, walking—and relatively little work on the table," she explains. "Every Alexander teacher varies in her approach to teaching. My atti-tude is that if anyone has pain or discomfort, my goal as an Alexander teacher is not to address his pain directly and take it away from him, passively, by mas-sage or joint manipulation, but to teach him to use his body in better ways that will help to relieve the cause of the pain. I find that working exclusively on the table encourages a sense of passivity—the student feels that he is here to be 'fixed'—and I want him to accept more responsibility for taking care of him-self. All of my students are people who come to me with specific, often severe, medical problems."

We begin with standing. I am fully dressed in my street clothes, including sneakers. Deborah has me stand erect, my head facing forward, eyes open. She asks me to become aware of everything within my field of vision as both she and I center ourselves. She holds my head gently between her hands, helping it and my neck to release, as she gently encourages me through her words to allow my neck to release back and my head to balance forward and up.

As she works with me, Deborah explains the basis of the Alexander Tech-nique. "The Alexander Technique engages both conscious and kinesthetic aspects of movement. You can read the theory in a book, but that is only part of it. You also need the experience of the feeling of the work, which involves the kinesthetic sense. I help you to develop this awareness by encouraging your body to assume a more efficient alignment, and you receive this message. You don't have to do anything. A lot of what the Alexander Technique is about is learning not to perform a habitual movement."

For instance, Deborah points out how I have a tendency to pull my head back and down, tilting my face upward in the process. This shortens my neck, causing it to contract in back. She asks me to release the muscles in the back of my neck. This allows my head to freely rotate forward slightly and ease up in relation to my neck. Now my eyes are pointing more directly ahead, rather than up. This feels awkward to me; it is not what I think of as "up." I've always associated correct posture with my parents' command to stand up straight. This meant I strained to make myself straight and pulled my head backward (which I thought was up) in the process. Deborah is letting me see that what I had thought of before as length was actually a shortening of my neck.

"People will say to me, 'How can the Alexander Technique make someone taller?'" Deborah shares. "And I'll explain to them that it doesn't actually make you physically longer, but it undoes the shortening that most people do to themselves."

This has to do with inhibition. "F.M., which is what we affectionately called Alexander," Deborah explains, "found that even after he had discovered what he was doing wrong—shortening his neck muscles by throwing his head back, just like you and most of the world do—he was unable to implement a new pattern just by willing it. He discovered that he had to go through an intermediary step, which he called inhibition, where he consciously decided not to engage in the old shortening pattern. He found that if he focused on inhibiting the old pattern rather than on trying to recite well, the old pattern disappeared *and* he was able to recite without straining his voice.

"F.M. was way ahead of his time in this regard. People warned him that his term of 'inhibition' would be misunderstood. 'Freud is on the horizon,' they exhorted, 'and people will not understand what you mean by inhibition.' But Alexander knew what he meant, and he knew that inhibition was the right word to use—we have to consciously intervene to stop our old patterned responses in order to allow another pattern to emerge. Alexander was brilliant. As one of the few Alexander teachers who is also a physical therapist, I found it immensely gratifying to study anatomy and physiology in detail and validate from the Western physiological perspective what Alexander understood empirically. From recent findings in neurology, we know that one of the functions of the most developed parts of the central nervous system is to inhibit unwanted activity. 'Inhibition' is the correct scientific word to describe our conscious decision not to perform an action."

Having taught me a little bit about inhibition and allowing me to feel somewhat longer in my head and neck, Deborah proceeds to teach me how to sit. She explains that Alexander really had four basic directions that he gave to people: (1) Think longer; (2) think wider; (3) let the back open; and (4) let the legs separate from the torso. All four principles, even though expressed in a linear, consecutive sequence, are meant to be done separately and together at the same time. And all four are required in the act of correct sitting.

Deborah coaches me to allow myself to sit in such a way that I maintain my spine long and wide while I do so (as opposed to my habitual tendency to throw my head back and shorten my neck). She also encourages me to feel that my torso and spine can move independently from my legs. She reminds me that there are large joints at the hip designed for just that purpose. Deborah has me practice sitting down, standing up, then sitting down again, a number of times. Her hands are alternately on my head, neck, and spine to encourage them to maintain their lengthened state as I move. I can feel, and hear, a cracking in my back as this subtle lengthening causes my vertebrae to shift. As my torso lengthens, Deborah's hands slide smoothly down my torso, one hand in front, one in back, almost as though she were putting the finishing touches on a freshly ironed shirt, to remind me how long my spine can be. She reinforces her tactile message by repeating, "Head forward and up; torso lengthening and widening." I can eventually feel it happening. Deborah will stop me in the middle of a movement, when I am half sitting, so I can experience what that movement feels like. She has me turn my head to look in a mirror on the wall, so that I can visually reinforce what I look like when my body is in correct alignment. And she punctuates her educational comments and coaching instructions with words of praise "That's nice!" "That's right!" "Good job!" "That's nice and long!" The experience of being in correct alignment feels pleasurable to me on all levels—intellectually, kinesthetically, and emotionally.

Deborah is ready to introduce some work on the table, and she asks me to remove my sneakers. She stops me halfway through my act of taking off the first sneaker.

"Feel what you're doing. Think about being long and wide. You don't have to throw your head back and compress your whole body to reach your shoe. You can allow your head to lead your spine into length. Now continue to lengthen as you use the flexibility of your spine to reach your shoe."

And I realize that my old patterns are still at work. Awareness, as Deborah explains, is a skill that develops over time. That is why work in the Alexander Technique generally requires a series of lessons spread out over a period of time.

Deborah has me lie fully clothed, except for my shoes, on my back on the table. She places a couple of books under my head to adjust it to a comfortable horizontal position relative to the table. She holds her hands under my head, neck, shoulders, and then legs, encouraging me to allow my whole body to be long and free. She reinforces the importance of inhibition.

"You can't 'make' your legs release away from your torso; you'd need muscles between your feet and the wall to pull your limbs out. But you can allow yourself to say 'no' to tightening your hip muscles. Then, as you think of releasing your legs away, your hip joints will be freer."

She explains that it's particularly important to allow the muscles in the buttocks to relax. "Many people don't realize it, but tension in this area puts a lot of pressure on the sciatic nerve and can cause a lot of the pain associated with low back pain. In fact, one of the major reasons I wrote my book on back pain was to get the word out on this—too many books encourage people with back pain to tighten these muscles, and that's exactly the opposite of what anyone should do."

As Deborah speaks, I do feel longer, lighter, easier, more flexible from my head down through my pelvis and out through the tips of my toes. Yes, indeed, I feel as though I have grown longer.

Deborah completes the lesson by instructing me in two other activities. First, she teaches me to walk. Even though I may have been doing this all my life, I realize I haven't been doing it in the most efficient way. She shows me how I can walk while allowing my head and spine to lengthen up and my legs to move freely.

Finally, knowing that I am a massage therapist and that I often feel tight and sore in my back after doing several massages in a row, she teaches me better body mechanics so I can use my body more intelligently and efficiently. "If you allow your head to remain forward and up and your torso to be long and wide, you won't feel so compressed in your back. Rather than feeling tired, you'll actually be strengthened and stretched after giving a massage. And you'll be able to communicate greater power, strength, and relaxation to your clients.

"I frequently teach classes to physical therapists," Deborah explains, "to help them use their bodies more efficiently when they work. It's ironic: They go into physical therapy because they want to help other people feel better, but by misusing their bodies, they're tired and sore by the end of the day. At the end of my workshops, I have these students pair up and work on one another. The overwhelming comment is how much more relaxed and effective the person doing the work is and how much more comfortable and enjoyable the session is for the receiver.

"The Alexander Technique is wonderful for people who have to use their bodies in physically demanding ways. This is why it is so popular among dancers, actors, and musicians. I began my career as a professional dancer, and I found that my background in the Alexander Technique helped me tremendously."

"How many lessons does it take to develop the kind of awareness necessary to incorporate the principles of the Alexander Technique?" I ask Deborah.

"It varies from individual to individual, but as a general rule of thumb, an initial series would consist of about thirty lessons received consecutively at a space of one or two lessons a week. Following the initial lessons, students should take a break for a while and integrate the work. After that, they might want to receive a couple of lessons periodically to refresh and expand the work. Of course, when I first start to work with someone, I don't usually prescribe a set number of lessons. We have to see how the work goes and evaluate what progress we're making. And I have to ask the student how *he* feels about the work, if he feels he's benefiting. Other practitioners may be different and work more according to a prescribed schedule."

As I leave Deborah's office and float down the corridor outside her apartment, I feel taller, lighter, longer. The lesson definitely has done something for me. But I feel that if I really want to benefit from the work, I'll need to come back for more lessons. If I can improve the way I use my body so that I avoid pain in the future before it can start, I'm sure the lessons will prove valuable.

THE BENEFITS OF THE ALEXANDER TECHNIQUE

Alexander teachers do not attempt to diagnose illness or treat particular symptoms. Their goal is to help you improve your use of the self. However, experience has shown that if you use your self in a more appropriate way, you may often notice a corresponding improvement in your level of functioning, which may contribute to overall health and relief from pain and strain.

In developing improper body mechanics, we often cause muscle shortening and tension. Learning a more efficient use of the self can help release this contracted musculature. The Alexander Technique is frequently used by individuals suffering from back injury and chronic neck, shoulder, and back tension as well as abnormal spinal curvatures, such as scoliosis, lordosis, and kyphosis (some experts estimate that up to 80 percent of us suffer from back pain at one time or another). The Alexander Technique has been especially helpful for people who have undergone back surgery and, in some cases, has helped people suffering from slipped disks or lumbosacral strain avoid surgery.[12] It has also helped people suffering from arthritis; TMJ disorder; headaches; gastrointestinal complaints, such as spastic colon; and breathing disorders, such as asthma and emphysema. Performing artists—actors, dancers, singers, and musicians—whose livelihoods depend upon professional use of their bodies, swear by it. Moving with greater coordination can help reduce accident-proneness. Releasing physical stress can help individuals feel less stressed emotionally and psychologically. Learning how to exert control in physical movement can provide the greater freedom of choice that accompanies enhanced control of one's daily mental, emotional, and psychological activities. Nearly all people who receive Alexander lessons feel a greater sense of calm, lightness, poise, and vitality following a session. A frequent response to an Alexander lesson is "I feel taller," which is a natural sensation that accompanies the lengthening of the spine achieved by the technique.

The changes in conscious awareness and control brought about by the Alexander Technique can benefit anyone at any age. Lessons given to children can help prepare them to interact with their environment with the greatest amount of conscious awareness and freedom of choice. In the case of the middle aged and elderly, Alexander lessons can help restore coordination and vitality. John Dewey didn't begin lessons until he was fifty-eight, Aldous Huxley was in his forties when he started to take lessons with Alexander, and his wife and friends credited the technique for liberating his creative potential in ways that nothing else in his life had.[13]

Despite the fact that the Alexander Technique has been practiced for nearly a century, it still remains to be satisfactorily explained how it works. Frank Pierce Jones performed research on the physiological principles that might underlie the Alexander Technique. Over decades of extensive research, he was able to document a number of significant factors that bear upon Alexander's work: Our responses to stress and other environmental stimuli originate in the nerves and musculature of the neck and then spread to other parts of the body, and subjects who have undergone training in the Alexander Technique do show marked improvements in coordination and bodily functioning, which are not replicable by other techniques.[14] But the underlying mechanism by which all of this happens still remains to be explored.

The proof of the effectiveness of the Alexander Technique would seem to lie in the improvements that those who have taken lessons in it experience. Professor Nikolaas Tinbergen summed this up succinctly when he said in his Nobel acceptance speech: "Medical practice often goes by the sound empirical principle of 'the proof of the pudding is in the eating.'" He emphasized the importance of Alexander's method of empirical observation—of "watching and wondering." As he put it: "This basic scientific method is still too often looked down on by those blinded by the glamour of apparatus, by the prestige of tests, and by the temptation to turn to drugs."[15] We owe a debt of gratitude to F. Matthias Alexander for undertaking the painstaking observation of his use of his own self in order to point us on the way toward our own path of exploration and self-improvement.

CONTRAINDICATIONS TO THE ALEXANDER TECHNIQUE

Because the Alexander Technique uses gentle movements, there are no contraindications.

BACKGROUND AND TRAINING OF PRACTITIONERS

A number of training programs have been established to teach the Alexander Technique in the United States. Some of these programs were developed by teachers who were trained by Alexander while others have been established as nonprofit institutes grouping together diverse Alexander teachers and practitioners.

The primary professional organization for the Alexander Technique in the United States is the American Society for the Alexander Technique (AmSAT). AmSAT is an educational nonprofit organization that was formed in 1987 to educate the public about the Alexander Technique and establish and maintain standards for the training and certification of teachers. The official AmSAT mission statement is "To define, maintain, and promote the Alexander Technique at its highest standard of professional practice and conduct."

Alexander teachers undergo one of the longest and most selective training programs in the field of bodywork. The minimum standards of training required for certification by AmSAT as an Alexander teacher correspond to the minimum standards established by the Society of Teachers of the Alexander Technique (STAT) in London and adopted by other national organizations. These requirements consist of 1,600 hours of training over a minimum of three years; an average teacher-to-student ratio of 1 to 5; and 80 percent of training hands on. The American Center for the Alexander Technique (ACAT) in New York City, which has trained nearly half the Alexander teachers in the United States, limits enrollment to twelve new students per year.

While the background of Alexander teachers varies widely, many performers have been attracted to teaching the technique because they have found it to be so helpful in their own careers. Currently there are about five hundred certified Alexander teachers in the United States and additional practitioners worldwide.

FOR FURTHER INFORMATION

For further information on the Alexander Technique in the United States, including a list of practitioners in your area, a list of readings and supplemental materials, and training programs, you can contact AmSAT:

The American Society for the Alexander Technique
P.O. Box 60008
Florence, MA 01062
Tel: (800) 473-0620 or (413) 584-2359
Fax: (413) 584-3097
Website: www.amsat.ws (includes a list of AmSAT certified teachers)
E-mail: info@amsat.ws

Established in 1964, the American Center for the Alexander Technique is the oldest training center for the Alexander Technique in the United States. You can contact ACAT at:

The American Center for the Alexander Technique, Inc.
39 West 14th Street, Suite 507
New York, NY 10001
Tel: (212) 633-2229
Fax: (212) 633-2239
Website: www.acatnyc.org
E-mail: acat@acatnyc.org

For information on Alexander teachers in the rest of the world contact:

The Society of Teachers of the Alexander Technique
First Floor, Linton House
39-51 Highgate Road
London NW5 1RS, England
Tel: 0845 230 7828
Fax: 020 7482 5435
Website: www.stat.org.uk
E-mail: office@stat.org.uk

SUGGESTED FURTHER READING

F. Matthias Alexander wrote four books. They are all in print and are available from AmSAT books, though often hard to find elsewhere:

F. M. Alexander, *Constructive Conscious Control of the Individual* (London: Mouritz, 2004; first published by E. P. Dutton, 1923).

_____. *Man's Supreme Inheritance* (London: Mouritz, 1996; first published by E. P. Dutton, 1910).

_____. *The Use of the Self* (London: Orion Books Ltd., 2001; first published by E. P. Dutton, 1932).

_____. *The Universal Constant in Living* (London: Mouritz, 2000; first published by E. P. Dutton, 1941).

The following anthology of Alexander's writings is still in print:

The Alexander Technique: The Essential Writings of F. Matthias Alexander, ed. Edward Maisel (New York: Carol Publishing Group, 1995). This is an anthology of selected writings drawn from Alexander's four books, with a biographical and theoretical introduction by Maisel.

The following are books by others on the Alexander Technique:

Wilfred Barlow, M.D., *The Alexander Technique: How to Use Your Body Without Stress* (Rochester, VT: Healing Arts Press, 1990). This is an easy-to-read, thoughtful introduction to the Alexander Technique, written by a medical doctor who was trained by Alexander and who founded the Society of Teachers of the Alexander Technique in London.

Deborah Caplan, P.T., *Back Trouble: A New Approach to Prevention and Recovery, Based on the Alexander Technique* (Gainesville, FL: Triad Publishing Company, 1987). This is a concise explanation by a master teacher of the Alexander Technique, with emphasis on how it can be used to help relieve back pain and related complaints. It includes illustrated do-it-yourself exercises.

John Gray, *Your Guide to the Alexander Technique* (New York: St. Martin's Press, 1990). Gray trained with Wilfred Barlow, and his book is a good introduction to the Alexander Technique.

Judith Liebowitz and Bill Connington, *The Alexander Technique: The World-Famous Method for Enhancing Posture, Stamina, Health, and Well-being, and for Relieving Pain and Tension* (New York: HarperCollins, 1990). Liebowitz co-founded ACAT and taught at the Juilliard School for more than twenty years; Connington was chairman of the board of ACAT and a faculty member at Juilliard.

THE FELDENKRAIS METHOD AT A GLANCE

BASIC FACTS

- **The Feldenkrais Method is a comprehensive approach to movement reeducation that aims to restore and optimize a full range of human function.** The practitioner helps the client, called a student, become aware of habitual and limited movement patterns and provides the context for learning new skills.

- **This method was developed by Moshe Feldenkrais, D.Sc. (1904–1984).** A Russian-born Israeli physicist and engineer, Feldenkrais used his wide knowledge of science to reeducate himself to work after he suffered a severe knee injury.

THEORY

- **The Feldenkrais Method establishes new connections between the brain and body.** Feldenkrais maintained that we learn nearly our entire repertoire of movements during the first few years of life. These learned movement patterns constitute only 5 percent of the total possible movements of which we are capable. Habitual physical behavior patterns are mirrored in fixed ways of responding to emotional, psychological, sexual, and social situations as well. They lead to anxiety, strain, and pain.

- The central nervous system can be retrained. The Feldenkrais practitioner helps the student recognize improved patterns of behavior to replace old, inefficient habits. The practitioner's task is to create the conditions for learning that will expand the student's perception of choice.

- **Improved physical functioning leads to increased vitality and ease in daily life.**

TYPICAL SESSION

- **The Feldenkrais Method uses one of two formats:** Functional Integration (FI) lessons are private one-on-one sessions custom-tailored to the needs of the individual. Awareness Through Movement (ATM) classes are taught in a group setting.

- A Functional Integration lesson typically lasts forty-five minutes to an hour. The student lies on a low padded table and dresses in loose, comfortable clothing. The Feldenkrais practitioner uses his hands to communicate to the student new movement configurations.

- An Awareness Through Movement class lasts forty-five minutes to an hour.

Students wear loose, comfortable clothing and assume relaxed positions lying on the floor, standing, or sitting supported in a chair. A teacher verbally guides a group of students through exercises designed to increase awareness of movement potential.

- Expect to pay $50 to $90 for a Functional Integration lesson and $10 to $15 for an Awareness Through Movement class.

BENEFITS

- **The Feldenkrais Method aims to restore full physical function to the greatest extent possible.** Advocates of Feldenkrais claim relief from the pain associated with TMJ disorder and other joint disorders; headaches; and neck, shoulder, and back pain.

- **Practitioners report particular success in treating muscular disorders,** such as cerebral palsy and multiple sclerosis as well as stroke and accident cases, offering relief from pain and helping restore range of motion where other treatments have provided little or no comfort.

- People from many different walks of life, including athletes and performing artists, have found Feldenkrais to be a powerful method for achieving greater freedom of movement and increased performance.

CONTRAINDICATIONS

- Because Feldenkrais lessons involve gentle movements performed without strain, there are no contraindications.

BACKGROUND AND TRAINING OF PRACTITIONERS

- **All certified practitioners complete a professional Feldenkrais training program.** Training consists of approximately 800 hours of theoretical and practical study over a period of four years. Halfway through training, a student is authorized to teach Awareness Through Movement classes.

- There are more than thirteen hundred certified practitioners of the Feldenkrais Method in the United States, with additional practitioners in Australia, Canada, Europe, Israel, and South America.

CHAPTER 4

THE FELDENKRAIS METHOD: AWARENESS THROUGH MOVEMENT

What I'm after isn't flexible bodies, but flexible brains. What I'm after is to restore each person to their human dignity.[1]

—MOSHE FELDENKRAIS, D.SC.

WHAT IS THE FELDENKRAIS METHOD?

The Feldenkrais Method is a comprehensive approach to movement reeducation that aims to restore and optimize a full range of human function. The practitioner helps the client become aware of habitual and limited movement patterns and provides the context for learning new skills. Developed by a Russian-born Israeli scientist, Moshe Feldenkrais, D.Sc. (1904–1984), it aims to help you learn how to learn. In the process, you may become aware of unconscious patterns of movement that can be limiting, inefficient, and contradictory. The Feldenkrais practitioner calls the client a student. A practitioner aims to create the conditions within which learning and change can occur, thereby expanding a student's perception of choice.

The Feldenkrais practitioner utilizes one of two formats: one-on-one private lessons called Functional Integration (FI), where he gently touches the student's body to communicate newer and more efficient methods of movement, and group classes known as Awareness Through Movement (ATM), where a teacher verbally guides a class of students through a structured sequence of movement explorations that create new movement skills. As Feldenkrais practitioner Marcy Lindheimer, director of the Feldenkrais Learning Center in New York City, explains: "With the Feldenkrais Method, movement is an excuse for learning."

THE ORIGINS OF THE FELDENKRAIS METHOD

Moshe Feldenkrais was born in Russia and emigrated to Palestine at the age of thirteen. After earning his doctorate in science at the Sorbonne in Paris, he worked as a nuclear physicist and engineer. Feldenkrais was an early devotee of the martial arts and held a black belt in judo. He is credited with introducing this martial art form to the West through his founding of the Judo Club of France and the authoring of several books on the subject.

An avid athlete, Feldenkrais suffered a debilitating knee injury while playing soccer. Medical doctors gave him a fifty-fifty chance of recovery if he underwent surgery. Feldenkrais didn't like the odds. He approached this situation as a challenge: Through a synthesis of his knowledge of anatomy, physiology, psychology, neurology, biomechanics, physics, and martial arts, he developed a method by which he was able to regain complete function. He continued to refine this system over a period of forty years. At the age of fifty, Feldenkrais devoted his time exclusively to teaching his method, training hundreds of teachers to carry on his legacy before his death.

Feldenkrais originated his method in Israel. Through the sponsorship of Esalen, which helped bring many pioneers of bodywork to public attention, he began a series of public trainings in the United States in 1972. This led to the establishment of the Feldenkrais Guild in San Francisco to maintain standards of practice and serve as a training organization for practitioners.

THE THEORY UNDERLYING THE FELDENKRAIS METHOD

Feldenkrais believed that we learn nearly our entire repertoire of movement during the first few years of life. Patterning our movement after our parents' movement and responding to emotional and environmental stresses, we develop habitual, characteristic patterns of functioning, which we repeat compulsively to the exclusion of other patterns—even though other patterns might be freer and more efficient. We learn just enough to function adequately, to get done what we need to get done but not to move with the degree of ease, flexibility, and coordinated grace that characterize our human potential. So great is this tendency to use the same old patterns that Feldenkrais maintained we use only about 5 percent of our total potential movement ability. (If this figure seems astounding, consider the fact that most of our everyday vocabulary consists of words we learn by the age of two and that science, with all its advances, can still account for only about 10 percent of the functioning of the brain.)

The key player in the establishment of our learned movement patterns is our nervous system. When we are born, the nervous system is not yet fully developed, and we do not have control over many of our voluntary motor functions. Examples of this include an infant's difficulty in holding its neck and head erect, standing up, or using its vocal muscles to speak. As we grow, the nervous system learns to process sensory input received from the outside environment and directs the body to respond to those stimuli in learned movement patterns. As the nervous system develops, specific connections are made between discrete areas of the brain and specific muscles upon which they act. These connections are reinforced over time, resulting in habitual patterns of movement. The manner in which these connections are learned and maintained is a complex one involving psychological as well as physical factors. Among the most important of these is our dependence on the approval of our parents and the outside world for our sustenance and security, which results in the reinforcement of some behaviors to the exclusion of other prohibited behaviors.

The problem with this process, as Feldenkrais saw it, is that we compulsively repeat the same limiting patterns of movement and behavior even as we grow older. Because these patterns become so fixed over a lifetime of learning, we are unaware of them and of the wider world of freedom of movement that awaits us if we are willing to pursue it. To aid us in laying claim to our full movement potential, Feldenkrais developed a system that helps reeducate the body (through the nervous system) to act in a way that allows it to select the most appropriate action to accomplish a particular goal.

Feldenkrais's message is ultimately one of hope. Human behavior, which is formed primarily by personal experience of the world, is dynamic and can be changed. Our nervous and muscular systems are so flexible that we can reverse previously learned patterns. Even though we might have adopted inefficient patterns and used them for a lifetime, our bodies have a kind of inner wisdom that knows a more efficient action when it experiences it. The hallmark of appropriate behavior is a sensation of freedom and ease both at rest and in performing any action.

In the beginning, Feldenkrais worked exclusively in private sessions. He utilized one-on-one custom-tailored individual lessons to gently communicate movement through touch in order to teach this expanded repertoire of movement. These private lessons came to be known as Functional Integration. As his work progressed, however, Feldenkrais wanted to make his teachings available to a wider audience. This led to his development of Awareness Through Movement classes, which are taught in a group setting.

Feldenkrais considered both formats to be different ways of doing the same thing. Awareness Through Movement, by its nature, cannot be as specifically tailored to a particular individual's needs as a private lesson. Progress with individual lessons is, therefore, more rapid than in the group setting. Functional Integration lessons are also more productive for someone who has difficulty progressing in the class lessons.

The Feldenkrais Method has much in common with many other types of bodywork, especially those classified under the heading "Structural/Functional/Movement Integration." These approaches in general are based on the premise that we develop characteristic habitual patterns of holding in response to learned postural patterning and emotional and physical stress. Structural/Functional/Movement Integration methods, such as Rolfing and the Alexander Technique, seek to release these patterns of holding. Feldenkrais was a close personal friend of Ida Rolf and shared with her a background and interest in science, particularly biomechanics and engineering, which were strong factors influencing both practitioners to focus on the structural organization of the body. Additionally, Feldenkrais admired the work of F. Matthias Alexander and recommended Alexander's books, especially *The Use of the Self,* to his students.

What makes Feldenkrais's approach unique is the goal of his method: namely, to bring unconsciously driven movement into conscious awareness and provide other options that enable us to choose our pattern of movement and behavior. His work is to the body what psychotherapy is to the mind—he tries to bring movement from the realm of the unconscious to the conscious, just as a psychotherapist tries to bring unconscious thoughts into conscious awareness. Those readers interested in bringing the fullest degree of conscious awareness to movement might be especially interested in exploring the Feldenkrais Method.

THE TYPICAL FORMAT OF A FELDENKRAIS SESSION

A typical lesson in Functional Integration lasts about forty-five minutes to one hour. The client remains fully dressed, wearing loose, comfortable clothing. She lies or sits on a low padded table while the practitioner gently uses his hands to communicate movement so that new movement configurations can be learned. A practitioner does not always directly manipulate the specific area of an injury or difficulty. A Functional Integration lesson addresses the underlying patterns that maintain a student's difficulty and aims to create new conditions that support more dynamic patterns of movement. Unless new and better choices are available, an individual will continue to respond with her habitual repertoire of choices.

A typical class in Awareness Through Movement lasts about forty-five minutes. In these classes, students also wear loose, comfortable clothing, and sit or lie on the floor, stand, or sit in a chair. In beginning classes, students generally lie on the floor. That way the student does not have to fight gravity to stay upright. This position relaxes muscles that are normally contracted, such as the large muscles of the back, thereby reducing extraneous interference from muscular tension. By removing these distracting influences, the student is better able to focus full awareness on the particular muscles that are engaged during performance of the lesson. The teacher verbally guides the student through a sequence of small, precisely defined movements, such as turning the head to one side or raising an arm a few inches. The movements are small so that the student can focus fully on them. Feldenkrais believed that when the amount of tension present is small and we perform small movements, we can detect finer and finer changes. The exercises are performed slowly, without strain or pain.

Feldenkrais was careful to distinguish his exercises from traditional gymnastic exercises, or calisthenics. Calisthenics are designed to strengthen muscles by repetition with increasing speed and force. His exercises are designed to reeducate the student to widen and refine conscious control of bodily movements. Feldenkrais's goal is no less ambitious than teaching the student the art of learning how to learn.[2] With increased learning, we become able to make a wider range of choices. The Feldenkrais student learns to inhibit undesired movements and to perform new desired actions. This learning is achieved partially through a process Feldenkrais described as differentiation. Differentiation requires us to inhibit certain neuromuscular activities while activating others. Sensory motor reeducation can occur at the unconscious, or subcortical, level, as well as at the conscious level of awareness. Even repeating an exercise only one time can change habitual programming. "So smart is the brain, when we permit it," said Feldenkrais, "that even after doing something a million times the wrong way, doing it right even one time feels so good that the brain-body system *recognizes* it immediately as right [emphasis in the original]."[3]

In addition to directing the student to make physical movements, the teacher may guide the student to just visualize performing the action. Both methods help the student develop new connections between the part of the brain that is responsible for initiating movement and the muscles that it uses to accomplish this goal. Generally, a class focuses on one exercise out of a repertoire of more than one thousand lessons that Feldenkrais devised. The instructions for the full original series of exercises were developed in Hebrew; out of these, more than six hundred have been translated into English.

The aim of the Feldenkrais Method is to make us more aware of our movements, so it initiates a process that unfolds gently and gradually. This process requires time and patience, and for this reason, it is advised that a series of lessons be taken. In the case of chronic or serious physical dysfunction, a longer series of lessons may be recommended. Once the student has mastered the exercises in class, she can perform them on her own at home.

Awareness Through Movement classes are typically offered in a series of four to six sessions that meet once a week. Some teachers organize a series to concentrate on specific areas of reeducation, such as alleviating TMJ pain; learning how to sit with greater ease if you have a desk job (current research shows that stress on the spine can be 50 percent greater in a sitting versus standing posture); and learning general relaxation movements to reduce stress.

THE EXPERIENCE: AWARENESS THROUGH MOVEMENT

It is a crisp Sunday autumn afternoon, and I'm participating in an Awareness Through Movement class sponsored by the Feldenkrais Learning Center on Manhattan's Upper West Side. The Learning Center includes a faculty of nine Feldenkrais practitioners, who offer several classes a week in Awareness Through Movement. I've opted to take a workshop entitled "Freedom in Use of the Arms," which uses exercises designed to clarify the connection between chest mobility and the use of the arms. This is one of a menu of workshops with such diverse titles as "Sitting with Ease," "ATM for Dancers," "Feldenkrais and Self-Defense," "TMJ," "ATM and Vision," "Working out with Awareness," "Swimming with Awareness," and "Feldenkrais for Improved Running." A number of these workshops have several variations since there are a number of ATM lessons that can be practiced to bring awareness to a specific concern. There seem to be lessons geared to everyone's occupational and leisure-time needs.

I selected this particular workshop because I use my arms a great deal, both in writing and in performing massage therapy. Suffering from intermittent bouts of muscle tension and pain in my shoulders, arms, and chest, I realize I need to learn to use my body more efficiently to avoid strain. It turns out I'm not the only one whose profession stresses the oft-used muscles in the arms and chest: The class of twelve includes a computer keyboard operator and a pianist, both of whom develop chest and arm pain in performing their work. In addition, there are a number of people who suffer from chronic shoulder and chest pain and who are seeking a means of relief. The age of my fellow students ranges from a young woman in her mid-twenties to senior citizens. We're all dressed comfortably in loose-fitting clothing.

Our instructor is Lisa Wiener, a young, attractive, dark-haired woman who has gone through the extensive Feldenkrais practitioner-training program and who maintains a private practice in Brooklyn. As I arrive in the basement studio of the large apartment building where our class is to be held, several students are already lying on exercise mats on the floor. Lisa crawls on the carpeted floor as she moves from one student to another, answering preliminary questions. The first thing I notice about Lisa is her ease of movement, which seems to flow from a comfortable alignment and efficient use of all her body segments.

As the class begins, Lisa assumes a seated position at the front of the class. Her voice is soft and relaxed; her manner patient and nurturing.

"Feldenkrais is not exercise in the usual sense of the word. If you're used to thinking of exercise as working hard, doing large movements, that's not what Feldenkrais is about. The movements are small, even tiny. We do them slowly, many times, so you can begin to feel what you're doing.

"Some of you here today have shoulder or neck problems. Please do everything within your level of comfort. That means working within the range that is truly comfortable for you, without causing discomfort. If you have even a twinge of pain, do less. You can even visualize a movement and still learn. You don't have to feel like the ship has sailed and you're left behind.

"Make each movement easy, with as little effort as possible. Relax as much as you can and let go of the movement each time so each movement is new. Rest when you need to.

"And last but not least, the lessons are fun. They're meant to be a way for you to explore and learn. Think of them as not being too important. People seem to benefit more when they do the lessons without worrying about whether they're doing them right or not."

Having offered these general guidelines, Lisa explains that we'll be working on the floor, lying on our backs and on our sides. This will allow us to free ourselves from the tension imposed on our bodies by the weight of gravity and allow us to be more sensitive to what is going on in our bodies as we perform each movement.

Lisa asks us to be aware of how our backs meet the floor. Is there a hollow under them? If so, how does it feel? Does the left side feel the same as the right side?

Scanning my body, I become aware of it in a way that is absolutely novel. I realize how much I take it for granted. Even with my interest in, and respect for, the body, this simple exercise shows me how much of a stranger it is to me. By feeling my body for myself, with awareness, I establish a new relationship with it. I feel the tension on the right side of my body. I feel the curves of my back, the slight hollow under my low back as it arches toward the ceiling, the comforting relationship of support between my legs and the mat as they sink into the ground that supports them. I also realize there is no difference between me, which I think of as something inside my head that thinks, and my body: I am my tension; I am my curves. Only now I am aware of this dynamic relationship.

Lisa has us turn on our right sides, legs bent at a ninety-degree angle and lying on top of one another in front of us to support us so that we do not need to strain. She has us lift up our top, left leg to see how it feels. I'm amazed at how heavy it is; in effect, I'm lifting and carrying around this heavy mass of muscle, bone, and other tissue nearly every waking moment, and I'm not even aware of it. Lisa has us lift up our head as well to get a sense of how it feels. Again, I am amazed at how heavy it feels and at how hard my neck muscles must work to hold it up.

Next, we begin the movements related to clarifying the relation between arms and shoulders. The movements start small and gradually grow larger, though still small in comparison with the movements of many daily activities. We perform them slowly, gently, and with awareness. This means we are aware of how the movements feel, of which muscles we are using, of where our tension and strain is, of how we might be using our bodies to create this strain. Lisa, who remains seated at the front of the class, relays the instructions of the lesson to us in her calm, hypnotic voice. As the lesson progresses, she instructs us in one or two gentle movements, then has us return to a relaxed position, lying on our backs, so that we can rest and also be aware of any changes in how our bodies feel as a result of the movements we are performing. The movements are enjoyable, but I notice that they are also tiring, requiring concentration throughout their performance.

Lisa asks us to gently draw our left shoulder forward. We then reverse the movement and draw it backward. This is followed by a series of movements, punctuated by frequent rest breaks, that consist of drawing our left shoulder up toward our head, then down toward our left hip; rotating our shoulders in complete circles, forward and backward; drawing our left hip up toward our head, then down toward our feet; moving our hips forward and backward; moving our head toward our hip at the same time we draw our hip toward our head; and finally rotating our shoulders and hips in synchrony with one another and in opposite directions.

As we proceed with the lesson, I register a number of impressions. I become acutely aware of the places where I hold tension: in the lower part of my shoulder blade and in my neck. Lifting the neck, which I do all the time in my habitual activities without giving it a second thought, seems an immense effort. When this action is isolated from others and I bring my full awareness to it, I realize the tremendous strength and tension I am using to accomplish it. No wonder I (along with many others) develop such tension in the neck and upper shoulders. I'm also aware of how the muscles of one area are interconnected with the muscles of other areas. Moving my hip brings my shoulder muscles into action as well, exerting a pull and strain all the way up to my neck and head. It begins to dawn on me that I may not need to engage all these muscles: There may be a smarter, more efficient way of moving that would conserve rather than consume energy. I begin to think of alternatives to moving the way I habitually do that might involve less wear and tear.

What I notice most of all, though, is the powerful impact these movements are having on releasing the tension in the muscles of my shoulder, chest, and arms. Each time we finish a movement and return to the resting position on our backs, I'm aware of an increased sense of relaxation on my left side versus my unexercised right side. This feeling starts as a sense of general relaxation, then steadily grows, so that I feel as though the whole left side of my body is alive and glowing. I feel as though it has lengthened, expanded; it vibrates with a radiant energy that does not exist on the right side. In comparison, the right side feels tiny, constricted, atrophied, almost dead. My left side feels like Samson dwarfing the David that is joined to it on the right.

Lisa asks us to lift our leg and then our head, paying attention to how they feel. I notice how much lighter they have become. This dramatic change is the result of differentiation: My whole self rather than just individual parts has become involved in making these movements.

As we conclude the lesson, Lisa encourages us to rest on our backs for as long as we need, then gently roll over onto our sides to come to a seated position. We slowly walk around the room to become aware of how we feel. As we do, we look a bit like newborn babies taking our first steps, relaxed and learning all over again what it is like to move.

The tension in my shoulders is gone, particularly the left shoulder. It is amazing to me that such subtle, gentle movements can induce so powerful a release. I am aware of the imbalance between my left and right sides. The right still feels tighter, more constricted. Lisa explains that the lesson learned by the left side of the body will be transferred to the right side, often within as short a time as half an hour.

As I leave the class and return to the sidewalk, filled with bustling, if not frenetic, New Yorkers bent on weekend shopping, I feel incredibly relaxed, light, energized, and clear. My movements seem effortless. Later in the day, I take an aerobics and calisthenics class. I am struck by how ungraceful—even unhealthy—these large, jerky movements feel. I begin to sense how many of the movements that I routinely make are putting unnecessary strain on my body.

My feeling of relaxation and well-being outlasts the demands of my exercise class and stays with me throughout the rest of the day. Indeed, for the next few days, I continue to feel the relaxation and ease I achieved throughout my entire body, both right and left sides, in Lisa's workshop. And, most important, I am aware of how I feel. I can sense how this awareness, cultivated over time, will enable me to appreciate the inefficiency of my habitual movement patterns and help me to integrate more efficient patterns of movement into my daily repertoire.

I also have powerful dreams the evening following the class. Various issues regarding parts of my life that I've ignored, or whose importance I've denied, enter my awareness while sleeping. They come in such a way that I am able to see them clearly. Having become consciously aware of them, they no longer frighten me, and I am able to let them go. Awareness has penetrated more than just my movement.

THE BENEFITS OF THE FELDENKRAIS METHOD

The Feldenkrais Method aims to restore full physical function to the greatest extent possible. Advocates of Feldenkrais have reported relief from the pain associated with TMJ disorder and other joint disorders; headaches; and neck, shoulder, and back pain. Because Feldenkrais seeks to break up chronic habitual neuromuscular patterns and open up new possibilities, its benefits also include improved breathing and sleep patterns, greater mental clarity, and a heightened sense of vitality and freedom of movement. Some people even report feeling taller as contracted muscles relax to their normal length. Because Feldenkrais lessons effect a change in self-image, they can affect your overall feeling about yourself as well as the quality of your social interactions. As Feldenkrais noted, the only thing permanent about our behavior patterns is the belief that they are so.

Feldenkrais seems to work particularly well with people with muscular disorders, such as cerebral palsy and multiple sclerosis, as well as stroke and accident victims, offering relief from pain and helping restore range of motion and muscular control—in some cases where physical therapy provided little or no relief. In his book *The Case of Nora,* Feldenkrais recounts his inspiring experience in working with Nora, a Swiss woman paralyzed by a stroke. Feldenkrais was able to help Nora regain use of her motor functions through his method.

People from many different walks of life have found Feldenkrais to be a powerful method to help them achieve greater freedom of movement and increased performance. Athletes, musicians, dancers, and other active and creative individuals have appreciated the benefits of the Feldenkrais Method. Feldenkrais techniques have been used in many drama programs, including those at Carnegie-Mellon University, the University of Pittsburgh, and New York University. Professional ski instructors in the Vail, Colorado, area have attended Awareness Through Movement classes to help them improve their performance on the slopes.[4] Among his many admirers Feldenkrais counted the anthropologist Margaret Mead (who felt his method was especially beneficial in preventing and reversing deterioration of function in the elderly); the first prime minister of Israel, David Ben-Gurion (who dubbed Feldenkrais a "national treasure"); the director Peter Brook; and the concert violinist Yehudi Menuhin.

CONTRAINDICATIONS TO THE FELDENKRAIS METHOD

Because the Feldenkrais Method involves gentle body movements, there are no contraindications.

BACKGROUND AND TRAINING OF PRACTITIONERS

Only those practitioners who have been trained and certified by the Feldenkrais Guild of North America are entitled to use the service marks Feldenkrais, Feldenkrais Method, Functional Integration, and Awareness Through Movement, which are service marks of the Feldenkrais Guild of North America. Currently, there are more than thirteen hundred certified practitioners of the Feldenkrais Method in the United States and Canada.

The Feldenkrais Guild of North America approves all training programs. A recent schedule of classes shows courses being offered throughout the United States and Canada. The Feldenkrais training program is generally conducted over a period of four years, with several intensive sessions of several weeks' duration each year. The total four-year program constitutes a minimum of 800 hours of theoretical and practical study, spanning about 160 days. Halfway through the program, a student is authorized to teach Awareness Through Movement classes. At the completion of the entire program, the student is certified to become a practitioner. No specific background is required for acceptance into the Feldenkrais training program.

FOR FURTHER INFORMATION

The Feldenkrais Guild was established in 1977 by Moshe Feldenkrais to serve as the professional organization of practitioners of the Feldenkrais Method. The Guild maintains standards of practice, provides educational information, and sponsors research on the Feldenkrais Method. The Guild also oversees the training of practitioners of the Feldenkrais Method. You can obtain additional information on the Feldenkrais Method, including audio and videotapes and a free practitioner list, by contacting:

Feldenkrais Guild of North America
3611 S.W. Hood Avenue, Suite 100
Portland, OR 97239
Tel: (503) 221-6612 or (800) 775-2118
Fax: (503) 221-6616
Website: www.feldenkrais.com
E-mail: guild@feldenkrais.com

The best way to learn about the Feldenkrais Method is to experience it, either in a class or in a private lesson. However, if you are interested in trying some of the lessons on your own, you can obtain guided audio and video instruction tapes by contacting:

Feldenkrais Resources
830 Bancroft Way, Suite 112
Berkeley, CA 94710
Tel: (800) 765-1907 or (510) 540-7600
Fax: (510) 540-7683
Website: www.feldenkraisresources.com
E-mail: info@feldenkraisresources.com

SUGGESTED FURTHER READING

The following books are by Moshe Feldenkrais:

Moshe Feldenkrais, D.Sc., *Awareness Through Movement: Easy-to-Do Health Exercises to Improve Your Posture, Vision, Imagination, & Personal Awareness* (San Francisco: Harper & Row, 1972).

_____. *The Elusive Obvious or Basic Feldenkrais* (Cupertino, CA: Meta Publications, 1981).

_____. *The Potent Self* (San Francisco: HarperCollins, 1985).

The following book is by a Feldenkrais practitioner:

David Zemach-Bersin, et al., *Relaxercise: Ten Effortless Techniques for a More Flexible, Energetic, Pain-Free, Stress-Free Body* (San Francisco: HarperCollins, 1990).

PART III

OTHER CONTEMPORARY WESTERN BODYWORK PRACTICES

Not until we experience it is it more than just words. After we experience it, there is no need for words. The importance of words is to stimulate the desire to experience.[1]

—MILTON TRAGER, M.D.

Bodywork practices included in the following section represent syntheses of a variety of practices. These approaches are all united in their common goal of unifying body and mind, the unconscious and the conscious.

BASIC FACTS

- **Myofascial Release is a whole-body approach to healing that seeks to restore balance by releasing tension in the soft connective tissue known as fascia.** It results in relief from pain and improved function.

- **Myofascial (Greek *myo* for muscle and "fascia") Release was developed by John Barnes, P.T.** A physical therapist, Barnes integrated soft-tissue manipulative techniques with CranioSacral Therapy in a whole-system approach to releasing fascia.

THEORY

- **Myofascial Release removes constriction in the fascia.** Fascia can become constricted due to trauma, such as illness and other physical and psychological stresses. If it becomes tight, fascia can pull muscles and bones out of place, resulting in pain and lack of mobility. Fascia as well as muscle must be released for long-lasting effect.

- **Myofascial Release uses long, sustained pressure to stretch the fascia.** This removes tightness and associated pain and discomfort. Release of unconscious emotional material frequently accompanies release of the fascia.

TYPICAL SESSION

- **Myofascial Release sessions last thirty minutes to an hour and a half.** The client lies on a massage table and is dressed in underwear or a bathing suit. No oil is used.

- **Practitioners use surface areas of their bodies, such as the fingers, palms, elbows, and forearms, to elongate and stretch the fascia.** Strokes are deliberately slow—a minimum of 90 to 120 seconds, and at times as long as 5 minutes. Pressure is gentle but firm.

- It is suggested that initial treatment consist of several sessions.

- Expect to pay $100 to $150 per hour for treatment.

BENEFITS

- **Proponents maintain that Myofascial Release is especially effective in providing longer-term relief for chronic pain and dysfunction associated with muscular tightness.** Conditions treated include neck, jaw, and back pain; muscle tension; recurring injuries; scoliosis; and stress-related disorders.

CONTRAINDICATIONS

- Myofascial Release is completely contraindicated in the case of malignancy, aneurysm, and acute rheumatoid arthritis.

- Local contraindications (treatment may be given, but problem areas should be avoided) include bruises, open wounds, and fractures.

BACKGROUND AND TRAINING OF PRACTITIONERS

- **Many practitioners are trained by the Myofascial Release Treatment Center & Seminars.** The training program is offered in a series of intensive workshops and supervised clinical internships. Practitioners are generally health professionals who hold licenses or certificates in related disciplines.

- More than fifty thousand healthcare professionals have studied Myofascial Release.

CHAPTER 5

MYOFASCIAL RELEASE: PHYSICAL THERAPY JOINS HANDS WITH MASSAGE THERAPY

Mind-body awareness are two sides of the same coin, different aspects of the same spectrum, immutably joined, inseparable, connected, influencing, and communicating constantly. Myofascial release techniques and myofascial unwinding allow for the complete communication necessary for healing and true growth. I believe that the body remembers everything that ever happened to it.[1]

—JOHN F. BARNES, P.T.

WHAT IS MYOFASCIAL RELEASE?

Myofascial Release is a whole-body approach to healing that seeks to restore balance to the body by releasing tension in the fascia. Practitioners use long, stretching strokes to release muscular tension. This technique, which is generally gentle, has the effect of relieving pain and improving function.

THE ORIGINS OF MYOFASCIAL RELEASE

Myofascial Release is most frequently associated with John F. Barnes, P.T., who has pioneered this approach to healing over the past thirty years. Drawing upon his background as a physical therapist, Barnes integrated a variety of techniques drawn from soft-tissue manipulative and unwinding techniques designed to mobilize the fascia and facilitate movement. His approach also incorporates principles of CranioSacral Therapy in a whole-system approach to releasing fascia.

THE THEORY UNDERLYING MYOFASCIAL RELEASE

The term "myofascial" is derived from the Greek *myo*, meaning "muscle," and fascia, a thin layer system of connective tissue that surrounds, supports, and interweaves every muscle, organ, and bone in the body. It is referred to as the packing material of the body because of its omnipresence and supportive function. If you were to remove everything but the fascia from the body, the body would still retain its recognizable shape.

Because fascia gives strength, support, and form to the body, it plays a key role in any type of bodywork. In its natural state, fascia is elastic and relaxed. However, it can become constricted due to trauma, such as illness, physical injury, habitual poor posture, and emotional and psychological stress. If fascia becomes tight or distorted, it can pull muscles and bones out of place, resulting in pain and lack of mobility. Practitioners of Myofascial Release believe that in order to release tension in the body with lasting effect it is necessary to release the fascia. If a practitioner works only on the level of releasing muscles, a client may feel temporary relief; however, the tension will return if underlying constrictions in the fascia that binds muscles remain untreated.

Fascia is composed of a gel-like component, which has the ability to release when warmed. In Myofascial Release, a practitioner uses the surfaces of her body, such as the fingers, palms, and elbows, to slowly and steadily warm the fascia, thereby making it more malleable, somewhat like melting butter. This long, sustained pressure elongates and stretches the fascia, which becomes glue-like in feel. By lengthening the fascia, the practitioner removes the tightness and constriction that are the source of pain and discomfort. Myofascial Release seems to be accomplished by this gentle, sustained stretch and thermal effect and by the flow of the electromagnetic energies that all trained, sensitive therapists can produce. Along with the release of physical tension, clients frequently report a release of emotional material. As Barnes explains, Myofascial Release "seems also to reach underlying or hidden information in the subconscious."[2]

THE TYPICAL FORMAT OF MYOFASCIAL RELEASE

A typical session in Myofascial Release lasts thirty to ninety minutes. The client undresses down to his underwear and is draped on a padded treatment table. The practitioner applies a series of strokes that are deliberately long, slow, and steady—a minimum of 90 to 120 seconds per stroke and at times as long as 3 to 5 minutes. Because the practitioner wishes to use friction to her advantage in stretching the fascia, no oil is used. As a general rule, practitioners recommend that in the initial stages of treatment, a client experience several sessions a week, with frequency of visits diminishing as a condition improves.

THE EXPERIENCE: MY MYOFASCIA IS RELEASED

It is a sunny early spring afternoon, and I've just escorted Vicki Calpena-

Eklund, a Myofascial Release therapist, into my apartment. I obtained Vicki's name and phone number and those of several other practitioners from the Myofascial Release Treatment Center when I called for referrals to practitioners in the greater New York City metropolitan area. I contacted Vicki and several other practitioners and was particularly impressed with Vicki's professional manner, training, and experience.

Vicki is a New York State–licensed massage therapist whose background includes training in traditional Swedish, medical, and sports massage; CranioSacral Therapy; massage for women in their childbearing years; and Myofascial Release therapy. Vicki practices in a number of environments—her apartment in Manhattan's East Village; a professional space she shares with other therapists; a luxury Manhattan spa called Cãrapan; as well as home visits. I decided to treat myself to the luxury of a home visit and so arranged for Vicki to come to my apartment.

Vicki is young, attractive, vivacious. She is dressed casually in a sweater and jeans. Her air of inner quiet impresses me.

Vicki explains that she pursued training in Myofascial Release after working exclusively with Swedish massage for several years. "I would work on people with chronic pain, and they'd feel better for a while. But the pain would come back. After working with them for six months or so, I'd wonder if there wasn't a better way I could help them. I could feel things going on in their bodies, areas of holding, but I didn't know how to release them. A therapist friend told me about Myofascial Release, and I decided to try it. It's been a powerful tool for effecting long-term change in people with chronic pain. In my own case, I was able to get rid of sciatic pain I'd had for years through Myofascial Release treatments." Like Barnes, Vicki believes it is useful to draw on a variety of approaches to help people relieve chronic pain.

Following her encouraging introduction to our session, Vicki asks me to tell her how I'm feeling. I tell her I'm feeling tense in my back and shoulders; my legs are sore because I've been overdoing it with exercise; and I feel a little tired, experiencing a low level of energy that I associate with the change of season.

Vicki explains that she'll begin the session by assessing my body visually. She asks me to disrobe down to a pair of gym shorts, then stand facing her in a well-lit space. "And relax," she says. "Just let your body assume whatever position it feels it wants to sink into, without worrying about gravity." With that, I close my eyes and let my awareness sink into releasing my body.

Vicki stands several yards from me. "I'm noticing that your left shoulder is higher than your right. Your head is twisted toward the right shoulder. Your left hip is higher than your right. That causes a tightness in your right hip and leg and a turning out of your right foot. Your left leg is rotated slightly inward, with a twist at the knee. The height difference on the left hip is reflected in your high left shoulder. There seems to be a line of tension that travels across your diaphragm, from your left hip to your right shoulder. Your right arm hangs lower than your left, and the right elbow is twisted, moving the whole arm closer to your body. Your right ankle looks lower than your left. Is that a scar I see on your left leg?" she asks as she advances toward me to look more closely. "No," she says, "it's just a vein." She's sized me up in a minute or so.

Vicki asks me to turn in profile, then with my back to her. She notices an area of tight tissue on the right side of my midback, the area where I experience chronic pain. She approaches and runs her hands down the skin of my back to feel the quality of the tissue. "It's also tight in the low back," she reports.

Vicki explains that this visual full-body analysis will enable her to design a session addressed to my unique structure. By understanding areas of pull and constriction in my body, along with their corresponding compensations, she can prioritize the work to be done.

I lie down on my back on a padded massage table. (Because I have a massage table, Vicki did not need to bring one with her. Many massage therapists who make home visits carry portable massage tables with them, though.) Vicki goes to the foot of the table and places her hands over the front of my ankles. I feel heat emanating from her palms. She listens to the fascia of my body to learn where it is holding. By feeling the tissue at my feet and attuning to what it is telling her, she reports that she feels that the most compelling restriction is in my right hip. It is amazing she can know this just by feeling my ankles. Vicki's hands are extremely sensitized; because the fascia forms one continuous web throughout the body, she can feel distortions of pull at any point within the system. To confirm her findings, Vicki moves to the head of the table, where she sits down while placing her hands under my head. She is listening to the fascia covering my head and neck, which confirms her evaluation.

Vicki moves to the right of the table and places her hands on my outer right thigh. Her two hands are close together, providing full hand contact. She uses the heel of her palm as a stabilizer and gently rotates my leg inward. "I'd like to help this leg become less turned out, remove some of the tension here," she says. She holds for several minutes. I can feel the tension in my leg; her touch feels deep as it meets my leg, not painful but firm. "I'm allowing my hands to meet the resistance in your tissue," she explains. "It takes some time for the tissue to release. Sometimes ninety seconds or so; sometimes as long as five or ten minutes." She holds for what feels like several minutes, increasing the resistance on my tight muscles. I feel as though the resistance becomes stronger before the tissue releases. As the tissue releases, it feels like a strand of taffy that's been warmed and stretched out.

"That's good," Vicki encourages me as she releases my thigh and returns to my feet. "Very good," she says. "You're much more relaxed. Your legs feel longer and lighter. The right leg is still turned out, but less so."

Vicki next turns her attention to the pull she'd detected in my diaphragm. She places one hand under my back at the center of my bottom ribs while she places the other over my upper stomach and sternum. As she gently holds for several minutes, I feel as though the tissue that covers my stomach is turning, rotating to the right, then releasing and returning back to the left. I breathe a deep sigh as my diaphragm opens up. "I feel as though the fascia was being pulled to that tight right hip at first," Vicki corroborates. "Then it released and became more balanced."

As she worked on my stomach, Vicki became aware of a tightness in my right psoas muscle. This muscle, one of the toughest and often tightest in the body, runs from the bottom of the spine through the back of the abdominal cavity to insert on the upper inner thigh. Often after working out I feel a tightness in the lower right quadrant of my stomach, which is related to the tightness in my psoas muscle. To release the fascia related to this muscle, Vicki has me slide over to the right edge of the table. She places a bolster under my low back and asks me to let my right leg dangle loosely over the side of the table. She edges her fingers into the right lateral side of my stomach, her fingers resembling a bear claw, as she engages the fascia connected to the psoas muscle.

This area is sensitive. It hurts, not beyond my threshold for pain but to a point of discomfort. I tell Vicki it is uncomfortable, and she reassures me, "All you have to say is 'Halt' and I will." I don't feel the discomfort is great enough to stop. "Sometimes," Vicki explains, "an area that is tight doesn't want to let go, so it holds even more. You may want to shout out or you may feel a change in your breathing: Emotional release is often connected to physical release. Sometimes the discomfort increases before it releases. The discomfort can come from different sources. Tightness in the tissue can cause pain—where my hands are now I can feel scar tissue. My hands were led closer to the umbilicus by the movement of the fascia. Sometimes this scar tissue can go back to our birthing experience. In addition, the stomach is an extremely sensitive area, tied in to many emotional issues that can cause discomfort."

Vicki continues to hold while her fingers slowly glide back and forth over the knot of scar tissue. Simultaneously, she gently rotates my right leg to feel for areas of restriction. I feel the tightness in the fascia, the knot she's talking about, and then I feel a release taking place; the area feels like one of those lacquered Chinese hand fans that had been closed and now is fully opened. As the area releases, I find my thought processes releasing, too. I'd been thinking about some situations that had upset me—problems with friends, anxiety about impending deadlines. But suddenly, as the tension is removed from my body, my mind becomes less agitated, more settled. Those troubling thoughts seem like passing clouds that have drifted away. In fact, instead of regarding these situations as stressful, I become aware that I've been forming creative solutions to them.

Vicki spends five, perhaps even ten, minutes on the psoas release. It takes time to listen to the tissue and wait for release, she explains. Sometimes a therapist may treat only a few areas during an entire session.

Vicki looks at my chest. "You have much more color here now," she reports. "I also look for any vasomotor responses in the body, because they indicate changes that are taking place." She touches my chest and tells me it feels warm. "That's natural," she explains. "When energy that has been blocked in a place is released, it gives off heat." To enhance this change, Vicki places one hand under my upper back and the other over my upper chest. She holds for a few minutes. I feel my chest opening up. I'm aware of a greater fullness on the left side. As the tissue releases, my breathing deepens.

Vicki returns to my feet to listen again, to see which area of my body is calling out to her. I'm feeling a tightness in my low left back, which is what calls Vicki's attention, too.

Vicki asks me to roll onto my right side, and she places a pillow under my right waist and my head. My right leg is flexed on the table in front of me; my left dangles off the table. "I'm going to work on the fascia related to your quadratus lumborum," she says. This muscle, which runs along the lower back ribs, is responsible for much low back pain. She eases her fingers into the area between my left waist and low back. As she holds them there, I can feel the tightness in the tissue. She applies her forearm and elbow to the area to intensify the stretch. She holds for several minutes, then firmly grasps my left ankle with both hands for increased traction. I can feel the tension going from my left waist and groin area all the way up to my chest, even to the area around my left eye. The slow movements made over a period of time seem to allow me to become aware of my areas of greatest holding and to feel how they extend to other parts of my body. I feel the tension building up, then releasing. Vicki feels it, too. She stops the traction and returns to the side of the table. Her arms are crossed as she applies a slow, deliberate stretching stroke to the left side of my torso, her hands gradually spreading farther away from one another. I feel a lightening and lengthening of my entire torso.

"I'd like to do a little work on your shoulders and back before our time is up. Could you kindly turn over onto your stomach?" she asks. I obediently comply. "Nice," Vicki says. "Not too much tension in your shoulders. There is some tissue tightness along your right midback, though."

Vicki executes a variety of soft-tissue mobilization techniques designed to release the superficial tissue covering my back. These strokes are more rapid than the previous release techniques, and many of them emphasize use of the fingers rather than the full hand. She applies pressure with several fingers in the direction of tightness over my shoulder blades, twisting her fingers at the end so that the stroke forms the shape of the letter *J*. She places her fingers perpendicularly into the tissue at the top of my back and moves them slowly back and forth over muscle and fascia, as though strumming the string of a guitar. She moves her fingers along the skin that lines either side of the spine, picking up folds of fascia that lie in the spaces between the vertebrae. Where the tissue is tight alongside my spine, she applies a technique known as finger rolling: She picks up the skin and rolls the tissue under it between her fingers, moving rapidly up and down in quick passes that form straight lines parallel to my spine. I experience a pinching, burning sensation as she works. When she approaches my low left back, the pain intensifies. Vicki confirms: "Yes, it's especially tight down here." She explains that ideally this should feel loose like the skin of a dog. By the time she finishes with my back, it does. She admires my back and says, "Now, that's nice."

Vicki completes the session by evaluating and balancing the flow of cerebrospinal fluid that circulates through the spinal column from the head to the sacrum. This draws on techniques used in CranioSacral Therapy. She asks me to assume the fetal position and places some pillows in front of my chest for me to hold on to for support. She sits by the side of the table facing my back and places one hand on my sacrum, the other on the occiput of my head. She's feeling for the smooth, even flow of fluid. After holding for several minutes, she reports that initially she felt an obstruction in the flow in my low back. By holding with the intention to help my body balance itself, she was able to facilitate a releasing of this area of constriction. Fluid then flowed more smoothly. "I'm just here to help your body heal itself," Vicki explains as she concludes the session with a smile.

I look at the clock and note that Vicki worked on me for nearly an hour and a half. "I feel that there's still more we could do—to release the constriction in your low back and also some residual tension in your quadriceps," Vicki confides. "But we can't do everything in one session. I usually recommend that new clients begin with two or three sessions of Myofascial Release. Then we reappraise and see if more sessions would be beneficial."

That night, I realize the benefits of the session extend beyond the physical release of tension. I have a number of vivid dreams that help release me from fears dating back to childhood. I wake the next morning feeling peaceful and less anxious.

The next day, I notice that my chest feels wide and open, my head and neck longer. When I visit the gym, I'm delighted to realize how relaxed my muscles feel. I can lift more weight than usual with greater ease and without the feeling of tensing I normally feel. I'm feeling released.

THE BENEFITS OF MYOFASCIAL RELEASE

Proponents of Myofascial Release maintain that it is especially effective in providing longer-term relief for chronic pain and dysfunction associated with muscular tightness, including neck, jaw, and back pain; muscle tension; recurring injuries (including sports injuries); scoliosis; and stress-related disorders.

CONTRAINDICATIONS TO MYOFASCIAL RELEASE

Myofascial Release therapy is contraindicated in the case of malignancy, aneurysm, and acute rheumatoid arthritis. Local contraindications (which means that treatment can be given but problem areas should be avoided) include bruises, open wounds, and fractures. Barnes recommends that a diagnostic workup be performed by a physician prior to treatment. Additionally, the therapist should complete a comprehensive evaluation before treating.

BACKGROUND AND TRAINING OF PRACTITIONERS

Myofascial Release is performed by practitioners with a variety of backgrounds. John Barnes established the Myofascial Release (MFR) Treatment Center & Seminars to provide training in his approach. In addition to sponsoring training workshops, this organization operates clinics in Paoli, Pennsylvania, and Sedona, Arizona, for client treatment and practitioner training. More than fifty thousand healthcare professionals have studied Barnes's method in seminars conducted around the country. Many massage therapists, as well as physical therapists and doctors, practice Myofascial Release.

There is no separate national licensing for Myofascial Release. This practice is taught in a series of intensive, graded workshops, generally to health professionals who already hold licenses or certificates in related disciplines. As in selecting a practitioner of any type of bodywork, you should investigate the overall background and training of any therapist you may consider consulting.

FOR FURTHER INFORMATION

For further information on Myofascial Release, including books and audiovisual aids, a list of practitioners in your area, and a schedule of trainings, contact:

MFR Treatment Center & Seminars
222 West Lancaster Avenue
Paoli, PA 19301
Tel: (800) FASCIAL (327-2425) or (610) 644-0136
Fax: (610) 644-1662
Website: www.myofascialrelease.com
E-mail: paoli@myofascialrelease.com

SUGGESTED FURTHER READING

John F. Barnes, P.T., *Myofascial Release: The Search for Excellence, a Comprehensive Evaluatory and Treatment Approach* (Paoli, PA: Myofascial Release Seminars, 1990). This book is a comprehensive presentation of the foundational principles and techniques of Myofascial Release.

_____. *Healing Ancient Wounds: The Renegade's Wisdom* (Paoli, PA: MFR Treatment Centers & Seminars, 2000). This book explores intuitive awareness and the dynamic mind/body healing principles of Myofascial Release.

THE TRAGER APPROACH AT A GLANCE

BASIC FACTS

- The Trager Approach utilizes nonintrusive pain-free hands-on touch and exercises to release deep-seated psychophysiological areas of holding. As areas of blockage release, an individual is freed to move and pain and dysfunction disappear.

- The Trager Approach was developed by Milton Trager, M.D. (1908–1997). As a teenager, he recognized his special gift for healing and used his approach to treat his own congenital back pain and his father's sciatica.

THEORY

- **Physical discomfort and pain begin in the mind.** Through the nervous and neurochemical communicating systems, the mind maintains muscles in chronically contracted and inflamed positions.

- **The Trager Approach reeducates the nervous system in more relaxed, less painful patterns.** Through informed technique and intuitive awareness, a Trager practitioner communicates with the unconscious aspect of the client. The Trager Approach bypasses the conscious mind to effect permanent change.

- **The Trager Approach accesses a state that Trager called hook-up.** This is a deeply meditative state in which a practitioner hooks up to the flow of energy all around her to actively facilitate release.

TYPICAL SESSION

- **The Trager Approach to psychophysical integration is practiced in two formats.** Individual bodywork treatment is commonly referred to as tablework. A companion program of Mentastics (Trager's coined term for "mental gymnastics") movement exercises are performed at home or in class to reinforce the message given to the client's unconscious during a tablework session.

- A typical tablework session lasts sixty to ninety minutes. The client lies on a massage table, in a warm, comfortable environment, wearing swimwear, briefs, or additional clothing. No lotion or oil is used. The practitioner uses gentle, rhythmic rocking, kneading, shaking, vibrating, and stretching movements to increase range of motion and induce relaxation.

- A Mentastics class typically lasts thirty to ninety minutes. Longer workshop formats are available, too. Students perform simple dancelike movements that utilize relaxed stretching, rocking, and shaking. Mentastics are designed to show how free and light the body can feel. Mentastics exercises are often given as homework following a private tablework session.

- Practitioners recommend that individuals begin treatment with a series of individual sessions for maximum benefit. Subsequent periodic reminder sessions can be helpful.

- The fee for a typical Trager tablework session can range between $45 and $120 depending on the geographic location of the practitioner. A Trager session can last from one hour to an hour and a half. The fee for a group Mentastics class ranges from $10 to $15 per hour.

BENEFITS

- **While this approach is not a medical treatment, Trager reported success in treating a wide range of physical ailments.** These include polio; muscular dystrophy and other degenerative muscular disorders; multiple sclerosis; chronic pain syndromes, such as low back problems; emphysema; migraine headaches; and asthma.

- The Trager Approach is used by a number of trainers and athletes to enhance athletic performance.

- **Individuals who experience the Trager Approach report an increased sense of relaxation, vitality, mental clarity, and creativity.** They experience what they describe as a place beyond relaxation: "peace."

CONTRAINDICATIONS

- Because the Trager Approach is gentle and involves no deep manipulation, there are few contraindications. Situations where movement may not be advisable include broken bones; blood clots; fever; joint, bone, and disk disorders, including recent surgery; problem pregnancies; and use of drugs that alter perception.

BACKGROUND AND TRAINING OF PRACTITIONERS

- **Trager practitioners are trained in a curriculum administered internationally and certified by one of the national Trager associations of the practitioner.** The training program includes formal courses in theory and practice, fieldwork, and private tutorials. Practitioners are certified upon completion of 409 hours of supervised and unsupervised (sessions given and received) training. Practitioners maintain their professional status by completing annual continuing-education requirements.

- **There are approximately one thousand Trager practitioners, represented in nearly every state and in many foreign countries.** More than four thousand students have learned the Trager Approach, and six hundred students are currently in training in areas as diverse as the United States, Canada, Western Europe, Israel, Australia, and Japan.

CHAPTER 6

THE TRAGER APPROACH: MEDITATION IN MOTION

Many times after a real good session with a patient, I get so moved by their face that I must take them by the hand, take them to a mirror, and say "I want you to meet this person." Sometimes they say, "I haven't seen her in 25 years." What I feel is that this is actually the soul of the individual uncovered.[1]

—MILTON TRAGER, M.D.

WHAT IS THE TRAGER APPROACH?

The Trager Approach is a method of movement education and bodywork that utilizes nonintrusive pleasurable hands-on touch (tablework) and a program of do-it-yourself exercises (Mentastics) to release deep-seated psychophysiological areas of holding in the mind and body. As areas of blockage release, an individual is liberated to move freely and pain and dysfunction dissipate. "Since these blocks are released at the source (the mind)," Trager explained, "the patient can experience long-lasting release and relief from fixed patterns."[2]

THE ORIGINS OF THE TRAGER APPROACH

The Trager Approach was developed by Milton Trager, M.D. (1908–1997). In the mid-1920s, at the age of eighteen, Trager was an aspiring young boxer. Trager recognized his innate gift for healing when he gave his trainer a massage and received this awe-filled response: "Hey, kid. Where did you learn how to do this? . . . I'm telling you, you've got hands."[3] Subsequent experience confirmed this: Trager proved able to facilitate healing in people with disorders ranging from polio to sciatica, not to mention his own congenital low back dysfunction. Trager developed his signature approach to healing and practiced it relatively quietly for a period of nearly fifty years. Along the way, in 1955, at the ripe young age of forty-seven, he earned his M.D. degree and combined his practice of medicine and physical rehabilitation with his own personal method. While pursuing his medical degree in Guadalajara, Mexico, Trager experienced a particularly dramatic incident. Using his approach to healing, he was able to help restore movement to a young polio patient. Nuns fell to their knees in prayer, and the hospital dedicated a wing for Trager to pursue his work. In 1975, the Trager Approach gained widespread recognition when Trager was invited to present his technique at Esalen. In 1977, Trager retired from medical practice to respond to students' demands that he devote full-time attention to training practitioners in his work.

THE THEORY UNDERLYING THE TRAGER APPROACH

For Trager, physical pain and dysfunction begin in the mind. It is the mind—through the nervous and neurochemical communicating systems of the body—that maintains muscles in chronically contracted and inflamed positions. "Tight muscles could be caused by many things, but the pattern of the tightness is all in the mind," Trager explains.[4] The Trager Approach releases blockages at the source so that the client can experience long-lasting relief of physical symptoms.

Trager referred to his work as psychophysical integration because it utilizes feeling and physical touch to bring about change in deep-seated psychophysiological patterns in the mind and body. These patterns, which block the flow of movement in the body, are responsible for pain and physical dysfunction.

In a tablework session, using informed technique and intuitive awareness, the practitioner communicates with the unconscious aspect of the client to reeducate the nervous system in more relaxed, less painful patterns. The Trager practitioner's hands silently repeat on an unconscious level the following questions to the client's tissues: "How should this feel? What is softer? Lighter? Freer?" The Trager practitioner does not try to change the condition of tissues with his hands, but to communicate a quality of feeling to the client's mind by way of the nervous system. A Trager session is a lesson in teaching the unconscious of the client, which is the real agent of change. Because it accesses the unconscious, adherents maintain that the changes it evokes are permanent.

In order to enter into a deep level of touch communication involving his own unconscious as well as that of the client, the practitioner enters a state Trager describes as hook-up. In this state, which resembles a meditative state, the practitioner hooks up to the flow of energy all around him. Unlike meditation, though, which can be a solitary experience, the practitioner actively uses this heightened state of awareness to facilitate releases in the client. During hook-up, the practitioner establishes a deep level of rapport with the unconscious of the client.

The companion program of Mentastics exercises is designed to reinforce the pleasurable message given to the client's unconscious during a tablework session: "Yes, I can be lighter, freer, more flexible, and it feels like this." Mentastics help the body to maintain the openness achieved during tablework and even to enhance that feeling over time.

THE TYPICAL FORMAT OF THE TRAGER APPROACH

A typical Trager tablework session lasts sixty to ninety minutes. The client lies on a padded massage table in a warm, comfortable environment. He wears swimwear, briefs, or additional clothing, and no lotion or oil is used. Unlike massage and forms of deep manipulative work, the practitioner does not apply long flowing strokes or deep manipulations. Gentle, rhythmic rocking, kneading, shaking, vibrating, and stretching movements are used to increase range of motion and induce relaxation. These movements are designed to educate the client by reminding him what it feels like to have a free and open body: The pleasurable experiences felt during the session help to replace negative habitual patterns.

Following an individual Trager session, the client is given homework exercises called Mentastics. Mentastics, which is the expression Trager coined for "mental gymnastics," are likened to mindfulness in motion. Mentastics are simple dancelike movements that utilize relaxed stretching, rocking, and shaking. They differ from traditional calisthenics in that no force or effort is used.

Trager recommended that, in the beginning, a series of Trager sessions be given for maximum benefit. Reminder sessions administered from time to time can also be helpful. The client can perform Mentastics on an ongoing basis to maintain and amplify the sense of freedom imparted by the initial bodywork on the table. Mentastics can be practiced either on one's own or in a group setting.

THE EXPERIENCE: I GET "TRAGERED"

I arrive at the office of Trager practitioner Roger Tolle, whose name and telephone number were kindly provided me when I contacted the Trager Institute in search of a practitioner in my area. In addition to being a practitioner, Roger is also a teacher of the Trager Approach.

Roger works out of his spacious, sprawling apartment on Manhattan's residential Upper West Side. His work space is in the sun-drenched living room, where he has set up a massage table in the middle of the room. Roger is a young, attractive man with short black hair, a mustache, and a kindly face that exudes energy and concern. His carriage is erect, and he moves with a grace and ease that betray his previous career as a dancer. He confides that it is his fascination with movement that drew him to the Trager Approach.

As I sit on a comfortable sofa, Roger begins our session by asking me a few basic questions about my medical background and any relevant issues regarding my body. I explain that I am in good health but suffer from routine tension in my neck, shoulders, and back. Roger can easily understand this. "Working as you do as a writer, you're hunched over a desk, which puts strain on your shoulders, neck, and even your eyes. Typing at a computer stresses your hands and arms, too. Working over a massage table also tends to make people hunch their shoulders forward and puts added stress on the hands," he shares.

"The Trager Approach helps us better understand our bodies and how we're feeling in them," Roger continues. To demonstrate this, he asks me to remove my shoes and stand in front of him, feet securely placed on the floor. He asks me to bring my awareness to the left side of my body as I allow my left arm and hand to dangle by my side. He asks me to gently jiggle that arm until I become aware of the position and presence of my left thumb. As I focus my awareness I'm surprised, and delighted, to feel how I can differentiate the feeling of my thumb from my other fingers. I had never really thought about this possibility before. Roger asks me to bring my awareness to each of my fingers in succession; as I do so, I become aware of a kind of vibration or pulsation in each one. Roger then asks me to see if I can focus my attention on the individual bones inside my hand. I've studied anatomy and physiology and know intellectually where all the bones of the hands lie, but I've never actually tried to feel them inside my hand. It is an exciting moment for me as I realize I can become aware of what the *inside* of my hand feels like. By the end of this portion of the exercise, my hand is full, alive, vibrant, glowing. It feels as though it has grown.

Roger asks me to see if I can become aware of the bones in my forearm. Roger performs the exercise with me. He seems to be experiencing the exercise for his own sake as well as acting as a guide for me. Up until now, I've been jiggling my hand gently back and forth along my side. Roger asks, "If I wanted to feel the bones in my forearm, how would I do this? Maybe I'd want to bring my arm up to my shoulder, swing, jiggle, dangle, toss it, whatever movement works, in larger circles. All the while doing this, I might also ask myself, 'What feels best? What do I need now? What feels lighter?' I sometimes think of myself as a butterfly caught in a spider's web and wonder what it might feel like to have my wings free. Maybe today big movements will make me feel lighter while at another time smaller movements might make me feel lighter. It's important in Trager to become aware of how we're feeling and what the body seems to need now."

Following his verbal cues, I experiment with various ways of moving my arm, in large circles, all the while jiggling and vibrating my hand and arm, then in smaller circles. I feel my whole limb grow alive with pulsating fullness. After this exercise, Roger asks me to pause. "Compare the feeling in your two arms. How do they feel?" he asks. The left arm, which I've been experimenting with, feels big, large, light, pulsating with energy. The right arm, by comparison, feels thin, small, almost shriveled. Roger assures me that this imbalance will not persist: The brain strives to equalize the feelings within the body. Already I can begin to feel a vibrant sensation spreading to my right arm.

"Trager called these types of exercises Mentastics, which is short for 'mental gymnastics,'" Roger explains. "While performing them, the brain is making new connections that allow one to be lighter and freer. The movements are meant to be playful and pleasurable. We use pleasure to reeducate the nervous system and tissue toward more comfortable ways of being. This involves working with the neurochemical balance in the body. Recent studies have shown that various sensations within the body are connected to specific chemicals. The chemicals associated with feelings of pleasure can boost the functioning of the immune system. One of the things we're doing is concocting a kind of chemical cocktail that has more of the ingredients associated with pleasure.

"In the Trager Approach, the practitioner does not try to force any set response on a client. Whatever the client feels is an appropriate response and true for that client. What is important is the awareness that is achieved. Once we have a new awareness of our bodies, we often begin to respond to the world differently. Others begin to respond to us differently, too, so all our relationships change. We approach the world from a place of peace and balance," Roger explains.

"It's important for people to do the Mentastics exercises on their own, to maintain their awareness and prevent tension from building back up to the point where it becomes painful or uncomfortable. Mentastics are just as important as the tablework we do. In a way they're more important. What we do in the individual session is just a starting point in helping us to become aware. As we take our awareness into daily life, we become aware of every action we make." To demonstrate this point, he picks up a decorative pillow from the sofa and continues. "Even in a simple action such as this, we can be aware of how we have to move in order to pick up a pillow; what the pillow feels like; how it meets the hand; how much it weighs. Everything we do can become imbued with awareness. Sometimes I have clients who don't want to do exercises on their own; they just want to come once a week for me to fix them. I have to evaluate whether or not I want to work with them because they're really not going to get the full benefit of the Trager Approach."

Having shared these insights with me, Roger asks me to disrobe down to my underwear. I lie down on my back on a padded massage table covered with a sheet. Roger places a blanket over me to keep me warm. My feet extend off the table several inches; Roger places a large bolster under my knees that both supports my low back and makes my legs feel more comfortable.

Roger asks me to let him know if I should feel uncomfortable at any time or chilled on this winter afternoon. When he places his hands on my heels, I do not feel chilled at all. I feel intense heat coming from his hands, which warm me all the way from my feet up through my spine. Roger gently jostles my legs for a few moments, then says he will begin the session by working first on my hands. He walks over to the right side of the table and gently begins to play with my right hand and arm. He picks up my forearm and jostles it back and forth, in circles, in figure eights. He lifts it up, vibrates my arm, pulls gently on my fingers. He is creating movement throughout. I ask him what he is feeling for, and he tells me a quality of free flow of circulation and energy throughout the tissue. As he works with my hand, I become aware of the enormous tension I've been holding there. Using my hands all day at the computer and performing massage, they are full of hidden tension. As he encourages flow within the tissues of my hand, it feels alive and glowing. Roger performs the same movements on my left arm, bringing about the same change in tissue quality.

I ask Roger if he usually begins tablework with the client's hands. There is no set protocol, he explains. In deciding the order of a session he takes into account a number of factors, such as areas of sensitivity reported by the client or areas where he is intuitively drawn as well as taking into account how well he knows a client. With new clients, it's often easier to start with the hands or feet because it's less invasive.

Roger moves to the head of the table and sits on a chair. He begins to roll my head from side to side. At first the motion is subtle, but soon it becomes a pulsing vibration, rocking my whole body, down through my torso to my pelvis and out my legs to my feet. Roger is rocking, too, rolling his body in a kind of playful dance, to make mine vibrate. The sensation is novel. I feel as though I'm floating on a rubber raft in a pool of water that has just been shaken by a large wave. The feeling is one of pleasant movement, with just a bit of a rolling jar to it. I feel as though this motion is creating a kind of confusion throughout my body and nervous system. I'm no longer in control of my body and its habitual responses to stimuli. I am literally being shaken up; in that place of confusion I become aware of new possibilities for reacting. As he works on me, Roger is supporting me with verbal cues. When he encounters an area of holding that he's encouraging to release, he may take an audible deep, long breath accompanied by a sigh. This has the almost hypnotic effect of inducing the same deep relaxed breathing in me, as though my breath was following his, like one wave in the ocean following another. When I release an area of tension, Roger reinforces the change with short exclamations like "Good!" "That's great!" and "That's nice!"

As Roger works on my neck, I become aware of the silence in the room. While many massage therapists play gentle background music while working, there is none here. Roger explains that he generally works without music in the background because there is no music that has the variety and subtlety of rhythms to keep pace with the rhythms of the work we are doing. In addition, music can be a distraction to awareness of the changes that are taking place during the session.

After releasing my neck, Roger asks me to feel the quality of the tissue in it. He guides my hands to gently caress the nape of my neck. I feel how soft and pliable the tissue feels. Not rigid and tight as I would have expected, but warm and soft. He asks me to remember the feel of this relaxed tissue.

Next, Roger places his hands over my face. His fingertips gently press into the skin of my face as though it were clay and he were gently contouring it. He moves down to my jaw and vibrates it vigorously between his two hands, and I feel a tremendous release. I realize how much tension I've been holding in my jaw. I'd recently become aware that I've been building up some TMJ tension. My jaw would be slightly stiff in the morning, as though I'd been grinding my teeth at night. When I visited my dentist last week, both he and his oral hygienist had remarked that there seemed to be more tension in my jaw than usual. I hadn't thought to mention this to Roger, but his knowing hands seemed to have picked it up regardless. He explains to me that he realized there was a holding in my jaw that needed to be released before he could continue with his work. "It's as though your jaw were saying to me, 'Wait a minute. Hold on. Don't go so fast. We're not ready to release here yet.' So I stayed longer and worked with the tissue until it had more flow." I can feel my jaw releasing as I become more present to it. As Roger is working on this area, I hear his telephone ring. Only a few short rings, promptly terminated by the noiseless efficiency of his answering machine recording the call. But in the moment of the initial ring, I feel myself tensing my jaw. I become aware of my normally unconscious response to unexpected noise and stress in the environment. No wonder my jaw is tense. If such a slight ring of a telephone can make me set my jaw, I can begin to appreciate the cumulative effect of all the other stronger stresses I'm subjected to each day.

Roger pauses for a moment (as he will periodically throughout the session) to enable me to take stock of any changes I feel. It seems as though he is also taking the time to peruse my body to evaluate its present condition before deciding what to do next. Roger stands up and walks back to the foot of the table. He asks me to scoot back up the table a few inches so that my feet are on the table. He places a pillow under my head and removes the blanket from my right leg so that he can work more easily with it. He picks up my right leg and holds it straight while jostling and swinging it a few times. He seems to be getting a feeling for the amount of tension there at the same time that he is already beginning to increase the flow of circulation. He detects some tension in my right hip and asks, "I wonder if this hip could be freer, lighter; if the low back could be more relaxed?" His question is a rhetorical one, but I quickly respond, "I'm sure they could be." "And I wonder what that would feel like," he muses. The answer is already apparent. Between the jostling, relaxing movements of Roger's hands and his verbal suggestions for me to relax with awareness, the tissue of my leg, hip, and low back are releasing. "Good," Roger says. "Very good!"

With my hip open, Roger begins a series of movements with my right leg that feel especially pleasurable, even playful. He picks up my right foot, bends my right leg toward my torso, gently pushes my right knee in toward my left knee. He allows it to move on its own momentum, eventually swinging back out and down to the table, with his hands providing gentle support. I feel as though my leg is like a kid on a swing, and Roger is gently pushing it out and letting it swing back and forth on its own. This is one of the most enjoyable sensations I've experienced in bodywork. It makes me aware of the body's potential for pleasure in small acts of playful spontaneity. Roger is helping me remember what it's like to play—a luxury I'd forgotten.

Roger asks me to notice the difference between my right and left legs. I report that my right leg feels alive and full. I can feel it pulsing with energy, flowing freely throughout, from my foot up through the bowl of my pelvis to my spine. I feel that my thigh has grown as large as Arnold Schwarzenegger's. My left leg feels small, contracted. I feel a buzz of energy around my ankle and realize that energy seems to be pooled there, limiting circulation to the rest of the limb.

"I bet you'd like your left leg to feel more like the right one," Roger says. He walks to the left side of the table and repeats the series of movements he has just performed on my right leg. My left leg now feels fully alive.

Having worked with my extremities, Roger proceeds to the center of my body. All other things being equal, he explains, Trager practitioners generally work first with the extremities, relaxing them, then progress to working with the central, deeper structures of the body. "Of course, even when we work with the extremities, we're also affecting the center. For instance, when I jostle your foot, that motion is setting up a reverberation that goes all the way to your shoulders, even your head moves," he clarifies. I had observed that when Roger sat at the head of the table and rocked my shoulders and neck, he set up a strong rolling action throughout my entire body, down to my toes. And when he stopped that rolling, I felt a large release in my solar plexus as my stomach swelled up like a bellows and my breathing capacity expanded.

Roger begins a series of firm stretches to my torso. Up to this point most of his work has involved gentle rolling, rocking, and vibrating movements. Now he is gently pumping the area of my pectoral muscles, the large muscles that cover the upper portion of the chest. His movements are moderately quick as he rhythmically pumps my chest with the palms of his hands. I feel as though this is loosening areas of holding. I feel as though I am crying silently inside as he does this, as though I've been carrying an unacknowledged store of grief and sorrow in my bosom. Roger initiates a series of wringinglike movements as he rotates my shoulder, increasing mobility in the shoulder girdle. One of the insights Roger had shared at the beginning of our session was that he would like to help me open my chest so I could feel wide and long. He's doing it.

Roger proceeds to my abdomen and the area between my hip bones. He initiates a strong rolling motion as he rocks my hips from side to side. I become aware of a feeling of sexuality as I tune in to my sexual energy. It's as though my pelvis, home of the sexual organs and much of my feelings about sensuality, has been locked and rigid. The sheer physical force of these strong vibratory movements cannot help but make me present to this part of my body, including both the physical organs located there and my feelings about them. This growing awareness comes without any conscious effort on my part. It comes precisely because I am not trying to lead my consciousness anywhere. Roger concludes treatment of the front of my body by rubbing his hands across my abdomen in a crisscross scissors-like movement that also serves to increase my sense of awareness of this inner core that houses my vital organs.

Roger asks me to roll over gently onto my stomach. He takes the pillow from under my head and places it under my chest to provide support for the curvature of my chest. I feel much more comfortable this way. While I am in this position, Roger spends most of his time working on my back, especially the area around my shoulders. He begins on my right side, initiating strong vibration movements in my right shoulder. This jostling is very stimulating and I feel revitalized. This is not the sensuous relaxation of a flowing Swedish massage effleurage stroke, but a deeply energizing motion. Roger explains that I have a tendency to hold my tension in my shoulder; this tension has caused a pooling of circulation, and he is using these energetic movements as a way of increasing flow to the area, including the flow of blood and other fluids and nutrients. I can feel a release of tension as he does so. Roger swings my arm back and forth, along the side of the table, increasing flow in the tissue there. He applies some compressing, rhythmic pumping motions and stretches to the long expanse of my back as he elongates the tissue. He sets my whole body rocking, then steps back to admire his handiwork, complimenting me on the wonderful fluidity of the movement. I can feel the change as my body rolls with greater ease. Roger performs the same movements on my left side.

Roger concludes the tablework portion of the session by jostling my feet a little, which moves my entire body, then gently stroking my head. He asks me to rest for a few minutes as he leaves the room. This gives me time to compose myself while I appreciate the newfound ease in my body.

Roger returns to the room and asks me to roll over into a seated position on the table. I do so, without great finesse, bringing myself into a taxing sit-up position to do so. I know it is much easier on the body to roll over first onto the side, then gently rise while supporting oneself with one's arm. I teach this to my clients all the time. Yet when I perform the same movement I do so clumsily, inefficiently. This session in psychophysical integration is making me more aware.

To help me refine my awareness even further, Roger asks me to stand up and walk around the table a few times. He asks me to describe what I'm feeling. I tell him I'm groggy, as though I've just woken up. No, wait a minute; I feel energized. I feel both relaxed and energized at the same time. Then I realize I'm not quite sure of what I'm feeling. Somehow my mind seems to have reached a point where it realizes it is not separate from my body. I need to experience what I'm feeling to express it. This is a turnaround for me. Normally, words come easily to me and I describe how I feel quickly, effortlessly. But I realize that's often because I'm relating what I'm thinking I'm feeling or felt some time ago; I'm not really present to what I'm experiencing at the moment. I luxuriate in the experience of being aware in the present. What am I feeling? I feel some tension in my low back. Funny, I was never in touch with that before. I feel lightness, tallness, wideness in general throughout my body. I feel clearer in my mind, less anxious.

Roger has me stand in front of him and offers an exercise for me. "Wriggle your hips as though you were shaking your tail," he suggests. "Now pretend there are tassels hanging from the tips of your shoulder blades and you want to wriggle them, too, so that the tassels come all the way down the side of your body to your hips. As you do this, allow your breastbone to rise up and your shoulders to become wide." I try this experiment and feel a sense of ease and lightness rising up through the midline of my body. Roger reports that an air of clarity radiates from my face as I achieve this state of ease. "I feel that you hold a lot of tension in your shoulders and upper back, in the area where the cervical vertebrae of the neck join the thoracic vertebrae of the upper back. This exercise will help release some of that tension."

I leave Roger's apartment feeling much lighter, more at ease. I realize that the Trager Approach is a powerful method of enhancing well-being and awareness in the body. I can appreciate how repeated tablework sessions in this practice coupled with performance of the Mentastics exercises could help reduce patterns of holding and alleviate or prevent the onset of pain.

Later that afternoon, I take an aerobics class. I feel that my body is moving with greater flexibility. Even more important, I feel more empowered to experiment with my movements. I improvise my own steps in rhythm to the music and the instructor's directions. I realize my hands and legs can dangle and flow in new ways. I feel as though I've gained a new awareness of my ability to react in unhabituated ways—an exciting discovery.

The evening following my session with Roger I am very tired. I feel that part of this fatigue is the result of the Trager session, that somehow the constant, repeated movements (which practitioners say can involve up to six thousand moves during a typical session) resulted in near sensory overload, which enabled the release of many areas of chronic holding. While exhilarated, I also feel tired, as though toxins that had pooled in areas of holding have been released into the bloodstream and are now circulating on their way to elimination through the kidneys. I respect this feeling of fatigue by spending a quiet evening at home, drinking lots of fluids and going to bed early. The following morning when I awake, I feel taller, lighter, softer. As I pass beneath the door frame of my apartment, I'm aware that my head comes closer to brushing its top beam.

THE BENEFITS OF THE TRAGER APPROACH

Trager practitioners have reported success in treating a wide range of physical ailments: polio; muscular dystrophy and other degenerative muscular disorders; multiple sclerosis; Parkinson's disease; poststroke trauma; chronic pain syndromes, such as low back problems; emphysema; migraine headaches; and asthma, to name some of the more prominent applications. While the Trager Approach is not a medical treatment, Trager elicited feeling from paralyzed limbs, and many clients have felt relief from chronic pain after only one session.

The Trager Approach is used by a number of trainers and athletes to enhance athletic performance. Professional athletes have availed themselves of the Elite Athlete Program in Austin, Texas, to incorporate the Trager Approach into their regimen of mental and physical training to maximize peak performance.

Individuals who experience the Trager Approach report an increased sense of relaxation, vitality, mental clarity, and creativity. They experience what they describe as a place beyond relaxation: "peace." Many find that as the physical blockages in their bodies are removed, they feel emotionally freer, too. As body and mind become better integrated, the client feels better balanced and whole.

CONTRAINDICATIONS TO THE TRAGER APPROACH

The Trager Approach is gentle and involves no deep manipulations. Absolute contraindications to the Trager Approach are extremely few and include active thrombophlebitis (blood clots) and recent (less than three months) surgery on joints. Those in a severely debilitated state who are extremely frail or who have experienced a recent hospitalization for severe illness should consider these conditions possible contraindications as well. Caution should be exercised in cases of bone cancer, inactive thrombophlebitis, severe degenerative conditions of the spine or disks, joint replacements, pain on motion of any joint, known problem pregnancies, and individuals taking any drugs that might alter perception.

BACKGROUND AND TRAINING OF PRACTITIONERS

All Trager practitioners in good standing have been trained through the Trager International curriculum and certified by one of the Trager national associations of the practitioner. In the United States, the United States Trager Association provides this function. All national association contact information can be found on the Trager International website (www.trager.com). The original Trager Institute was incorporated in 1980 in California to provide training, and the training program consists of formal courses in the theory and practice of the Trager Approach as well as anatomy. Additional fieldwork, including practice sessions, private tutorials, and practitioner evaluations are required. Practitioners are certified upon completion of 226 hours of supervised training and 183 hours of unsupervised (sessions given and received) training. An optional Senior Practitioner status is granted upon completion of a total of 500 hours of supervised training.

The training program constitutes minimum requirements for certification. To maintain certification, practitioners must remain active members of a national Trager association and participate in a regular ongoing program of continuing education. There are approximately one thousand Trager practitioners—represented in nearly every state and in many foreign countries. More than four thousand students have learned the Trager Approach, and seven hundred students are currently in training in areas as diverse as the United States, Canada, Western Europe, Israel, Australia, and Japan.

For Further Information

The Trager Institute was established in 1980 to further the work of Dr. Milton Trager. In 2001, the organization restructured to become Trager International and eleven national associations primarily in North America and Europe. All levels of the organization serve as professional communication and support networks, sponsor research projects, and provide a referral service for Trager practitioners. In addition, Trager International or any of the national associations can provide a list of articles, videotapes, and books on the Trager Approach.

You can obtain further information by contacting:

Trager International
P.O. Box 3246
Courtenay, British Columbia
Canada V9N 5N4
Tel/Fax: (250) 337-5556
Website: www.trager.com
E-mail: admin@trager.com

United States Trager Association
Website: www.trager-us.org
E-mail: admin@trager-us.org

Trager Canada
Website: www.trager.ca
E-mail: admin@trager.ca

Trager UK
Website: www.trager.co.uk
E-mail: enquiries@trager.co.uk

Suggested Further Reading

Books

Milton Trager, M.D., with C. Guadagno, Ph.D., *Trager Mentastics: Movement as a Way to Agelessness* (Barrytown, NY: Station Hill Press, 1987).

Jack Liskin, *Moving Medicine: The Life and Work of Milton Trager, M.D.* (Barrytown, New York: Station Hill Press, 1996).

ARTICLES

Kimberley A. Foster et al., "The Trager Approach in the Treatment of Chronic Headache: A Pilot Study," *Alternative Therapies in Health and Medicine,* Sept/Oct 2004, Vol.10, No.5.

Deane Juhan, M.A., "An Introduction to Trager Psychophysical Integration and Mentastics Movement Education," published by the Trager Institute, 1989.

Richard Leviton, "Moving with Milton Trager: An *East West* Interview with a Bodywork Pioneer," *East West Journal,* January 1988.

Shirley Vanderbilt, "A Softer, Lighter Mind-Body: Trager Approach and Breast Cancer," *Massage & Bodywork,* Oct/Nov 2004.

The Trager Journal, Vol. I, Fall 1982; Vol. II, Fall, 1987. There are diverse articles on the Trager Approach in this journal. Available from the United States Trager Association office.

RUBENFELD SYNERGY METHOD AT A GLANCE

BASIC FACTS

- The Rubenfeld Synergy Method is an educational approach to healing that combines touch with verbal expression. It promotes healing by unifying body, mind, emotions, and spirit.
- Rubenfeld Synergy was developed by Ilana Rubenfeld as a result of her search to heal complaints resulting from her training as a musical conductor. It integrates her eclectic background as a teacher of the Alexander Technique and Feldenkrais Method with training in Gestalt practice and Ericksonian hypnosis.

THEORY

- **The body, mind, emotions, and spirit are one.** They interrelate and affect one another. A Rubenfeld Synergist (as a practitioner is called) must address all aspects of the client in a unified paradigm.
- **Through a combination of gentle touch and verbal dialogue, clients become aware of areas of holding.** Once areas of holding are detected, the Synergist engages the client in verbal dialogue and movement to understand the cause of that holding. Through Gestalt practice, the client's unfinished business is addressed.
- **Synergists coach clients to a more pleasurable and integrated way of being.** The resulting relaxation is often accompanied by spontaneous alleviation of pain and resolution of emotional issues.

TYPICAL SESSION

- **A Rubenfeld Synergy session typically lasts forty-five minutes.** The client remains fully clothed and lies on a comfortable padded table.
- **The Synergist uses very gentle touch, verbal expression, and movement to detect areas of emotional holding and tension.** Through dialogue, the Synergist helps the client become conscious of the causes of holding. In addition to gentle movement, the Synergist may address the client's breathing patterns and postural habits or incorporate visualizations. At times, no touch is involved, and the Synergist may merely help the client become more self-aware.
- Because Rubenfeld Synergy involves a gradual unfolding process, it can require a number of ongoing sessions. The time period averages anywhere from six weeks to several years.

- Rubenfeld Synergy workshops and groups, which can last from one and a half hours to weekends and five days, include body/mind movement exercises, individual Rubenfeld Synergy demonstrations, and hands-on techniques for learning how to use gentle touch, self-care, and group process.

- Expect to pay $50 to $150 for an individual Rubenfeld Synergy session. Group and workshop formats vary in price depending upon length of time and location.

BENEFITS

The goal of Rubenfeld Synergy is to explore the cause of a problem that appears physically and help the client unfold its resolution, much as in psychotherapy and psychophysical education. Relief of physical symptoms and increased emotional and psychological openness often result.

CONTRAINDICATIONS

- Because Synergists use gentle touch and can work with awareness without using touch, there are no standard contraindications to Rubenfeld Synergy. If there is concern for any psychological or medical problem, consult your Synergist before beginning treatment.

BACKGROUND AND TRAINING OF PRACTITIONERS

- Rubenfeld Synergists are certified by Ilana Rubenfeld and master Rubenfeld Synergists through a program conducted by the Rubenfeld Synergy Center. The Rubenfeld Synergy Training Program consists of 1,600 hours. It meets three times a year (seven intensive days each time) with regional weekends in between over a period of four years, with the fourth year being an internship. Theoretical and hands-on practice during the training are supplemented with supervised field practice. There is a ratio of one teacher to every four to six students.

- Approximately five hundred Rubenfeld Synergists practice worldwide.

CHAPTER 7

RUBENFELD SYNERGY METHOD: TOUCH THERAPY MEETS TALK THERAPY

The client's innate healing potential already exists, waiting to be actualized. . . . Change cannot happen without awareness.[1]

—ILANA RUBENFELD

WHAT IS RUBENFELD SYNERGY?

Rubenfeld Synergy is an educational approach to healing that integrates touch with verbal expression. It was originated and developed by Ilana Rubenfeld as a synthesis of her own individual style and background, which includes training in the Alexander Technique, the Feldenkrais Method, Gestalt practice, and Ericksonian hypnotherapy. Rubenfeld Synergy is an excellent example of a new generation of body/mind work that is being developed by innovative practitioners who, schooled in a variety of methods, blend their own unique synthesis of techniques. Rubenfeld calls her work "synergy" on the recommendation of Buckminster Fuller, who recognized that her work evokes a greater wholeness than the sum of the individual techniques that make up its repertoire. As Rubenfeld's teacher, the innovative Moshe Feldenkrais, remarked, "There is no genius whose followers have not improved on him."[2]

THE ORIGINS OF THE RUBENFELD SYNERGY METHOD

Ilana Rubenfeld's background is eclectic. Born of Russian immigrants in Palestine, she moved to the United States at the age of five. While still a student at the Juilliard School, where she began her career as a musical conductor and assisted the legendary Leopold Stokowski, she learned something she hadn't counted on: How physically demanding the life of a conductor is. Standing four and five hours at a time, her shoulders hunched over a music stand, arms whirling like airplane propellers, she wreaked havoc on her spine and back. Debilitating pain sent her to seek relief in the form of lessons in the Alexander Technique with Judith Liebowitz, grande dame of Alexander teachers. (Liebowitz would later become chair of the Alexander Department at Juilliard, and executive director of the American Center for the Alexander Technique.) Judith's movement lessons were gentle yet powerful. Indeed, they elicited such a strong emotional response that Ilana burst into tears.

"I can help you with your physical problems, but not your emotional ones," Liebowitz explained, and referred Rubenfeld to a psychoanalyst to deal with emotional matters. Rubenfeld sought therapeutic help and was told by her analyst, "I can help you with your emotional issues, but I can't help you physically, and I definitely can't touch you." One talked and wouldn't touch; the other touched and wouldn't talk.

Rubenfeld soon realized a great divide existed between bodywork, which involved touch, and psychotherapy, which involved talk. Her life work, spanning more than forty-five years, has been consumed by her mission to develop, practice, and train others in her singular method of dynamically integrating the body, mind, emotions, and spirit. Along the way, she supplemented her education with certification as a teacher of the Alexander Technique and the Feldenkrais Method—signing up for the first U.S. training course offered by Moshe Feldenkrais himself. Training with Fritz Perls led her to incorporate Gestalt therapy into her method, which was later complemented by Ericksonian hypnotherapy.

THE THEORY UNDERLYING RUBENFELD SYNERGY

Rubenfeld Synergy is meant to explore, not cure, the cause of a problem. "This is contrary to what is generally valued in our society," Rubenfeld explains. "The person who can cure a problem most quickly is the most highly admired and rewarded financially. Rubenfeld Synergy aims to help the individual in his process of self-discovery." Underlying this approach is a four-stage metaprocess involving awareness, experimentation, integration, and reentry, which occur simultaneously.

Rubenfeld Synergy is based on the premise that the body, mind, emotions, and spirit are one. They interrelate and affect one another. Therefore, the Synergist must address all aspects of the client in a unified paradigm. Rubenfeld believes, as do many other body/mind therapists, that the body retains emotional memories at the tissue, and even cellular, level. From her background in Gestalt therapy, she seeks to find the here-and-now state of the client and the relevance to the present of unfinished emotional business. She believes that the body does not lie. For instance, though a client may say she's feeling one thing, such as relaxed, her body may be saying something else: that she's tense and rigid, like an iron rod. A sensitive, trained Synergist can discover through an open and listening hand what the body has to reveal.

As a conductor, Rubenfeld learned to talk, listen, and move her hands and body all at the same time, an ability she tries to develop in her students. She believes an individual changes through pleasure not pain. Therefore, a Synergist uses a gentle touch, which is not invasive and does not inflict pain, to encourage a client to a more pleasurable way of being. Humor is important, and Rubenfeld Synergy often involves playful verbal exchanges with the client. Rubenfeld firmly believes that change without awareness is not lasting and that a client must want to change. Her work is aimed at promoting increased awareness as clients change to more optimal ways of functioning. In approaching a client, the Synergist emphasizes establishing a sense of safety and boundaries. "Client and Synergist meet in a sacred healing space," Rubenfeld underscores.

THE TYPICAL FORMAT OF A RUBENFELD SYNERGY SESSION

A Rubenfeld Synergy session typically lasts forty-five minutes. The client remains fully clothed and lies on a firm, padded table. The Synergist uses very gentle touch, verbal expression, and movement to detect areas of emotional holding and tension. The Synergist then dialogues with the client to evoke the unconscious emotional issues that are vested in that holding. Through the Gestalt technique of addressing these issues in the here and now, the Synergist helps the client become conscious of patterns and causes of holding. These techniques are complemented by work with breathing patterns, body posture, kinesthetic awareness, and visualizations. At times, no touch is involved, and the Synergist may merely help the client become more self-aware.

Rubenfeld Synergy, like psychotherapy and psychophysical education, initiates an ongoing process of change that unfolds over time. The amount of time this process takes can vary, but on average entails a series of sessions over a period of six weeks to several years. Immediate changes are often apparent as the client gains in self-esteem, increased relaxation, and a greater sense of confidence.

THE EXPERIENCE: I GET TOUCHED AND TALK

It is a sunny spring afternoon in April. I arrive at the apartment of Rob Bauer, a practitioner and senior instructor of Rubenfeld Synergy. I obtained Rob's name and phone number through the Rubenfeld Center. After talking with him on the phone about me and my needs, I felt comfortable with him and made an appointment to see him. Rob trained and practiced as a psychotherapist before becoming a Synergist. He was drawn to Rubenfeld's method because he felt he was able to accomplish his therapeutic goals much more quickly and dramatically by working with touch as well as verbal communication. Rob divides his practice between New York City and the Glens Falls/Saratoga Springs area of upstate New York. I opted to see him in the city at his apartment, which is not far from my own.

Rob greets me at the door. His manner is gracious and sincere. Locks of gray curls frame his caring face. Rob's studio, set off a courtyard in Manhattan's Greenwich Village, is light and airy. Its distance from the street gives it an atmosphere of peace and tranquility. I hear birds chirping on the branches outside as sun streams through the window. I have a sense of calm and safety in this space.

Rob shows me into his living area. He asks me to sit down in an armchair accented with a patterned throw cover while he sits opposite me. He takes a few minutes to get to know me, to ask me what he can do for me. Because I'm already familiar with the history and theory of Rubenfeld Synergy, he doesn't need to spend time explaining that to me. He also knows that my interest is in experiencing this healing approach directly, so he makes as much time during the session available for experiential work as possible. He explains that in some cases, much of the initial session might be concerned with doing a preliminary intake.

Rob asks me what issues are going on for me, in the here and now. What can he do to help me? What are my burning issues? I explain that I'm in a period of great transition. I'm arriving at a point in my life where I'm completing a number of projects that have been consuming my time for the last several years. I feel a great sense of relief at this for I've been aware of the pressure, deadlines, and other stresses involved in completing these projects. I also feel a great sense of freedom. I've been feeling tied down. A major segment of my life is coming to completion; I'll be free to entertain other projects. I'm also thinking about moving, leaving the apartment in which I've been living and using my new-found freedom to drift for a while and take stock of my life. I'd like to travel the globe—Paris, India, Nepal, Central America. The idea, while exciting, is also stressful. I've lived in my present apartment for seven years. I feel secure and grounded there.

Rob explains that what I've shared gives us plenty of material with which to begin our hands-on work. He explains that I'll be lying down on a padded massage table in the middle of the room. I will remain clothed during the session. I've dressed in layers of a T-shirt and sweatshirt and worn loose-fitting sweat pants to be comfortable during the session. Rob asks me to remove my watch and anything I may have in the pockets of my pants.

I lie down on my back on the table and close my eyes while Rob stands at the head of the table. He asks me whether I prefer to be called Tom or Thomas. Rob's seemingly simple question immediately unearths a conflict: I go by both Tom and Thomas. Family members and friends who have known me for a long time call me by my childhood name of Tom. I now prefer to be called Thomas, which is the name I use professionally. In response to Rob's query, I reply "Thomas."

Rob asks me to begin the session by becoming aware of my body and any sensations I may be experiencing. He asks me how my body feels as it meets the table. How does my head feel? Does it have a tendency to fall to one side? Is it as relaxed as it can be? What about my shoulders, my back, my arms? As he asks how my arms feel, I experience a feeling of tightness around my eyes. I wonder if he senses this when he asks his next question: "How does your face feel? Notice your breathing, not to change it but just how it feels. Is it deep, full? How do your hips feel? Your legs? Your feet?" He asks me to become aware of all these sensations without trying to change anything and without judgment. Rob's voice is hypnotic as he talks. He seems to be both lulling me into relaxation as well as heightening my awareness. I am silent as I internally scan my body and feelings.

"I'm going to begin by gently touching your head," Rob says. He takes his hands and cradles the back of my head, just holding. "I'm just greeting you," he says. "I'm saying hello to you, and you're saying hello to me. We're getting to know one another on the level of touch. When you first came in, we got to know one another through talk. Now we're meeting through touch."

Rob lightly cradles my head for a short time, then he gently rolls it from side to side. He asks me to share with him what I'm feeling.

I explain that when I turn my awareness toward my body, I become conscious that the left side of my body seems to sink more deeply into the table. It feels more relaxed and open. My neck also feels as though it was pulled toward the left, not relaxed but stiff. When Rob puts his hands on my head, I feel an incredible feeling of support. Rob's simple gesture of intentional, caring touch, just holding and listening, without doing anything, feels wonderfully supportive. It makes me feel that everything is all right. I realize as he does this how much I worry, am fearful and anxious about doing things right, of being perfect. In the simple embrace of Rob's touch, I feel like everything is okay. It is okay for me just to be here, now, as I am.

"Just to be here, now, as you are, it's okay just to be here, now, as you are," Rob repeats. "Did you feel anything else that you want to share?"

I explain that I felt a stiffness in my neck. As Rob rolled my head from side to side, I didn't feel as though it rolled easily. It felt stiff, tight, not elastic.

Summing up my impressions, Rob asks, "Is it fair to say that one side of your body feels more open and free; the other more cautious and guarded? And if so, does that mean anything to you?"

I hadn't really thought of myself that way before. What Rob says seems to fit, though. It is obvious to me that my body is certainly saying that. And when I think about my particular situation, I feel it's true, too. One part of me wants to be free, open, like a child playing outdoors on this idyllic spring day. Another side of me says, no, you can't do that; you have to stay inside and work. You can't be free. Part of me wants to uproot myself and travel the globe; another part says, no, you have to stay put, you need security, you can't move.

Rob advances to the foot of the table. He gently rolls each of my legs. He asks me how they feel. I note how they feel heavy and leaden, like pieces of dead wood. I feel the same difference between right and left sides here, too: The right leg feels deader than the left.

"So the legs are telling us the same thing—one side is more open than the other," Rob says. He moves to the left side of the table. "Before we go any further, I'd like to make a contract with you. If anything feels at all uncomfortable to you, you're to let me know. Is that okay?"

The contract seems simple and more than fair to me. Rob continues, "I'm going to begin to work with your left side. Since that side is more open, it'll be easier to start there. I'm going to make a hip sandwich," he says, the humor of his comment causing me to grin. "I'm going to put my hands on either side of your left hip." And Rob places his left hand on top of my hip, his right under it. He holds for what seems like several minutes, then asks me to verbalize my feelings about what's happening. "You might experience these feelings as images, colors, or physical sensations, like the texture of the tissue. Whatever comes to you is okay."

"I'm feeling heat," I report. "When you first put your hands on my hip, I felt tremendous heat coming from your hands. But I also feel heat between them, in my own tissue. I'm feeling as though the tissue is expanding, that a tightness that was held there is releasing. It feels fuller, denser. I also feel my breath becoming much deeper. Almost as soon as you put your hands on my hip, my abdomen swelled up with deeper breath. Especially the lower abdomen, below the navel in the pelvic basin. It felt like a big football swelling up."

Rob says, "You felt the heat of my hands and you felt the warmth of your own tissue. It felt denser to you." He releases his hands and jostles my hip a little as it opens onto the table. He takes his hands and passes them down my left leg in a broad, sweeping, whooshing motion. When he gets to my feet, he jostles my left leg gently back and forth and asks me how it feels.

I see an image of my leg as a chicken leg. It feels like the leg of a chicken after it's been cooked and the flesh is loose and tender, and you can rotate the bones around one another easily. Before it had felt like the leg of a chicken before it's cooked, with the bones firmly embedded in the flesh. My leg feels free and open.

Rob moves to my right side and makes a hip sandwich around my right hip. He asks me to share what I'm feeling there. I can feel the heat of his hands and the area filling up. But what I'm most aware of is how empty this area feels. Even with the heat and sense of growing fullness, it seems caved in, hollowed out, in relation to my left hip. My right leg has a tendency to turn out, and I can feel how flat this makes the area around the hip feel, almost flat like a piece of plywood, as opposed to the roundness and fullness on my left side.

"Where do you feel this flatness?" Rob asks me. "Just in the hip or in other parts of your body?"

I feel it all the way down to my knee, which also turns out and feels flat on the table. I feel it up through my waist area to my right shoulder, too. I'm aware how the muscles and tissue of the body are connected, and how the tightness in my hip moves through my whole right side.

Rob releases my right hip, whooshing down to my foot again. He jostles my right leg from the foot, then my left leg. He asks me what I'm feeling.

Both legs feel very different. They feel alive, vibrating, pulsating with energy. The right side still feels more restricted relative to the left leg, but both legs feel much more open than they did at the beginning of the session.

"So one side still feels more open; one side more cautious," Rob summarizes. "If you had to say which one felt more open, more willing to explore, travel, let go, and which one felt more guarded, wanting safety, which would they be?"

My left side is the more open and free; the right feels more tied down.

"That's the second time you've used the phrase 'tied down,'" Rob says. "It must mean something to you. If you were to say something to your hip, which one would you want to talk to and what would you ask?"

I ponder for a moment. "I'd talk to my right hip. I'd ask it why it felt tied down. Why it feels tight and restricted."

"Then why don't you try asking it," Rob urges. "Ask it: Hip, why do you feel tied down? Why are you tight and restricted?"

"Why do you feel tied down, right hip? Why are you tight and restricted?" I ask.

"The body is wise," Rob counsels. "Maybe it has an answer for you. Why don't you see if it has an answer."

I feel a little self-conscious talking to my body in this way. At the same time, I'm beginning to feel a closer connection to my body. I feel as though it's offering answers at the same time I'm asking it questions.

"It tells me it's feeling left out, ignored," I explain. "It's always wanted to be free, to run and play."

Rob says, "If you're willing, perhaps you could ask it more questions, request more information."

All the while he's talking to me, Rob is moving his hands slowly, purposefully, noninvasively. His tone of voice and quality of touch convey both concern and gentle, caring support. Now his hands are under my back, noodling in gentle pressing motions the muscles that run alongside my spine. At times he seems to be just listening and patiently waiting. As he reaches the area under my right shoulder blade, I'm aware of the tension and pain in my muscles. This is the area where I tend to hold my habitual tension, the place where I feel my aches and pains. Rob's touch is firm, resisting against my tissue. It doesn't hurt physically, but I'm aware of a pain and sensitivity in the tissue. It feels like a burning sensation. I can't tell whether this pain is new, brought on by this session, or whether I'm just becoming aware of a pain that's always been there. Rob takes my right arm and tractions it up and out in a long stretching motion. My awareness of the burning sensation in my right side intensifies. I associate this burning sensation with the discomfort I might feel in stretching a tight muscle in order to help it release. I share these impressions with Rob.

"Often, people become aware of pain during treatment. Many people expect to feel relaxed and good. But I explain to them that this work often brings up pain. It's more like psychotherapy, making us aware of ourselves, than manipulating the body for relaxation and ease."

I listen to my body, to the pain and restriction I feel. I ask my right side why it feels tied down, restricted, ignored. It tells me that this feeling goes back a long way, to my childhood, to the days when feelings didn't yet have the words to express themselves. It's connected to my feeling that I couldn't be who I am, just be me. My parents' love always seemed qualified, as though they were telling me, "You can be anybody you want to be so long as it's what we want you to be."

"So your right hip got tied down," Rob says. "Because you couldn't be who you wanted to be, it got tied down."

Rob asks me to roll over onto my right side. He's manipulating my right torso and shoulder area from underneath my body in this side-lying position.

"What would you like to say to your right side?" Rob asks.

"I'd like to tell it that it's okay to be just who it is, without any limitation or precondition."

"Then try it," Rob suggests. "Try saying it to your right side."

I say to my right side, "It's okay to be who you are, just as you are. I'll love you anyway."

"How does that feel?" Rob asks.

My right side doesn't believe it. I've said the words, but I don't feel it in my body. It still feels tight. I want to believe that telling my body I love it and accept it just as it is will make it feel better, but it's not so easy. My body doesn't buy it.

"Maybe this part of your body doesn't trust what you say," Rob said. "Maybe it's been lied to before. Maybe your parents told it they loved it just as it was, but then didn't let it be who it was."

What Rob, or my body, is saying to me is very powerful. I realize all the mixed messages I've gotten. How many conflicting memories and feelings about myself are recorded in my body's tissues. I've been through many years of talk psychotherapy with several talented practitioners. I know many things at the intellectual level. But now I'm feeling them in the tissues of my body, and they don't lie. They won't accept something they don't believe.

Rob is working on my right shoulder. He stretches my arm in a circular rotating motion. I'm aware of how tight it feels, how my arm doesn't really want to go above my collarbone.

"What do you feel here in your right shoulder?" Rob asks. "What's going on for you?"

I tell him how tight this shoulder feels. "Yes," he agrees. "Why don't you try asking your shoulder what's going on, what it's feeling, why it's so tight?"

I ask my shoulder and it replies, "I can't even give you an answer because I've never been allowed to think for myself. I'm tight because I haven't been given the freedom to think."

"Your shoulder can't even think, and you want to make it go around the world with you?" Rob jokes. "No wonder it's confused. Why don't you ask it how it feels about that?"

I ask my shoulder, and it replies, "That's absurd. It's absurd that a grown man feels he can't think for himself, that he's going off around the world anyway. It's absurd, but true."

As I talk, Rob continues to hold. He employs gentle jostling, stretching, twisting motions to my body. I'm aware of a pain, a tight painful tissue, that stretches from my right hip all the way to my shoulder blade. It crosses the area where I feel the habitual pain in my right midback. It seems somehow connected to this pain I'm feeling. Rob reinforces my awareness that the pain I feel is not only in the hip; the holding is connected to a larger pattern of holding throughout my body. He asks me to roll over onto my left side. He continues gentle stretching, jostling motions to my right torso and shoulder as he continues to dialogue with me.

"What would you like to say to your right shoulder?" he says. "Maybe this holding is related to a child inside of Thomas, to the child Thomas," Rob suggests. "Is there anything the adult Thomas would like to say to the child Thomas?"

"The adult Thomas wants to tell the child Thomas it's okay for you not to think. It's okay for you just to be. Not to know what's going to happen next. To accept the fact that it's okay not to be perfect. That there's no one right way of doing anything. To trust in the universe."

"Maybe the child Thomas is afraid, afraid that the adult Thomas is going to give up all his security and run off around the world. But maybe the child Thomas doesn't understand that the adult Thomas is responsible, that he's not going to take any risks that would hurt the child Thomas. That it's okay to be free and open, responsibly, without being hurt."

As Rob offers these suggestions, I feel a plethora of images and impressions welling up inside me. They are difficult to express because they feel physically to be inside me, contained in the cellular level of the tissues running between my hip and shoulder. As Rob speaks, I can feel and see the child Thomas. Somewhere in the tissue of my body I see a small but bright white light, the child Thomas, who's afraid. I realize this is a part of myself that I've ignored all these years. What is so powerful about connecting with this part of myself is the immediacy of the feeling. Through talk therapy, I know that my parents, like many parents, were controlling; that they put limits on my behavior and attitudes. But that is an intellectual knowing. Here I'm going back inside the feeling in my tissue. My parents are out of the way and I'm dealing one on one with my free and spontaneous child self. The one who's afraid of expressing himself. And I know that he exists because I can feel him in the tissue beneath Rob's hands—as Rob touches these sensitive areas I can feel the child within. I realize I have an opportunity of establishing a partnership with my child self, that the adult Thomas and the child Thomas can support each other. That they can travel together, in security and not fear. This is a long-awaited moment of homecoming.

Rob concludes work on my shoulder by stretching the area between it and the pectoral muscles of the chest. This is an area of chronic holding, where I feel the roundedness of my shoulders, the sunkenness of my chest. It feels releasing to have it opened so wide. I associate the chronic holding and protection in this area with the fear the child Thomas has been holding all these years.

Rob asks me to roll onto my back again. He moves to the foot of the table and jostles my legs. They feel really free, open, and full now—like I imagine the Pillsbury Doughboy's must feel. He lifts my legs to position them at a 45-degree angle to my body, so that my low back is supported. He places one hand on my lower stomach, the other on my breastbone in what seems like a final balancing act. He asks me when I'm ready to open my eyes and share any feelings with him.

As I open my eyes, I notice the pale rose color of the paint on his ceiling. It mirrors the sense of peace and calm I feel. I tell Rob how much more relaxed I feel, especially my neck. How my body has melded into the table. How my low back makes much deeper and more secure contact with the table. How appreciative I feel to have met the child Thomas, to have the opportunity to get to know him better.

Rob asks me to gently roll over onto whatever side beckons me as I rise to a seated position. I move onto my right side, the poor, ignored child side, much more in tune with it. Rob suggests I sit quietly for a moment to allow myself to readjust to the vertical. He then asks me to walk around the room a bit to see how I feel.

What I'm most aware of is how much more I feel I'm inhabiting my lower body. Often after bodywork I feel very light and uplifted, almost ethereal. My awareness is often in the upper part of my body. Now I feel very grounded, my buttocks and legs feel heavy, my feet deeply rooted in the earth. "As though you're less airy and more grounded?" Rob inquires. Yes, that's right. I tell Rob I feel as though this is just the beginning of a process, though, and that there is still much work to be done.

"Of course, it's just the beginning," Rob agrees. "I work with some clients for weeks or months and others for years. Often as we work, different issues from the ones that brought the client to see me in the first place emerge, and we work on them. I work a lot with survivors of abuse," he adds.

I ask him how long a treatment period he would recommend for me. "I'd suggest that if you wanted to continue the work, we might make an agreement to work for, say, six sessions. At the end of that time, we could reevaluate."

Rob reassures me that the issues raised during our session are not unique to me. My feelings, such as that of not being loved for who I really am, reflect universal human concerns. And I feel further healing power through my connection to the greater pool of humanity.

In parting, Rob says, "I hope your work pressures aren't so great that you can't allow yourself to process what we've done, and enjoy. Remember the part of yourself that wants to do that."

When I leave Rob's apartment, I notice that the day is still warm and brilliantly sunny. This is the first warm day after what has seemed the longest and coldest winter in decades. I allow myself the spontaneous freedom to enjoy a stroll in the sun, secure in the knowledge that I will be responsible enough to make the time later to accomplish whatever work goals I might have.

Following the session, I feel much freer. I feel that it's okay to be just me and not worry that I should be perfect. Later that day, I give a massage to a client whom I see each week. This sense of openness is reflected in my work. I feel more free to improvise, not worrying about a preset treatment plan but moving with the flow of the moment. My client notices it, too: "Is it the day or is it you?" he asks. "I'm absolutely melting into the table. This is one of your best massages—you'll have to record it and duplicate it again." Without divulging my recipe, I take credit for the smoothness and flow of the work.

That evening, I dream about moving. I dream I've rented out part of my house to another man, a brother or a twin. I'm ready to move, but he isn't. He still needs a place to stay. The dream resolves itself in our agreeing that we will support one another wherever we may happen to be.

THE BENEFITS OF RUBENFELD SYNERGY

The goal of Rubenfeld Synergy is to explore the cause of a problem and help the client to unfold its resolution, much as in psychotherapy. The Synergist aims to make the client conscious of unconscious emotional and physical material that limits expression in the present moment. As this material becomes conscious, the client may experience greater relaxation and ease, with spontaneous alleviation of pain and increased emotional and psychological openness. Individuals who have sought treatment include those suffering from physical problems, performers, and health professionals. Rubenfeld Synergists are currently undertaking research to apply their approach to treatment of a variety of clients, including the aged, individuals suffering from chronic pain syndrome, people with AIDS, those seeking help with substance abuse and codependency issues, individuals desiring to enhance self-esteem and self-awareness, and those dealing with inner-child issues.

CONTRAINDICATIONS TO RUBENFELD SYNERGY

Because Synergists use gentle touch and can work with awareness without using touch, there are no standard contraindications to Rubenfeld Synergy. Individuals with specific psychological or medical concerns are encouraged to consult with a Synergist before beginning treatment.

BACKGROUND AND TRAINING OF PRACTITIONERS

Training in the Rubenfeld Synergy Method, which is currently overseen by senior faculty members, was developed by Ilana Rubenfeld. The 1,600-hour training course, which consists of three seven-day training periods each year for four years with regional weekend meetings in between, combines theoretical and hands-on work in body/mind integration. The fourth year of the training program is an internship. There is a ratio of one teacher to every four to six students. Each student is required to experience a minimum of twenty sessions with certified Synergists as part of the training. There are more than five hundred certified practitioners of Rubenfeld Synergy throughout the world.

FOR FURTHER INFORMATION

In addition to professional training, Rubenfeld and her staff present introductory workshops in Rubenfeld Synergy throughout the country at such well-known institutions as the Kripalu Center for Yoga and Health, the Omega and Esalen institutes, and many conferences, such as the Association for Humanistic Psychology (AHP), which awarded its 1994 Pathfinder Award to Ilana Rubenfeld. In 2002, Ilana Rubenfeld was awarded the lifetime achievement award by the United States Association of Body Psychotherapy (USABP). For further information on the Rubenfeld Synergy Method, introductory workshops, or the training program, or for a list of certified Synergists in your area, contact:

The Rubenfeld Center, Inc.
104 Bush Street
Ashland, OR 97520
Tel: (877) RSM-2468 (776-2468)
Websites: www.ilanarubenfeld.com (for information on training and itinerary)
www.rubenfeldsynergy.com (for information on graduates and practitioner referrals)
E-mail: rubenfeld@aol.com

SUGGESTED FURTHER READING

Ilana Rubenfeld, "Beginner's Hands: Twenty-five Years of Simple Rubenfeld Synergy—The Birth of a Therapy," *Somatics,* Spring/Summer 1988.

_____. "Gestalt Therapy and the BodyMind: An Overview of the Rubenfeld Synergy Method," in *Gestalt Therapy: Perspectives and Applications,* ed. Edwin C. Nevis (New York: Gardner Press, Inc., 1992).

_____. *The Listening Hand: Self-Healing Through the Rubenfeld Synergy Method of Talk and Touch* (New York: Bantam, 2000). This is the inspiring account of the Rubenfeld Synergy Method, presented by its pioneer, complete with guided body/mind exercises and practices.

_____. "Ushering in a Century of Integration," *Somatics* Autumn/Winter 1990–91.

Mirka Knaster, "Ilana Rubenfeld: Our Lady of Synergy," *Massage Therapy Journal,* Vol. 30, No. 1, Winter 1991.

Vicki Mechner, *Healing Journeys: The Power of Rubenfeld Synergy* (Chappaqua, NY: Omniquest Press, 1998). The author, a Rubenfeld Synergist, allows real people to tell the stories of their own experience with Rubenfeld Synergy.

BASIC FACTS

- **Rosen Method is a healing approach that uses gentle touch and verbal support.** It assists clients in unlocking old memories that might have prevented them from becoming who they really are.

- **Rosen Method was developed by Marion Rosen, a physical therapist.** Born in Germany, Rosen also studied sensory awareness, movement, breath, relaxation techniques, and massage.

THEORY

- **Old forgotten emotions and memories lie stored in the body.** A practitioner's gentle touch can help a client relax and surrender conscious holding. In this state, unconscious material that might have been causing pain can surface.

- **Breath is the gateway between the unconscious and the conscious.** A change in a client's breath is a signal of important unconscious emotional material. The practitioner facilitates a state of relaxation where unconscious emotional material can become conscious.

- **Practitioners are midwives to a process of self-discovery.** They offer encouragement and support for clients to trust their own processes of self-transformation.

TYPICAL SESSION

- **A Rosen Method session lasts an hour.** Typically, the client is dressed only in underwear, although more clothing may be worn if desired. The client lies covered with a warm blanket on a massage table. No oil is used.

- The practitioner uses gentle noninvasive touch to detect areas of muscle tension. Pressure is applied slowly to meet resistance in tense muscles. The practitioner pays particular attention to shifts in muscle tension as well as breathing patterns. The practitioner may make short nonintrusive comments to facilitate client awareness.

- Expect to pay $50 to $110 for a one-hour session.

BENEFITS

- **The goal of Rosen Method is to prevent the development of illness.** Rosen maintains that many illnesses could be prevented if people were to become more aware of unconscious chronic tension and take appropriate steps to relieve it.

- **Rosen Method induces relaxation.** Clients often report alleviation of symptoms related to muscle tension and stress, including muscle pain, headaches, fatigue, and irritability.

CONTRAINDICATIONS

- Because it has the power to unlock unconscious material, Rosen Method is best used in conjunction with psychotherapy for individuals in a state of serious emotional crisis or who have a history of psychosis.

BACKGROUND AND TRAINING OF PRACTITIONERS

- Rosen Method practitioners are trained through one of fifteen centers worldwide and the Rosen Institute has certified each center. Training lasts usually over a four-year period and requires 250 hours of classroom work (a minimum of six weeklong intensives) and 350 hours of internship.
- There are over 900 Rosen Method practitioners worldwide. There are 350 practitioners in the United States, 450 in the Scandinavian countries, and the rest spread throughout the remaining centers. There are training centers in the United States (five), Canada (one), Western Europe (seven), Russia (one), and Australia (one).

CHAPTER 8

ROSEN METHOD: LISTENING TO THE BODY

If you bring forth what is within you, what you bring forth will save you. If you do not bring forth what is within you, what you do not bring forth will destroy you.[1]

—MARION ROSEN'S UNOFFICIAL MOTTO,
FROM THE GNOSTIC GOSPEL OF THOMAS

WHAT IS ROSEN METHOD?

Rosen Method is an approach to healing that uses gentle touch and verbal support to assist clients in unlocking old memories that might have prevented them from becoming who they really are. In the process of becoming aware and letting go of suppressed emotions, individuals often report a release of chronic muscular tension and an improvement in physical, emotional, mental, and spiritual well-being.

THE ORIGINS OF ROSEN METHOD

Rosen Method was developed by Marion Rosen, who was born in 1914 in Nuremberg, Germany. Coming of age in the Nazi era, she was denied entry to Germany's universities. She privately studied therapeutic practices combining movement, breath, relaxation, and massage with Lucy Heyer, a student of Elsa Gindler, a celebrated pioneer in the field of body relaxation and breathing based on sensory awareness. Heyer's husband, Gustav, was a psychotherapist who had been trained by Carl Jung, and the two women would administer body-relaxation treatments to Dr. Heyer's patients before he treated them with psychotherapy. From this early partnership, Rosen learned the powerful benefits of combining body therapy with verbal interaction. Fleeing the Nazis,

Rosen studied physical therapy in Sweden before emigrating to the United States. She completed the Mayo Clinic's physical therapy program and established a private practice as a physical therapist in Oakland, California.[2]

Over the years, Rosen noticed that many of her physical therapy clients kept coming back with the same problems. She realized that physical therapy temporarily relieved their symptoms but did not reach the root cause of their pain and discomfort. Rosen began to observe those clients who showed more permanent improvement: As she worked on their bodies, they reached a level of physical and psychological relaxation that enabled them to access the repressed emotional traumas that had given rise to their physical symptoms. While in this state, clients would talk about their unconscious sources of stress. Verbalization enabled them to let go of their patterns of holding, thereby facilitating their healing.

Working out of her basement office, Rosen gained a reputation in the medical community for being able to help people who suffered from psychosomatic disorders. In 1977, she taught her method to her first student, whose brother Rosen had cured of asthma. In 1980, the first training class in Rosen Method formed. Early graduates of these classes formed the Rosen Institute to oversee the training of Rosen Method practitioners.

THE THEORY UNDERLYING ROSEN METHOD

Rosen maintains that old forgotten emotions and memories lie stored in the body and that these memories are the source of constriction, which leads to physical dysfunction. A practitioner's gentle touch can help a client relax and surrender conscious holding. Supportive verbal exchange helps the client become more aware of the source of tension.

From her experience as an asthmatic, Rosen learned firsthand the importance of relaxed breathing. Rosen Method emphasizes the role of breath, which is seen as the gateway between the autonomic and central nervous systems, between what is involuntary and voluntary, between the unconscious and the conscious. When a client relaxes, he enters a state in which he can integrate unconscious material that might have been causing pain, and so release both the repressed memories and the attendant pain. Breath can be an important indicator of what is happening in the client's process. For instance, shortness of breath could indicate areas of tension and holding while deep breathing could be an indicator of relaxation and release.

Rosen considers practitioners midwives to a process of self-discovery. Rather than acting as psychotherapists, which they are not trained to be, practitioners offer encouragement and support for clients to trust their own processes of self-transformation.

THE TYPICAL FORMAT OF A ROSEN METHOD SESSION

A typical Rosen Method session lasts about an hour. The client disrobes down to his underwear (although additional clothing may be left on if the client feels more comfortable). The client is covered with a warm blanket and lies on a padded massage table. The practitioner applies no oil and stands or sits next to the massage table.

Treatment usually begins with the client lying on his stomach. The practitioner uses dialogue and gentle noninvasive touch to detect areas of muscle tension. (As the session progresses and the client becomes more relaxed, the practitioner uncovers portions of the body to be worked on.) Next the practitioner has the client roll over on his back in order to release the diaphragm and to enable full deep breathing. Pressure is applied slowly to meet resistance in tense muscles. The practitioner uses one hand to feel for muscle tension while the other hand remains still and listens. The practitioner pays particular attention to shifts in muscle tension as well as breathing patterns. These shifts usually signal an emotional release. If appropriate, the practitioner may make a brief nonintrusive comment (such as "Yes" or "What are you experiencing?") to indicate that she has noticed a shift. The practitioner does not try to interpret the meaning of such shifts, but is solely helping the client become aware of them. In this way, issues that have remained unconscious can become conscious.

In addition to individual bodywork sessions, Rosen developed the Rosen Method of Movement. Refined over a period of thirty years, this method is a system of range-of-motion and stretching exercises designed to lubricate the joints, expand the chest, and loosen the diaphragm. Taught in class settings, the Rosen Method of Movement has helped many senior citizens retain flexibility and vigor.

THE EXPERIENCE: I LISTEN TO MY BODY

I arrive at the home/office of Heather Brown, a practitioner of Rosen Method. Heather lives in a large loft apartment in Manhattan's mixed residential/commercial Flatiron district. I received Heather's name and phone number when I contacted the Rosen Institute in search of a practitioner in my area. When I called Heather to discuss her work, I was struck by what I felt was a tone of honesty and caring in her voice, and I scheduled an appointment to experience Rosen Method with her.

Heather is an attractive woman. She wears no makeup; her pale complexion is tinged with rose, which seems to reflect good, open circulation. Her eyes are bright and her manner sincere. She is dressed in a long-sleeved loose-fitting tunic sweater and baggy floral pants.

Heather has been practicing massage therapy for nearly twenty years. A former dancer, she studied living anatomy and energetic bodywork with Bonnie Bainbridge Cohen as well as learned the Alexander Technique. She completed training in Swedish massage before becoming interested in Rosen Method in the early 1980s. At that time, one of her dance colleagues, who was the sister of Rosen's first student, invited her to attend a demonstration of Rosen Method. The demonstration included a videotape of Marion working on a client. "I was impressed with the way Marion was able to elicit powerful change from her clients while remaining relatively still and using gentle movements. I'd never seen anything like that before," Heather relates. She was so impressed that she signed up as one of Rosen's earliest students, training with her in Berkeley, California. Since that time, Heather has devoted her practice entirely to Rosen Method.

Heather shows me into her work space, a small room with a massage table, a sofa, a few chairs, and assorted pillows scattered about. It's a cold northeast winter afternoon, but sun streams in through the south-facing window. Heather asks me to sit down on the sofa while she takes a few minutes to get to know me. She asks me to tell her anything I wish about myself and how I'm feeling.

I tell her that normally I feel pretty energetic, but today I'm dragging. The winter has been a long, hard one and has had a cumulative depressing effect. I've had trouble sleeping of late. Last night I saw *The Piano*, the film in which Holly Hunter plays the role of a mute woman struggling to express her will. I found the story of a vital woman silenced and victimized by the society around her disturbing. The day before, I took a strenuous class in yoga, the Eastern practice designed to unite body and mind. I'm not sure what it did for my mind, but I know it made my body feel achy. I've also been working hard, drinking a lot of coffee, and feeling some anxiety and stress.

Heather explains that the work we will be doing has the potential to tap into a lot of early childhood memories and that it will be helpful for me to tell her about my own early experiences with touch and what they meant to me. I search my mind for my childhood. I can't remember a great deal of touch. My parents, whose families originally emigrated from northern Europe, were very reserved people. They were self-contained and didn't show a lot of affection on the outside or engage in much physical touch. I tell Heather that, if anything, my early childhood seems noteworthy for its lack of touch. I add that that's probably why I've made it my life's mission to find out and share as much as I can about touch.

A significant element of the work we'll be doing together is breath. My breathing, including differences in its quality from one area to another, can be a meaningful indicator of what is happening in the underlying tissue. What is important is simply to be aware of the breath, and not to try to force it. Rough, shallow, jagged breathing is just as valuable in providing information about what's going on as deep, full, rhythmic breathing. I tell Heather this is interesting because I had some trouble breathing this morning. I would find myself gasping for air at times, a kind of response I associate with stress and drinking too much coffee.

Heather explains that during the session, it might happen that when we're talking about associations, memories will come up. She reassures me that I should feel comfortable at all times, both physically and emotionally. If I don't feel like talking about something or feel that my personal boundaries are being threatened, I should let her know. She then asks me to disrobe down to my underwear. "If you're uncomfortable with that," she adds, "you can keep on whatever additional clothing you wish." She leaves the room to provide me some privacy.

I take off all my clothes except my briefs, then call out to Heather that I'm ready. She enters the room and asks me to lie down on my stomach. She surveys my body before placing pillows under my ankles to relax my body. She asks if I would be more comfortable with a pillow under my chest to support it. I try this out and feel it is more comfortable. Heather asks if I would feel warmer with a blanket over me. Since there's still a bit of a chill in the air, I assent and she covers me with a light cotton blanket from my heels up to my shoulder blades.

Heather stands at the side of the table to my left. She places her hands on top of the blanket and makes smooth gentle stroking motions down the length of my back, from my neck to my hips. It's almost as though she's ironing out wrinkles. I feel that as Heather is stroking my back, she's doing some exploring, like a puppy in a new yard, sniffing out the terrain in innocent discovery.

As she continues to work, Heather stretches my muscles in a wringing motion, her hands working in a synchronous rhythm. While they may move in different directions at times, they seem to relay information as if one hand was sent to explore and the other hand was a listening station.

While Heather's hands glide gently along, I become aware of tension in my low and midback. "Yes, that's right," she says, as her listening hands tell her that I'm aware of the tension she's feeling. Slowly, she lowers the blanket to my waist. She is now free to work directly on the surface of my skin. Heather uses no oil or lotion. Her hands move slowly, gently. I'm more aware of areas of tension because her pressure is firm and her touch is deliberately slow. This lets me feel more clearly the difference from one area to another, and because she is not working too deeply, my muscles do not guard in pain. Through her firm, noninvasive pressure, my awareness penetrates deep through what feels like many layers of tissue to contact a pain that seems as ancient as my very being.

"That's good," Heather encourages. "Try to feel what's going on." I feel how much guarding there is in the muscles of my back, how much protection these tight muscles have been providing me all these years. Usually I don't think about my back—"Out of sight, out of mind," as the adage goes—but now I am acutely aware of my back and the tension in it. I tell Heather I feel that this pain is about protection. I realize how much tension I've put into my back in an attempt to protect myself. "Very good," she says. "I feel as though this part of your body is saying to me, 'I don't want to let you in.' See if you can feel what that protection is about."

"Fear," I reply. I feel as though I've been contracting the muscles of my back out of fear. But what is this fear about? I can't identify it with any one particular fear. It's more a general feeling of insecurity, of not being able to protect myself or provide for myself. Usually, I associate pain with some injury or wrong that's inflicted on someone. I can't remember anyone hitting me or physically abusing me in a way that would cause me to armor myself. If anything, this protection seems to be arising from a lack: a lack of feeling loved, of feeling I can be loved only if I'm a good boy, a perfect boy. But since I can never be perfect, I'm doomed to be unloved. The depth of this sadness is nearly overwhelming. As this awareness enters my consciousness, my breath deepens. I exhale long and fully. I feel that with that breath I'm exhaling my image of myself as a bad boy, my fear of not being loved. I realize how arbitrary the labels "good" and "bad" are: I just am, and it's okay to be who I am. I can be no less and no more. Somehow, this realization seems to afford me more space—the space to be myself, the space to breathe more deeply. I feel my back widening, expanding.

"That's nice," Heather responds. She moves her hands along either side of my torso and slides them under my rib cage. I suddenly become aware of how the muscles of my back are connected to the muscles of the front of my body, of how the tightness I feel in my back spreads around to the front of my body. The large muscles of my back feel like octopi tentacles wrapped around the front of my body. This inhibits my diaphragm, making it harder for me to breathe. I had never realized how strong this holding could be and how much it could affect my whole being.

Heather places her hands on the thick surface of my back and elongates the tissue in a long stretching motion. In my mind's eye, I see an image of tectonic plates, shifting beneath ocean beds. I feel that my muscles have become as hard and stiff as bedrock. Yet even so, movement is possible; these muscles can be rearranged; the pressure can be released. Heather is doing this with the simple yet firm movement of her hands.

Heather returns to my midback. Her thumbs glide back and forth over the thick ropelike tissue of the erector spinae muscles that run along either side of and parallel to my spine. She is feeling the tightness and holding there. I feel it with her as it slowly releases. The tissues feel as though they are vertical strands of fabric being pulled apart to make more space.

Heather asks me to roll over gently on my back, and she covers me again with the blanket before beginning to work on my diaphragm. First, she works through the reassuring cover of the blanket. I feel as though this area has been partially warmed up and relaxed through the work she's already done on my back. After several minutes, Heather removes the blanket from my stomach and works directly on my skin. Her hands make large stretching and crisscross motions along the surface of my torso from my abdomen to my shoulders.

As Heather touches the front of my shoulders, I become aware of tension. The area feels tight, as though it's impinging on my breathing, so I try to breathe deeply into the area to relax the tissue. Heather encourages me not to try to force my breath in order to relax. She feels that I'm working to relax.

"I feel such a strong pulse of vitality inside of you, yet I feel you are working to control your breath to make it long and deep. If you can, just let it flow naturally. If that means breathing shallowly, worrying that you may suffocate, gasp for breath, that's okay," Heather suggests.

I listen, too, for what this tissue is saying. To help me, Heather seems to be increasing the pressure of her hands in the area. Because she is using no oil, I can feel the full firmness and pressure of her hands directly on my skin. Through her resistance, I am becoming aware of the holding and resistance in my tissue. As she does so, I pay attention to my breath. It is not deep and relaxed, but short and shallow. My controlled breathing casts an air of false self-composure over feelings of inner turmoil, much as I have kept my feelings hidden behind a facade of calm. It is not easy to contact this deeper level of consciousness. I am so used to working at my habitual ways of being that it is hard to let go and just trust what will happen. I realize how my chest is tight and constricted, cutting off my air supply. In a near dreamlike state, I see the image of Holly Hunter in *The Piano* as she is pulled into the ocean by the cable tied to her piano. She gasps for breath as she faces suffocation. I experience this feeling of suffocation, the suffocation of a small child denied fulfillment of his longing to be loved. But the feeling tone of the moment begins to change. Owning this pain, it is no longer so frightening. Despite this sadness and pain, I'm alive and well. I realize I can fend for myself; yes, even love myself. I no longer feel as though I'm being suffocated. Instead, a hole is being bored through my chest, a space opens that allows my breath to go deeper into my lungs. Simultaneously with this deepening of breath, I feel the surface tension of the outer muscles covering my chest release. My chest expands and I breathe deeply—not through learned, controlled breath, but spontaneously. "Good," Heather says. "Very good." I ask her why she makes this comment; what is she experiencing? She tells me she feels a strong opening taking place, echoing my own inner feelings and images.

Heather completes her work on my body by moving to the head of the table, where she sits and applies some long tractioning motions to my neck. I feel tightness in my neck and a general relaxation as she stretches the muscles. Heather places one hand over my forehead and the other over the center of my chest, slowly disengaging her hands from my body. She covers my chest with the blanket and asks me to rest quietly for a few minutes. Heather leaves the room, giving me time to compose myself. She explains that she'll be back in a few minutes to answer any questions I may have.

As I lie on the table, I take stock of the session and share my feelings with Heather when she returns. This has been an unusual, at times disturbing, experience for me. Often massage and bodywork are about relaxation. While this session has left me feeling relaxed with a healthy glow to my complexion, it has also left me contemplative, more in tune with my body and wanting to make sense of it, including my patterns of tension. Rather than urging me to float off in a state of luxurious oblivion, Heather has asked me to come more into my body. She has encouraged me to feel my shortness of breath and my pain. Heather relates the experience of a friend of hers, whom she sent to Rosen for treatment. Her friend also expected an experience of peace and relaxation but instead felt volcanoes erupting inside her. Because that was what was going on with her.

I feel as though Heather has taken my hand, led me to a mirror, stood me squarely in front of it, and said: "Look, Thomas, this is who you are. No more, no less. See clearly who you are. Accept who you are, without feeling you need to control, deny, or change." And somehow, as a result of this experience, I feel better about myself. I realize I don't have to be perfect. I can feel content and comfortable to be who I am. With that realization, I feel tremendous space opening up within. The space of becoming who I truly am.

THE BENEFITS OF ROSEN METHOD

The goal of Rosen Method is not to cure a particular illness but to prevent it from developing in the first place. Rosen believes that if individuals are more in touch with their bodies and take measures to reduce the unconscious and chronic tension they carry, many illnesses could be prevented. Because of the physical relaxation that Rosen Method induces, clients often report alleviation of symptoms related to muscle tension and stress, such as muscle pain, headaches, fatigue, and irritability, and experience heightened vitality. As unconscious memories become conscious, it can also aid healing of emotional and psychological issues.

CONTRAINDICATIONS TO ROSEN METHOD

Because Rosen Method has the power to unlock unconscious material, it is most appropriately used in conjunction with psychotherapy for individuals who are in a state of serious emotional crisis or who have a history of psychosis. Individuals with addictions or who are being medicated by a psychiatrist should consult with a practitioner before beginning treatment.

BACKGROUND AND TRAINING OF PRACTITIONERS

Rosen Method practitioners are trained through one of fifteen centers worldwide and the Rosen Institute has certified each center. Training lasts usually over a four-year period and requires 250 hours of classroom work (a minimum of six weeklong intensives) and 350 hours of internship. There are over 900 Rosen Method practitioners worldwide. There are 350 practitioners in the United States, 450 in the Scandinavian countries, and the remaining are spread throughout the rest of the world.

FOR FURTHER INFORMATION

The Rosen Institute is located in Berkeley, California. Training in Rosen Method is offered through one of fifteen training centers located in the United States (five centers), Canada (one), Western Europe (seven), Russia (one), and Australia (one).

Because each of its centers operates independently, the best way to obtain further information on the Rosen Method is to visit the Rosen Institute's website. This site has all the contact information for each of the centers and includes information on their individual websites. In addition, by using the organization's e-mail address, you can seek information about training and practitioners, or ask a question about the Rosen Method. The Institute does not have a direct phone line.

For information on Rosen Method workshops, certification programs, and practitioner referrals, contact:

Website: www.rosenmethod.org
E-mail: info@rosenmethod.org

SUGGESTED FURTHER READING

The following books, written by Marion Rosen with Sue Brenner, provide a basic introduction to Rosen Method:

Marion Rosen with Sue Brenner, *Rosen Method Bodywork: Accessing the Unconscious through Touch* (Berkeley, CA: North Atlantic Books, 2003).

————.*The Rosen Method of Movement* (Berkeley, CA: North Atlantic Books, 1991).

The following articles are about Rosen Method:

Robert Calvert and Judi Calvert, "Exclusive Interview: Marion Rosen," *Massage,* Issue 32, July/August 1991.

Bevalyn Crawford, "The Healing Touch of Rosenwork," *Yoga Journal,* March/April 1990.

Sandra Wooten, "Rosen Method," *Massage,* Issue 44, July/August 1993.

PART IV

ASIAN BODYWORK:
PRACTICES WITH EASTERN ROOTS

"If my body," said Shun, "is not my own, pray, whose is it?"

"It is the bodily form entrusted to you by Heaven and Earth. Your life is not your own. It is a blended harmony, entrusted to you by Heaven and Earth," replied Ch'eng, his tutor.[1]

—CHUANG-TZU

Asian bodywork is comprised of a wide range of healing practices that trace their origins to the Far East. This category encompasses traditions originating in China, India, Japan, Korea, and Thailand. Generally speaking, Asian disciplines are based upon a concept of a vital life force energy, variously called *ch'i, qi, ki,* or *prana,* which practitioners believe animates the body as well as all of creation. Asian bodywork attempts to modulate, or balance, the flow of this energy through physical pressure and manipulation. Several methods are used to evaluate the quality of the flow of vital life energy. Some of the most well known of these are derived from the principles of traditional Chinese medicine. Also included in this section are some modern practices that are related to ancient Asian healing traditions.

BASIC FACTS

- **Shiatsu ("finger pressure therapy") is an Asian healing method in which a practitioner applies pressure to specified points on the body.** It aims to restore energetic balance to the body, mind, and spirit.

- **Shiatsu was developed in Japan.** It traces its origins to a type of healing massage developed in China several thousand years ago.

THEORY

- **Shiatsu is based on the principles of traditional Chinese medicine.** This tradition maintains that every being is animated by a vital life energy called *ki*. This force circulates in the body through a series of channels called meridians.

- **Disease is caused by a disturbance or disharmony of the flow of *ki*.** The shiatsu therapist assesses a client's flow of energy. He then applies pressure to points that line the meridian pathways to balance it. These points are the same ones into which an acupuncturist inserts needles.

- **The goal of shiatsu is to balance the body.** The individual is then able to utilize her own powers of self-healing most effectively.

TYPICAL SESSION

- **A typical shiatsu session lasts from thirty to ninety minutes.** Traditionally, shiatsu is performed with the client (called a receiver) lying on a comfortable futon on the floor. The receiver generally remains comfortably clothed as this enhances the effect of friction strokes.

- The practitioner (called a giver) crawls around the receiver. He applies pressure from his thumbs, fingers, palms, elbows, and knees to pressure points on the receiver's body. Strokes are used either to build up areas of deficient energy or to disperse areas of excess energy. Pressure can range from gentle to deep. The giver may also stretch the receiver's body to facilitate circulation of energy.

- Expect to pay $30 to $120 per hour for treatment.

BENEFITS

- **The primary benefit of shiatsu is maintenance of health and prevention of disease.** Practitioners believe a balanced body is better able to withstand trauma from such sources as microbes, stress, and fatigue. Therapists see themselves as teachers who educate the client in more balanced living habits.

- **Shiatsu induces a deep sense of relaxation.** It is well suited to problems resulting from stress and psychosomatic disorders.

- **Shiatsu can stimulate circulation of the blood and lymph systems.** It can also help cleanse the body of toxins, such as lactic acid; stimulate the internal organs; and encourage the proper functioning of the endocrine and autonomic nervous systems. Practitioners report using shiatsu to treat ailments as varied as low back pain, nervous disorders, sinus problems, and constipation.

- **Stimulation to pressure points has been shown to result in the release of endorphins and enkephalins.** These are the body's natural painkillers.

CONTRAINDICATIONS

- Shiatsu is contraindicated in the presence of fever or any serious or contagious disease. It is also contraindicated in cases of cancer and weak or brittle bones. Shiatsu to the abdominal area is contraindicated in cases of high blood pressure or heart problems. People on cortisone treatment should seek a doctor's permission before receiving shiatsu. Because pregnancy affects a woman's energy and body, certain precautions should be taken: Pregnant women should consult with both their physician and the shiatsu practitioner before undertaking treatment.

BACKGROUND AND TRAINING OF PRACTITIONERS

- The background and training of practitioners vary widely.

- Some schools award certificates or diplomas upon successful completion of their curriculum. For instance, the Ohashi Institute, with more than thirty locations worldwide, awards a certificate upon successful completion of at least one and a half years of theoretical and practical study.

- It is impossible to estimate the number of shiatsu practitioners in the United States. There are many schools that teach shiatsu. There is no nationally recognized licensing or certification of shiatsu therapists, nor a single professional organization that includes every shiatsu practitioner.

CHAPTER 9

SHIATSU: ASIAN ACUPRESSURE AND OTHER BODYWORK PRACTICES

In Japan, we call shiatsu the echo of life. . . . The receiver becomes the giver and the giver becomes the receiver as their breathing becomes one. . . . I believe touch communication is love.

—OHASHI

WHAT IS SHIATSU?

Of all non-Western bodywork techniques, shiatsu is probably the most familiar to Westerners. Shiatsu, which literally means "finger pressure," is an Eastern healing system in which a practitioner (known as a giver) applies pressure from the palms, thumbs, fingers, heels of the hand, elbows, knees, feet, or other bony surface parts to specified points on a client's (called a receiver's) body that lie along channels of energy called meridians. These pressure points are the same points into which needles are inserted in the Eastern energy practice of acupuncture. For this reason, shiatsu is sometimes called acupressure. This name is somewhat misleading, however, because acupressure literally means "needle pressure." No needles are used in shiatsu, and so some shiatsu therapists refer to their work as acupuncture without needles.

The principles upon which shiatsu is based stem from traditional Chinese medicine. This tradition maintains that a life force energy, *ki*, animates the body as it flows through the meridians. By artful manipulation of points along the meridians, a giver can rebalance the flow of energy so as to promote health and well-being. Shiatsu can also involve gentle stretching of the receiver's body parts through which the meridians pass in order to improve the flow of energy.

THE ORIGINS OF SHIATSU

While some people may consider shiatsu a New-Age phenomenon, it is far from new. It represents a time-tested synthesis of principles drawn from the diverse healing practices and martial arts of Asia, including China, India, Japan, and Tibet. Scholars trace its origin to the treatment principles of traditional Chinese medicine presented in the classic Chinese text *The Yellow Emperor's Classic of Internal Medicine (Huang-Ti Nei Ching Su Wen)*. This seminal book, which was compiled between 100 and 300 B.C., codified a rich tradition of healing and body manipulation that is believed to have originated during the reign of the legendary Yellow Emperor (2697–2595 B.C.).

The Chinese system of medicine made its way to Japan about a thousand years ago, giving rise to a tradition of massage and manipulation of the body known as amma, or anma ("rubdown"). At the turn of this century, the Japanese government set out to control the practice of amma by establishing licensing laws. This reflected the growing influence of Western medicine, which emphasized a scientific approach to the body and healing. The new licensing laws also attempted to control a situation in which amma was straying from its therapeutic origins and gaining a reputation as being a dubious form of relaxation.

In response to these developments, some legitimate massage practitioners began to call their work shiatsu. They hoped primarily to bypass the new laws regarding the practice of amma. More significantly, though, they infused renewed vitality into massage by giving it a new name and focus that emphasized its therapeutic benefits, just as massage therapists have done much to raise public awareness of the therapeutic benefits of massage in this country in recent years.

The practice of shiatsu was nearly exterminated in Japan in the years following World War II when General Douglas MacArthur banned as unscientific the practice of many traditional Asian healing arts. Massage in Japan had customarily been performed by the blind, to whom it afforded a livelihood and whose touch was considered particularly sensitive. The Japanese Blind Association contacted Helen Keller for help. She responded by petitioning President Truman, who reversed the ban.

One of the most influential popularizers of shiatsu was Toru Namikoshi, who trained many shiatsu practitioners at his Nippon Shiatsu School in Tokyo. Namikoshi extended the profession of massage to include not just the blind; Westernized its theoretical framework, so that it was no longer based on traditional Chinese medicine; and simplified the technique to follow the lines of tendons, muscles, and nerves in the body. He did much to elevate the prestige of massage in Japan. Namikoshi's approach is the predominant form of shiatsu practiced in Japan today.

Some practitioners, like the medical doctor Katsusuke Serizawa, continued to base their work on traditional Chinese medicine. Others expanded their practice to include not only the principles of traditional Chinese medicine but also a wider concern for the psychological, emotional, mental, and spiritual factors that impact an individual's life and express themselves through the energy of the body. This awareness is responsible for the development of what has come to be called Zen shiatsu—linking shiatsu to Zen Buddhism and by association to a meditative, spiritual, and holistic approach to healing.

Shiatsu in the United States has, to a great extent, become synonymous with Japanese massage. Consequently, practitioners distinguish the emphasis of their work by descriptive adjectives, such as Namikoshi shiatsu, macrobiotic shiatsu, Ohashiatsu, and Zen shiatsu.

Shiatsu first began to gain adherents in the United States in the 1970s, following President Richard Nixon's visit to China. During this exciting and closely observed trip, James Reston of *The New York Times* had a much-publicized appendectomy and reported on the use of acupuncture for anesthesia. This led to widespread interest in the field of acupuncture. It also coincided with the growth of the human potential movement, which popularized bodywork. The person who did the most to bring shiatsu to prominence in the West is Wataru Ohashi, who had such clients and supporters as Henry Kissinger, Martha Graham, Gay Talese, and Halston. Ohashi originated the term "Zen shiatsu" in 1975 while collaborating on the classic text *Zen Shiatsu* with his teacher and mentor, Masunaga. Ohashi developed his own signature style of shiatsu, known as Ohashiatsu, which integrates body, mind, and spirit and which he has taught to thousands of students worldwide through the Ohashi Institute. This is the style of shiatsu in which I have been trained and practice. It provides the background for my understanding of shiatsu and is representative of the prevailing approach to shiatsu as practiced in the United States today.

THE THEORY UNDERLYING SHIATSU

Shiatsu is based upon an understanding of the body and health that stem from traditional Chinese medicine. This system is based on the concept that a vital energy or life force (called *ki* in Japanese; *ch'i* or *qi* in Chinese; *prana* in Sanskrit) permeates the universe. Ki, which literally means "air," surrounds and animates us. We derive ki from several sources: A certain predetermined amount, called prenatal ki, is given to us at birth by our parents. To this ancestral energy, we add ki from our environment through the air we breathe and the food we eat. Ki circulates through the body and is responsible for protecting each individual from negative external influences, such as bacteria and viruses, dampness, and wind. It also keeps the organs operating smoothly and maintains the body's internal temperature.

According to traditional Chinese medicine, ki manifests in the world through two opposite yet complementary aspects known as yin and yang. Yin is associated with quiet, dark, passive, inner qualities, and is often identified with feminine energy. Yang energy is expansive, light, active, and outward-directed; it is identified with masculine energy. Everything in creation contains both yin and yang, coexisting side by side, and transforming one into the other, just as the night turns into day. Thus, each individual contains both yin and yang qualities, female and male characteristics, with the balance of one to the other changing over time.

Ki expresses itself through five basic physical elements, according to what is known as the "Law of the Five Elements." Called *Wu Xing* in Chinese, this expression, which literally means "five movements," defines a theory that describes five forms, patterns, or phases that ki can assume as it enters the material world. Traditional Chinese medicine developed within the context of a rural lifestyle, where man lived in close harmony with nature. The Asian practitioner observed the functioning of the elements around him and noted five basic elements from which all objects in the physical world are composed: wood, fire, earth, metal (which is related to air), and water. Each element is associated with a season (in traditional Chinese medicine, there are five seasons—the fifth being *Do Yo,* or the period of transition between seasons) as well as with other characteristics, such as a unique color, taste, sound, smell, body part, feeling, planet, and even a dream.

Because change is a basic condition of life, the five elements are constantly undergoing a dynamic process of cyclic transformation. For instance, wood, when ignited, becomes fire. Fire forms ashes, from which the earth is made. Metal is formed deep within the earth. Mineral beds give rise to water, which in turn nourishes wood. In the Eastern world view, the human being is inextricably linked to his or her environment. Man is seen as a microcosm of the entire universe. All of the elements that we find in the material world are reflected within us. Our internal rhythms are governed by the same factors that govern the elements and the seasons, which propel us on dynamically through life.

Ki flows throughout the body within an orderly energy system comprised of twelve meridians consisting of six pairs. Within each pair, like a married couple, is a yin meridian and a yang meridian. The yin meridians, which are associated with the female, or earth, element, run from the ground up, or from earth to heaven. The yang meridians, which are associated with the male element, like the sun, run from the sky downward, or from heaven to earth.

All but one meridian is referred to by the name of an organ in the body, even though the system of energy to which the meridians relate is invisible. This association is made because the energy within each meridian shares the quality and supports the function of the organ after which it is named. The yin meridians are lung, spleen, heart, kidney, heart constrictor, and liver. The yang organs are large intestine, stomach, small intestine, urinary bladder, triple heater, and gall bladder. In traditional Chinese medicine, the spleen comprises not only the function of the spleen but also the pancreas. The heart constrictor relates to the pericardium, the sac that encloses and protects the heart. The triple heater has no corresponding physical organ in the body, and its concept is foreign to Western thought. Asians reasoned that there must be some mechanism in our bodies that maintains the heat of our internal environment, and they assigned this function to the triple heater.

When considering the names of the meridians, it is important to realize that they refer to the energy of the meridian and not necessarily to the organ itself. For instance, if a practitioner were to say a person's liver meridian was weak, this would not necessarily imply physical damage to the liver, only that the qualities of energy related to this meridian needed strengthening.

Each meridian is considered to have a peak time period of two hours, during which it is most active. Since there is a successive flow of energy from one meridian to another, all twelve meridians circulate in one complete cycle during each twenty-four-hour day.

Besides the meridians, the energy system is also made up of two main vessels—the conception and governing vessels—in addition to extraordinary vessels and organs, such as the brain. The conception and governing vessels (believed to be present from conception and to be the ancestral energy channels from which all twelve meridians are derived) regulate the balance of energy throughout the meridian system. So in the event of a serious impairment of energy flow in the meridians, they would provide energy to the entire body. The meridians and channels comprise a system of pathways that run from superficial to deep in the body.

Along each meridian are small areas, or points, called tsubos ("jars"), where the energy of the meridian is particularly close to the surface of the skin. (Scientific studies have demonstrated that tsubos correspond to areas of particularly high electrical conductivity in the body.) A tsubo is like a small cup-shaped vessel that provides a point of direct access to the internal energy system of the body. For this reason, tsubos are sometimes poetically described as windows to the world.

Think of the overall meridian system as the subway system of a large city: Each meridian is like an individual subway line and each tsubo like one station on that line. Shiatsu practitioners learn to manipulate the tsubos to better balance the overall energy of a particular meridian as well as the entire energy system in the body. While there are more than 360 tsubos in the body, in practice only about one-third of them are routinely used in shiatsu therapy.

Tsubos are defined by anatomical location in the body, but their precise location varies by individual. A shiatsu practitioner has enough experience to detect the appropriate points on each body. Often, a sensation of tenderness is felt when the site of a tsubo is pressed. Each tsubo has a descriptive name in Japanese, which helps the practitioner understand its location and purpose. For instance, the first tsubo on the kidney meridian, located on the sole of the foot, is called gushing spring. Its name denotes that it starts at the bottom of the body (it gushes upward) and that it is related to water (spring). Pressing this point can help vitalize a stressed-out body, so stimulating it can activate a gushing spring of energy.

Some meridians flow through a relatively small area. The heart meridian, for instance, originates in the armpit and runs to the tip of the little finger. Other meridians course through large regions of the body. The urinary bladder meridian, the longest in the body, starts at the inner crease of the eye, runs up the forehead, over the head, and down the back and legs, to terminate at the tip of the small toe.

The energy of a meridian can be affected at any point along its pathway. Therefore, a shiatsu therapist can treat a problem area in the head by working a tsubo in the foot. Meridians are bilateral, which means each meridian runs on either side (right and left) of the body. If your right arm is too sore to touch, a practitioner can treat it by working a tsubo in your left arm.

When ki circulates smoothly, we are in balance and enjoy harmony with our surroundings. Imbalance can cause ki to stagnate or pool in a particular area or tsubo of the body. This, in turn, can cause vital energy to back up and congest throughout the body.

Using the subway system analogy again, if a subway train were to become stalled in one station for any reason—a motor breakdown or a malfunctioning signal—this would cause a backup of all trains on that line and could affect the circulation of trains in the entire system. When the flow of ki is interrupted for any reason—physical trauma, infection, psychological stress, and so on—the flow of energy through the meridians is disrupted and an individual suffers an imbalance.

If an imbalance is permitted to remain for any period of time, it can grow more serious and lead to physical disease. It is a fundamental principle of Eastern medicine that disease is a manifestation of imbalance. If left unattended, imbalance can have a domino effect, progressing from emotional and/or psychological stress to a state of disease within the vital organs of the body. The all-important role of the shiatsu therapist is to encourage the restoration of balance in the receiver's body. Energy balance leads to inner well-being and physical health. From an Eastern perspective, the two are one and the same.

Each meridian in the body is related to one of the five elements. By knowing the associations of the five elements (the color or the sound associated with each, for example), the shiatsu practitioner can help pinpoint more precisely which meridian is out of balance. The wood element, which includes the gall bladder and liver meridians, is associated with the color green, the emotion of anger, and the tendency to control. If a client with a greenish cast to his skin (associated with jaundice, often a sign of liver disorder), who has a tendency toward shouting when speaking and behaves like a control freak, presents himself to a practitioner, the shiatsu therapist tunes in to a potential imbalance in one or both of these meridians.

The shiatsu practitioner spends a great deal of time learning the correspondences of each element. This takes many years to master because the only way to truly understand them is by first committing them to memory and then by practicing the theory with numerous clients. Shiatsu is an art that can be mastered only with experience.

In a healthy individual, yin and yang are balanced and ki flows freely. Total balance, however, is an ideal and if ever truly realized would represent death because it would mean lack of movement. To be alive and human means to be subject to change, and we are constantly being thrown off balance by the vicissitudes of life. The challenge to the shiatsu practitioner is to facilitate change so that we do not become stuck in a fixed energy pattern.

When our energy is out of balance, we can suffer from one of two conditions: We can have an excess of energy (which is referred to as a state of *jitsu* in Japanese) or we can lack energy (a state of deficiency termed *kyo*). Jitsu is generally considered a yang manifestation while kyo is considered a manifestation of too much yin energy.

As a rule, we are most aware of our jitsu areas. Since they are characterized by excess energy, they often feel tight, irritated, or painful when touched. They are the symptoms that draw our attention to the fact that we are out of balance. Because the kyo areas remain hidden, the shiatsu therapist must be a kind of detective on the lookout for them. He then attempts to build up, or tonify, the energy in the kyo areas. The body as a whole is a single balanced energy unit. If energy is added in one area, it will be taken from another—in this case, from any jitsu areas—and so will automatically result in a release, or sedating, of the excess energy of the jitsu areas. The individual becomes better balanced.

In the traditional Eastern model of healing, the practitioner plays a very different role from that of a medical practitioner in the Western model of healing.

The Western physician looks for the signs and symptoms presented by a patient in an attempt to determine and categorize the nature of a disease. He compartmentalizes the symptoms into a specialty area and uses standard objective measuring devices (such as laboratory tests or x-rays) to arrive at a diagnosis. His goal is to alleviate the symptoms of discomfort, which he does by interrupting the body's natural adaptive mechanism. The disease is a challenge to the doctor, who intervenes and acts to control the body's natural process, focusing on a specific remedy for a specific ailment. This relationship encourages passivity on the part of the patient while handing over power and authority to the medical establishment. The ultimate goal of such a healing approach is to prevent the progression of disease and, ultimately, death.

The Eastern model approaches healing in a different way. In the East, evaluation is used to understand illness as a process composed of various elements that came together to create it. Disease is seen as an expression of an individual and her lifestyle as well as a challenge to her to improve her lifestyle and thereby grow and regain health. The healing practitioner's role is to support the body's natural adaptive healing process. Because Eastern medicine focuses on the individual's own ability to heal herself, it encourages the patient to take control. To this end, the practitioner educates the client in ways that will help her lead a healthier and more balanced lifestyle. The goal of medicine in this model is to restore the natural vital functioning of the body. It is an empowering approach to healing.

The Eastern healer acts as a kind of healthcare practitioner, teacher, spiritual adviser, nutritional consultant, and coach. Because of the intuitive nature of the evaluative process, the unique artistry of the practitioner is very important. He must earn the client's respect and trust on a subtle healing level. This contrasts with Western medicine, which as a whole is much more standardized.

We live in an exciting period of cross-fertilization, when the best of both systems is increasingly available for us to choose what most suits our individual needs. Practitioners in the West are becoming more attuned to the benefits of Eastern approaches to healing arts, and Eastern practitioners are respectful of the power and efficacy of such Western contributions to medicine as antibiotics and surgery.

THE TYPICAL FORMAT OF A SHIATSU SESSION

A typical shiatsu session lasts thirty minutes to an hour and a half. Often the practitioner refers to himself as the giver, and to the client as the receiver. Traditionally, the receiver lies on a towel or blanket covering a futon, rug, mat, or other padded surface on the floor. Shiatsu is performed on the floor because it permits the practitioner to allow his full body weight to sink into the client, thereby providing a deeper level of pressure and feeling of connectedness and support. The receiver remains fully clothed and no oils are used, which lets the giver maximize use of friction in the pressure strokes that are utilized during treatment. As the practice of shiatsu evolves, some therapists are beginning to incorporate the use of a table in their treatment, so that the client lies on a raised padded surface; some practitioners also suggest that the client disrobe partially or completely to feel more free and natural.

The shiatsu practitioner begins a session by assessing which meridians are kyo and which are jitsu. He does this through a combination of four methods of evaluation: *bo shin* ("looking"), visual observation; *bun shin* ("listening/ smelling"), observation of the client's speech and body odor; *mon shin* ("asking questions"), direct questioning; and *setsu shin* ("cutting through"), manual palpation.

When evaluating by palpation, shiatsu therapists most frequently feel for the quality of energy in the client's solar plexus area, known as the *hara* in Japanese. The hara refers to an individual's vital energy center, where she feels her gut reactions. All twelve meridians pass through the solar plexus, which serves as a central storehouse of energy. Each meridian has a particular area in the hara associated with it, like the hour numbers on the face of a clock. By feeling the quality of the energy in the hara, a practitioner can evaluate the quality of energy in each of the twelve meridians. Palpation can also be performed on designated areas of the client's back or torso (which are also associated with specific meridians) as well as at any point on a meridian. A therapist can palpate the pulses in both wrists to evaluate the quality of up to twenty-six variables in a client's body.

Once a practitioner has determined which meridians are most jitsu and which most kyo, he devises a treatment strategy to balance the client's flow of energy. He accomplishes this by manipulating the tsubos of the affected meridians. The practitioner works with both hands. One hand, the "mother" hand, often remains stationary to provide support and receive information on the client's state while the other, "messenger," hand actively manipulates the client's tsubos and gathers information to relay to the mother hand. In general, it is most important to tonify the kyo problem areas first. Strengthening weak areas will automatically disperse, or sedate, excess energy that may have backed up in jitsu areas. In addition to using his hands and other body surfaces to exert pressure on the tsubos, the practitioner may also stretch the client in order to further open up the flow of energy in a particular meridian.

Because the shiatsu therapist is concerned with the whole person, he often concludes a session by providing a few suggestions on things a client might do on her own. For instance, the practitioner might demonstrate some stretches to be done at home to release tight muscles; make recommendations on diet; or suggest lifestyle changes, such as getting more rest, socializing, or having fun more often.

THE EXPERIENCE: BALANCING THE PATHWAYS OF ENERGY

The following is an account of a shiatsu session I gave to Karen Anderson. Karen is a talented massage therapist who specializes in Swedish massage. I thought it would be helpful to present the perspective of an informed colleague. Here is Karen's description of her shiatsu treatment:

I made my appointment with Thomas several days before our session. Thomas and I know one another because we studied Swedish massage together. I chose him for this shiatsu session because I know that in addition to traditional massage studies, he completed advanced studies in shiatsu with Ohashi and has many years' experience in this practice.

I arrive at Thomas's apartment for my session about fifteen minutes late, feeling a little rushed and harried. Thomas greets me at the door dressed in a *gi,* a freshly pressed white tunic and pants. This attire reinforces a sense of peace and serenity. Thomas ushers me into the living room, which is warm, open, and sunny. It is a bright spring afternoon, and sun streams through the large picture windows. A shiatsu mat is laid out in the center of the living-room floor. A clean white sheet covers this work area, and a large poster chart stands on the floor at the head of the mat. It depicts the human body with the pathways of the meridians of traditional Chinese medicine marked in brightly contrasting colors. The winding, intersecting lines of the chart remind me of a subway map. A piano with old black-and-white family photos and a wall of bookcases filled with books on healing and audiocassettes add to the warm and professional atmosphere of the space.

I sit on a couch situated between the shiatsu mat and the bookcase. Thomas offers me some lemon gingerroot tea. I am concerned that having the tea might cause an interruption during the session in case I have to get up. When Thomas explains that we can have just a small cup and that it might be calming, I agree. As he begins to ask some initial questions, we sip the tea together. I realize the tea is helping to break the ice and relaxing me.

Thomas asks me a number of questions, some about my health, including a brief medical history and checklist of any problems. I tell him I have some tension in my shoulders and neck area, and that my stomach is quite often sensitive from food allergies. Thomas also asks me some general questions—about my favorite color and season, whether I live with anyone or have any pets. He explains that the answers to these last questions will help him understand me and my personality better. When I tell him my favorite color is blue, I notice that I am wearing blue sweatpants. The preliminaries take about ten minutes, and we are ready for the session.

Before beginning treatment, Thomas excuses himself to wash his hands. I sit on the couch realizing how comfortable I feel. As a massage therapist, I'm aware that clients may feel awkward and uncomfortable at times. Massage is a very personal one-on-one experience. These fears don't concern me as I know I am in the hands of someone who takes his work seriously.

Thomas returns to the room and asks me to lie down on my back on the shiatsu mat. I am wearing loose clothing—sweatpants and an oversized cotton shirt. I know that Thomas will be stretching my arms and legs and I want to have lots of room to move.

Thomas kneels at my right side. He asks if I am comfortable and warm. He takes a moment to center himself, then stretches my right arm away from my side to give him access to my hara, or stomach area. He explains that he is going to begin by checking my hara to assess how to proceed. As I lie there, Thomas gently places his hands on my tummy. Since I informed him earlier that this is a sensitive and guarded area, he begins with soft palpation, asking me to let him know if anything feels uncomfortable. "Additional covers are nearby in case you get chilly," he adds.

Thomas explains what he is doing as he goes along. He starts with gentle circular compressive waving motions with the palms of his hands on my stomach. He then gently touches different areas of my stomach with his fingertips. Thomas says that each of these areas is associated with a separate organ for which there is a corresponding meridian. These areas can be read almost like the face of a clock to assess the quality of energy in each; for instance, whether it feels full or empty. What is to be accomplished during the session is a combination of calming and energizing that creates balance within the whole body.

I never once feel uncomfortable as Thomas gently touches each area of my stomach. He always keeps me apprised of his findings. He relates them to the theory of shiatsu and asks if what he is feeling corresponds to my own thoughts and awareness. As he speaks, I seem to go almost immediately into a deep relaxation in which my body feels heavy and limp. Not wanting to speak, I listen while he explains. Some parts feel more dense, energetic, jitsu; others feel soft, with lower energy, kyo; and some in between.

"Do you ever have trouble sleeping?" Thomas asks as he presses an area under my rib cage. "Do you have a lot of vivid dreams?" he continues. I tell him I have had some restless nights, during which I have had trouble sleeping because I got into uncomfortable and awkward positions. At first I tell him I don't dream, then realize I have been dreaming a lot lately. I don't remember my dreams last night, though, and that makes me out of touch with the fact that I have been dreaming.

"The area we're feeling now is related to the heart constrictor meridian," Thomas explains. "It feels active. In traditional Chinese medicine, it's associated with emotional stress and is often related to heart problems and trouble sleeping because of active dreaming. Oriental practitioners have always made this association. Only now, though, is Western science suggesting an association between dreaming and heart attacks. Most heart attacks take place during the early hours of the morning, when people dream most actively. An article in *The New England Journal of Medicine* reported that dream sleep is correlated with increased heart rate, blood pressure, and activation of the fight or flight response," he says. "This area feels a little jittery or jitsu to me. It points to a possible imbalance in the energy of this meridian. I noticed when you first phoned to schedule this appointment that you had a tendency to laugh and giggle a little. You're wearing a red shirt today. Both laughter and the color red are associated with the energy of the heart constrictor meridian."

Thomas explains his approach to me: "I think of us as setting off on a journey together to an unknown destination. Along the way, we discover landmarks and get our bearings. I'm sharing what I'm feeling and observing with you so that I can see if they correspond to what you're feeling and experiencing. Your feedback lets me know if we're on the right road."

Thomas continues to evaluate my hara. "Do you have a tendency to hold on to things, collect things, and not be able to let go of them? Do you ever suffer from constipation? The area I'm palpating is associated with the large intestine meridian. It feels full. The large intestine is involved with how we eliminate things, both psychologically and physiologically. I feel a holding here. This could also relate to the gastrointestinal discomfort you mentioned." I tell Thomas I've always been a collector of things. Lately, though, I've been trying to let go more. I do suffer from constipation.

"The stomach meridian, in contrast, feels a little empty. This could have to do with the sensitivity you feel in your stomach and may even reflect an underlying feeling of insecurity, maybe even some worry about finances." Thomas's comments seem appropriate. They reflect my situation as a freelancer, where business demands can ebb and flow.

"Reading the hara is like putting a jigsaw puzzle together," Thomas explains. "Once we see how all the pieces fit together, we can see a whole pattern and devise the most appropriate treatment strategy."

As he palpates my lower solar plexus, above the ridge formed by the pubic bone, he says, "This area is associated with the kidney meridian. I feel that it and the bladder meridian with which it is paired are a little weak; they could use more energy. When you arrived for your appointment, you were late. You looked rushed and a little anxious. These meridians are related to the water element and they have to do with fear. These meridians run down the back of the body, and often an imbalance in them reflects in people who are often late and feel like they're always behind. This results in stress. Physiologically, the kidneys and the adrenals have a lot to do with stress and how we handle it. Your fear of having to go to the bathroom during the session is probably related to the same meridians. These meridians are associated with the color blue/black. Blue is your favorite color and the color of your pants. You may not have noticed it, but you also have slight dark circles under your eyes, which correspond to the color black. They also indicate stress and an imbalance in the water element. Most clients I see have deficient energy in the kidney meridian as a result of the constant stress everybody is under."

Thomas places one hand slightly below my navel while keeping the other above my pubic bone. He holds for a minute or two. I feel myself becoming soft, relaxing into the floor. "I'm holding the areas associated with the large intestine meridian, which is the fullest, or most jitsu, meridian, along with the area associated with the kidney meridian, which feels the most depleted, or kyo. In shiatsu, we refer to this as the 'echo of life,' as the energy of the two meridians balances. If I've read a body accurately, the client usually experiences a subtle release as this balancing occurs.

"During our session, I'll work to tonify the energy in the meridians that feel most deficient—the stomach and kidney. I'll disperse, or release, energy in the meridians that feel fullest, the large intestine and heart constrictor. The other meridians feel more balanced, somewhere between full and empty. I'll also include some manipulative work to release the tension in your back, shoulders, and neck."

Thomas picks up my right leg, bends it at the knee, then stretches it toward my chest. "Before beginning to work on a meridian, I like to stretch it. We'll be working the stomach meridian first, which runs along the outer thigh. Stretching the leg like this helps open up and stimulate its pathway of energy." He rotates my leg at the hip, then gently returns it to the ground. He's placed pillow bolsters under my knees to relax my low back. It feels good.

Thomas places one hand on my hara. He works the palm of his hands down the outer top of my right leg, stopping at frequent intervals. He applies pressure for maybe ten seconds each time he stops. I tend to prefer deep pressure, and Thomas's touch at first is medium to light. I ask him if he can work deeper. "I generally start out more gently to relax the tissue, but I'll be happy to add pressure for you," he says. He makes several passes down my leg, using his thumb, then forearms, elbows, and knees to intensify the pressure.

I've had several other shiatsu sessions, at Japanese health clubs in New York City. The practitioners didn't check my hara. Their techniques were more vigorous and the pressure deeper. Their work reminded me more of Swedish massage. As Thomas works on me, I realize how varied the practice of shiatsu can be. I'm surprised to realize that pressure doesn't have to be deep: Even light touch can be effective, balancing, and comforting.

Thomas repeats his sequence of strokes on my left leg. I'm chilly and ask for a blanket. Thomas covers me with a light blanket as he crawls back to recheck my hara. He crawls up to my right shoulder, where he rotates my arm in a firm stretch. "I want to open up the arm before I work on the large intestine and heart constrictor meridians, which run through the arm," he explains. He palms along my arm, then presses with his fingers. The movements are quicker, sharper. "I'm using fast, deep movements to disperse the energy here," he explains. "In the legs, I used longer holding movements to build up the energy." He repeats the movements on my left arm.

Thomas cradles my upper body in one of his arms, then lifts my right knee with the other. He slowly rolls me onto my left side, exposing my right shoulder. He places a pillow under my head and one under my top knee, which he positions at a 45-degree angle to my body. I feel heavily sedated at this point, toasty warm in my blanket.

"I'm going to do some work on your shoulders and neck. When you're in a side-lying position like this, I can get right at your shoulder blade, even put my hands underneath it to apply friction to the adhesions that form there. We call this 'scraping the wings,'" Thomas explains. I feel totally relaxed, snuggly with my pillows supporting me, and zoned out.

Thomas repeats his sequence of moves on my left side. He then asks me to gently roll onto my stomach. He works the surface of the broad muscles of my back. I feel myself becoming more alert. I'd felt limp before, but now feel more wide awake. "I'm tonifying, or energizing, the bladder meridian, which runs along either side of the spine," Thomas explains. He uses his palms, then thumbs. "Would you like more pressure?" he asks. "No, this is okay," I respond. Thomas moves down to my legs and presses his palms into the midline of the back of my legs. He works his way down to the balls of my feet, then along the inside of the leg as he works his way back up to my buttocks. "This is the pathway of the kidney meridian," he explains. "We're tonifying it as well."

Thomas asks me to roll onto my back once more. He kneels above my head. He places both hands under my neck and tractions them along my neck, from my shoulders to the base of my skull. My neck feels like a wave rolling in the ocean. He turns my neck to one side and applies friction with his thumb to the muscles that run along the vertebrae in the neck. "I'm using a push/pull technique, pressing my thumb into your neck while pulling your head toward me. This allows for deeper pressure and more effective release," he explains. Thomas works both sides of my neck, then gently strokes my forehead and cheeks with the fingers of his hands, moving like windshield wipers. He crawls back to my side, places his hands together, then bows to me.

"Thank you so much for coming to see me today, Karen. This completes our session. I'll let you rest for a few minutes. Do you feel warm enough?" Yes, I'm warm and cozy.

Thomas leaves the room and reappears a few minutes later with a glass of water. "You may want to drink lots of fluids over the next day or so to help flush out any toxins that might have been released into the bloodstream," he suggests.

"In shiatsu, we try to help educate our clients in how to take better care of themselves. You're in very good shape. I can tell that you work with your body, because your muscles have a lot of tone. It might help to get a little more cardiovascular exercise, though. It would help your circulation and also offset some of the effects of stress. Since your life is so busy, full of appointments and running from one place to another, it could also be helpful for you to take some time for yourself, to plan some unscheduled time just for you. That also might help you feel less stressed out."

Thomas asks me how I feel. I feel both calm and uplifted. Lighter. The tension in my neck and shoulders seems to have vanished. I feel balanced.

"Often people feel more relaxed and better balanced after shiatsu. That's one of its great healing powers," Thomas says. "One young woman with whom I worked was suffering from a severe case of TMJ disorder. Doctors at New York University told her that she needed expensive surgery to correct it. During one of our sessions, I was working on her shoulder, and we both heard a sharp clicking sound. Her jaw had released and her TMJ problem disappeared. She avoided the surgery and has remained pain-free. In another case, I was working with a man. He returned after our first session together and said, 'What did you do last time? It made a big difference!' It turns out he'd been impotent and he'd experienced an improvement in his situation after our session. In both instances, I think shiatsu helped relax and balance these individuals so their own natural healing powers could assert themselves."

I leave Thomas's apartment and stop for lunch and a cup of coffee. I realize I don't need the caffeine, which would probably disrupt my sensations of calm and balance. My beeper goes off at the restaurant. A client wants a massage right away. After a Swedish massage, I usually feel so relaxed or tired I don't want to do anything. But now I feel centered, balanced, energetic. I have no trouble working. My mind seems clearer. The next day I am able to tackle paperwork I've been putting off for months. I feel better able to cope with my daily chores, and my day seems to have an easy flow to it.

THE BENEFITS OF SHIATSU

Because of its concern with maintaining proper balance in the body, the primary goal of shiatsu is to prevent the onset of disease. It is therefore recommended as an integral component of health maintenance. Oriental medicine teaches us that the time to take care of our bodies is before we have serious problems, not after. Because it balances our energy, shiatsu can also help us when we do have problems, especially when these problems are related to stress.

Shiatsu stimulates circulation of the blood and lymph systems; helps cleanse the body of toxins, such as lactic acid; stimulates the internal organs; and encourages the proper functioning of the endocrine and autonomic nervous systems. Stimulation to tsubos has been shown to result in the release of endorphins and enkephalins, the body's natural pain relievers. Shiatsu is an empowering modality. It makes an individual more aware of his body and better able to detect signals of stress and imbalance so he can take corrective action before illness develops.

Practitioners report using shiatsu to treat a host of chronic and acute ailments as varied as low back pain, nervous disorders, sinus problems, and constipation. In a study conducted at New York University, subjects suffering from traumatically induced spinal pain were administered a medically supervised program of shiatsu, Swedish muscle massage, and trigger-point suppression. The study concluded that this treatment was a cost-effective alternative to conventional pain management and recommended its use with both acute and chronic pain resulting from trauma.[1]

CONTRAINDICATIONS TO SHIATSU

A shiatsu therapist can probably deal with almost any problem since he can modulate his touch to range from deep pressure to the gentle reassurance of a caring hand. However, there are certain contraindications for any type of work using deep pressure. In general, you should not receive shiatsu if you are under the influence of alcohol or drugs; have a fever or a contagious disease (because infection is present and could be spread); have brittle bones or are on cortisone treatment (which can weaken bones); or have cancer. If you have high blood pressure or heart disease, no shiatsu should be given to the abdomen. If you have any of these conditions or are concerned about any other serious medical conditions, you should discuss them with your doctor before receiving shiatsu. Be sure to give your shiatsu therapist as much information about your general health as possible to aid him in devising the best treatment program for you. Because pregnancy affects both a woman's energy and body, certain precautions should be taken: Pregnant women should consult with both their physician and the shiatsu practitioner before undertaking treatment.

BACKGROUND AND TRAINING OF PRACTITIONERS

Shiatsu has come to encompass a broad range of styles, with such specialized designations as "barefoot shiatsu," "magnetic shiatsu," and "five-element shiatsu" recently coming into vogue. It is impossible to estimate the number of shiatsu practitioners in the United States because there are numerous schools that teach shiatsu; there is currently no nationally recognized licensing or certification of shiatsu therapists; and there is no single national professional organization that includes every practitioner.

There are certain recognized schools of instruction that award certificates or diplomas upon successful completion of the school's curriculum. For instance, the Ohashi Institute awards a certificate of completion for advanced studies in Ohashiatsu. This certificate is granted upon completion of approximately 350 hours of study and practice over a period of at least one and a half years, culminating in written and practical examinations. A certificate awarded by a school that is known for high standards can serve as an indication of technical competence and consistent quality. Additionally, the American Organization for Bodywork Therapies of Asia (AOBTA) (see listing at end of this chapter) certifies practitioners who have completed a minimum of 500 hours of study in Asian Bodywork Therapy. As with any therapy, check the background of practitioners to determine such factors as where and how long they studied and how long they have been practicing.

FOR FURTHER INFORMATION

If your curiosity about shiatsu has been piqued, you may want to do some further research on your own or treat yourself to a professional treatment. Here are some resources that can help you:

The Ohashi Institute is a nonprofit educational organization dedicated to the promotion and understanding of the Eastern healing arts since 1974. It awards a Certificate of Completion in Ohashiatsu upon successful completion of 347 hours (at least one and a half years of theoretical and practical study). The Ohashi Institute also offers a postgraduate instructor-training program that is 256 hours long and takes about a year to complete.

The emphasis of Ohashiatsu is on the communication and synergy between giver and receiver and the self-development of the giver, as well as the receiver, and on physical, psychological, and spiritual harmony for both. Ohashiatsu in particular among bodywork practices aims to maintain and improve the giver's posture, movement, and well-being.

The Ohashi Institute has over thirty locations worldwide. With more than 100 instructors, it has educated thousands of graduates in Ohashiatsu. For further information, contact:

The Ohashi Institute, Inc.
147 West 25th Street
New York, NY 10001
Tel: (800) 810-4190 or (646) 486-1187
Fax: (646) 486-1409
Website: www.ohashiatsu.org
E-mail: info@ohashiatsu.org

The Acupressure Institute offers a variety of acupressure programs. Practitioners it has certified have completed a minimum of 150 hours of training. It also offers 200-hour specialized programs and an 850-hour Acupressure Therapy training program. For further information, contact:

Acupressure Institute
1533 Shattuck Avenue
Berkeley, CA 94709
Tel: (800) 442-2232 (outside California) or (510) 845-1059
Fax: (510) 845-1496
Website: www.acupressure.com
E-mail: info@acupressure.com

Many traditional schools of massage are incorporating shiatsu into their curricula as interest in Asian healing arts grows. You might want to check with your local massage school for information on its programs.

SUGGESTED FURTHER READING

The Academy of Traditional Chinese Medicine, *An Outline of Chinese Acupuncture* (Beijing, China: Foreign Languages Press, 1975). This is a classic reference for the professional, providing detailed anatomical descriptions of all the meridians and tsubos.

Harriet Bienfield, L.Ac., and Efrem Korngold, L.Ac., O.M.D., *Between Heaven and Earth: A Guide to Chinese Medicine* (New York: Ballantine Books,

1991). Written by two American pioneers in acupuncture, this book provides an in-depth readable account of traditional Chinese medicine.

Dianne M. Connelly, Ph.D., M.Ac., *Traditional Acupuncture: The Law of the Five Elements* (Columbia, MD: Centre for Traditional Acupuncture, 1989). As director of the Centre for Traditional Acupuncture, the author draws on her rich experience as an acupuncturist to guide the reader on a poetic journey through the seasons and correspondences that make up the five elements.

Michael Reed Gach, *Acupressure's Potent Points: A Guide to Self-Care for Common Ailments* (New York: Bantam, 1990). The author, the founder of the Acupressure Institute, shows you how you can use your hands to relieve everyday aches and pains with acupressure.

Elson M. Haas, M.D., *Staying Healthy with the Seasons* (Berkeley, CA: Celestial Arts, 1981).

Ted J. Kaptchuk, *The Web That Has No Weaver: Understanding Chinese Medicine* (New York: Contemporary Books, 2001). This is a classic reference on traditional Chinese medicine.

Paul Lundberg, *The Book of Shiatsu: A Complete Guide to Using Hand Pressure and Gentle Manipulation to Improve Your Health, Vitality, and Stamina* (New York: Fireside, 2003). A teacher of shiatsu shows how you can release and stimulate the energy flowing through your body to awaken your body's natural healing abilities.

Wataru Ohashi, *Beyond Shiatsu: Ohashi's Bodywork Book,* 2nd Edition (New York: Kodansha America, 2003). This book presents Ohashi's signature approach to shiatsu, Ohashiatsu, complete with illustrations. It is helpful for both the beginner and professional bodyworker alike.

_____. *Do-It-Yourself Shiatsu: How to Perform the Ancient Japanese Art of "Acupuncture Without Needles"* 25th Anniversary Edition (New York: Penguin, 2001). This is a do-it-yourself book that provides a simple introduction to shiatsu, with diagrams and helpful tips on how to give a relaxing session and treat common ailments by using acupressure points.

_____. with Tom Monte, *Reading the Body: Ohashi's Book of Oriental Diagnosis* (New York: Arkana, 1991). Did you know that a red, swollen nose may be a sign of a weak heart from drinking too much alcohol? And that someone who first wears out the inside soles of his shoes may be off balance in his digestion or sex life? These are just some of the fascinating tidbits you'll find in this introduction to Oriental methods of evaluation.

Videos:

The Ohashi Bodywork Videos is a four-tape video series produced by Ohashi, in which he demonstrates how beginners and professionals can give shiatsu treatments with the receiver in different positions. This videotape series is available from the Ohashi Institute (see contact information above).

VARIATIONS ON SHIATSU: OTHER HEALING APPROACHES RELATED TO TRADITIONAL CHINESE MEDICINE

Shiatsu is a powerfully nurturing approach to healing. The physical contact of one human being to another communicates a sense of love and concern beyond words. Nothing can match the sensitivity of the fingers for making fine adjustments. As Ohashi affectionately describes it, shiatsu is "touch communication, touch for peace." However, there are a number of other healing methods based upon the energy system of traditional Chinese medicine that are worth noting.

Acupuncture is a method of working with the same energy system that is used in acupressure by inserting metal needles into the skin at acupressure points. This method of treatment is particularly effective in relieving pain. Chinese doctors are celebrated for performing complicated surgeries, like removing brain tumors, using only acupuncture as anesthesia, or using acupuncture in combination with a low dose of pharmaceutical anesthetic. Patients remain fully conscious and alert during surgery, reporting no pain. Acupuncturists claim to be able to treat a variety of ailments. Acupuncture should be performed only by a licensed acupuncturist, who undergoes a training different from massage therapists and bodyworkers.

Moxibustion lies somewhere between shiatsu and acupuncture. It is based on the application of heat to tsubos through igniting an herbal preparation. Moxibustion uses a dried herb called moxa, or mugwort, whose botanical name is *Artemisia vulgaris*. Mugwort is an herb that grows abundantly in northern China, where the use of herbs in treating disease is the method of choice. Dried mugwort is ground into a fine powder, which can be rolled into a large stick wrapped in paper that resembles a cigar in shape. A practitioner of moxibustion lights this stick and holds it close to the surface of the client's skin while rotating it around selected pressure points to stimulate the energy. Alternatively, the ground mugwort can be rolled into small cone-shaped pieces, which are then ignited, either directly on the skin or on pieces of wet ginger, onion, or little mounds of salt, all of which protect the skin from the intensity of the heat. When working on the navel, the skin is usually protected as this is a very sensitive area.

Adherents maintain that moxibustion stimulates the immune system by causing a local inflammatory response in the area of contact. Because they believe this irritation in turn causes white blood cells of the immune system to congregate and multiply at the area of inflammation, this type of therapy is sometimes administered to people suffering from weak immune systems. Because of the potential for burning and injury, moxibustion should be performed only by a skilled practitioner. Some shiatsu therapists are trained in this art.

Some experts maintain that acupuncture, because it uses needles, which are cold to the body, is best suited to the treatment of "hot," or acute, diseases while moxibustion, which uses heat, is best used with "cold," or chronic, diseases.

Acu-yoga uses yoga postures to release the energy in the pressure points used in shiatsu.

Electroacutherapy uses electrical equipment to provide electric shocks to acupressure points to stimulate them biomechanically.

Cupping is a technique of applying suction to shiatsu points by placing a heated airtight glass cup over a tsubo. **Sōtai,** developed by Keizo Hashimoto of Japan, is a technique for correcting body alignment using a system of active and passive exercises. Some Oriental practitioners use **ear seed acupuncture** in which seeds are taped to pressure points on the ear in order to stimulate them. For instance, seeds taped to certain points on the ear can be used to help someone kick the cigarette habit, forming a kind of acu-patch.[2]

Ear seed acupuncture is based on the practice of **auricular therapy,** which sees the ear as a complete representation of the human body, with all organs, glands, and body parts reflected in the ear. Auricular therapists view the ear as an upside-down embryo and believe they can treat the whole body by pressing selected points on the ear. Practitioners of **iridology** believe that the entire body is reflected in zones of the iris in the eyes. They examine the eyes to make a detailed evaluation of a person's health. Finally, **reflexologists** believe that all organs, glands, and body parts are reflected in discrete areas of the hands and, especially, the feet. They treat the whole person by applying pressure to the appropriate features of the hands and feet. Reflexology, which has become a popular form of treatment, is discussed in detail in the following chapter.

OTHER ASIAN BODYWORK PRACTICES

The world of Asian healing practices is vast. The variety of Eastern-based approaches available in the West is growing as diplomatic ties and cultural exchanges expand. The following approaches are gaining prominence in the United States today.

Amma Massage

Amma massage (which is distinct from amma, the traditional massage of Japan discussed in the section on shiatsu) is a unique synthesis of Eastern and Western healing traditions. Founded and developed by Korean-born Tina Sohn, it integrates the principles of traditional Oriental medicine to assess and evaluate imbalances in the energetic system with a Western approach to organ dysfunctions. Amma massage utilizes manipulative techniques to restore balance and harmony to the body. The Amma massage therapist works with the Eastern system of energy channels, applying pressure to traditional acupuncture points as well as to powerful energetic points discovered by Sohn. In addition, the therapist uses manipulative techniques to affect the body within the Western understanding of the musculoskeletal system. Amma massage has evolved over a period of more than thirty-five years to include dietary counseling; detoxification methods; the use of herbal, vitamin, and supplementary preparations; education in exercise; and such other aids as mild pressure devices and external herbal preparations.

FOR FURTHER INFORMATION

Tina Sohn has written two books on her work: *AMMA: The Ancient Art of Oriental Healing* (Rochester, VT: Healing Arts Press, 1988) and *AMMA Therapy: An Integration of Oriental Medical Principles, Bodywork, Nutrition, & Exercise* (Rochester, VT: Healing Arts Press, 1994).

Amma massage is taught at New York College of Health Professions, both as part of the core curriculum and as part of an upper division Bachelor's Degree Program in Advanced Asian Bodywork. For further information on Amma massage, including practitioners and training, contact:

New York College of Health Professions
6801 Jericho Turnpike
Syosset, NY 11791-4413
Tel: (800) 9-CAREER (922-7337) or (516) 364-0808
Fax: (516) 364-0989
Attn: Dean, School of Massage Therapy
Website: www.nycollege.edu
E-mail: info@nycollege.edu

Jin Shin Do Bodymind Acupressure

Jin Shin Do Bodymind Acupressure was developed by psychotherapist Iona Marsaa Teeguarden. Jin Shin Do (meaning "way of the compassionate spirit" in Japanese) acupressure combines gentle yet deep finger pressure on acupoints with verbal body focusing and emotional processing techniques to help release physical and emotional tension and armoring. This body/mind approach is a unique synthesis of traditional Japanese acupressure, classic Chinese acupuncture theory, Taoist philosophy, qigong (breathing and exercise techniques), Reichian segmental theory, and principles of Ericksonian psychotherapy. It promotes a pleasant trancelike state in which the participant can move out of the head and into the body, accessing emotional factors underlying the physical condition. As in shiatsu, the client remains fully clothed during a Jin Shin Do session. The physical pressure applied by the practitioners is slower than that used in shiatsu, each acupoint being held for one or two or more minutes, with an emphasis on deep release of tension. The practitioner holds two points simultaneously: one hand on a "local point" in a problem area and the other on a "distal point," which facilitates release and balancing of the qi (energy).

There are approximately six hundred authorized teachers and registered practitioners of Jin Shin Do in thirty-five U.S. states, six Canadian provinces and Austria, Brazil, France, Germany, Italy, Japan, Mexico, the Netherlands, New Zealand, Norway, Singapore, Switzerland, and the United Kingdom.

FOR FURTHER INFORMATION

Teeguarden has written three explanatory texts on her eclectic method:

Iona Marsaa Teeguarden, *The Acupressure Way of Health: Jin Shin Do* (New York: Japan Publications, Inc., 1978).

————. A *Complete Guide to Acupressure*, Revised (New York: Japan Publications, Inc., 2002).

————.*The Joy of Feeling: Bodymind Acupressure* (New York: Japan Publications, Inc., 1987; contact Jin Shin Do Foundation to order).

For further information on Jin Shin Do acupressure, including newsletters, training courses, charts, books, CDs, audio- and videotapes, and a directory of authorized teachers and registered practitioners, contact:

Jin Shin Do Foundation for Bodymind Acupressure
P.O. Box 416
Idyllwild, CA 92549
Tel/Fax: (951) 659-5707
Website: www.jinshindo.org
(Many authorized Jin Shin Do Teachers have websites, which are included in their listings in the directory on the Jin Shin Do Foundation website.)
E-mail: teegers@earthlink.net

Thai Massage

The traditional massage of Thailand, Thai Massage traces its roots to India some twenty-five hundred years ago. Influenced by both Chinese and Indian healing arts, the techniques used in Thai Massage resemble those used in shiatsu, with the practitioner applying pressure with the palms and fingers to release blockages and balance the energy along specified pathways in the body. The network of energy followed, however, is more closely related to the Hindu energetic system of nadis than to the Chinese system of meridians. In addition to pressure strokes, Thai Massage uses a series of passive stretching exercises to energize and increase range of motion. As more foreign massage therapists have the opportunity to visit and train in Thailand, Thai Massage is being introduced to the West.

FOR FURTHER INFORMATION

The International Professional School of Bodywork in San Diego, California, features training in Thai Massage; it has produced an educational videotape entitled *Traditional Medical Massage of Thailand*. For further information on this tape or training in Thai Massage, contact:

International Professional School of Bodywork (IPSB)
Student Services Office
1360 Garnet Avenue
San Diego, CA 92109
Tel: (800) 748-6497 or (858) 272-4142
Fax: (858) 272-4772
Website: www.ipsb.edu
E-mail: info@ipsb.edu

Tuina: The Traditional Chinese System of Manual Therapy

Tuina (pronounced "t-weigh na") is an ancient Chinese system of manual therapeutics that is based on the theoretical precepts of traditional Chinese medicine. It aims to facilitate healing by regulating the circulation of blood and ki, which controls body function and enhances resistance to disease.

Tuina encompasses an extremely wide range of techniques and indications. The practitioner applies various parts of his body to the client in techniques that range from light and soothing to strong and invigorating. Tuina derives its name from two of the hand techniques: *tui* ("to push") and *na* ("to lift and squeeze"), which are used to represent the system. While some practitioners report using more than 365 different hand techniques, strokes can generally be classified into the categories of pressing, rubbing, waving, shaking, percussion, and manipulating.

Refined over a period of two thousand years, Tuina is derived from the earlier practice of anmo (amma in Japanese). In China, it is regarded as a time-honored and venerable healing art. Many Chinese hospitals routinely offer massage treatment to their patients. For instance, the Beijing Special Massage Hospital has treated more than one hundred thousand patients a year. As professional exchanges with the People's Republic of China grow, knowledge and

practice of Tuina is expanding to the West. A number of acupuncture schools
have incorporated Tuina into their course offerings.

FOR FURTHER INFORMATION

An excellent educational video showing a Tuina treatment is available from the
China Academy of Traditional Chinese Medicine. For information on tours to
study Tuina in China or for a list of practitioners in the United States who have
studied Tuina there, contact:

China Academy of Traditional Chinese Medicine
U.S. Foreign Office
8839 Knox Avenue
Skokie, IL 60076
Tel: (800) 343-6030 or (847) 676-9891
Fax: (847) 676-9833
Website: www.china-usa.org
E-mail: info@china-usa.org

The American Organization for Bodywork Therapies of Asia (AOBTA) was
established in 1989 to serve as a professional organization representing practi-
tioners of the full spectrum of Asian Bodywork Therapy, including amma,
Amma massage, Jin Shin Do Bodymind Acupressure, Medical Qigong, shiatsu,
Thai Massage, and Tuina. Citing a current membership of fifteen hundred, the
AOBTA has established minimum entry-level standards for practitioners of
Asian bodywork. The professional level of a certified practitioner requires a
minimum of 500 hours of study in Asian bodywork.

For further information on Asian bodywork, including a list of practitioners
registered with the AOBTA, contact:

The American Organization for Bodywork Therapies of Asia (AOBTA)
1010 Haddonfield-Berlin Road, Suite 408
Voorhees, NJ 08043-3514
Tel: (856) 782-1616
Fax: (856) 782-1653
Website: www.AOBTA.org
E-mail: office@aobta.org

REFLEXOLOGY AT A GLANCE

BASIC FACTS

- **Reflexology is a technique of manipulating various reflex areas of the body, most often in the feet.** It aims to improve circulation, ease pain, and increase relaxation in the body.

- **Reflexology is related to ancient healing traditions.** It evolved from zone therapy, as developed in the early 1900s by William H. Fitzgerald, M.D., and elaborated on by physical therapist Eunice Ingham (1889–1974).

THEORY

- **Reflexologists view the foot as a microcosm of the entire body.** All body parts, organs, and glands are associated with specific areas, called reflex zones.

- **Illness and disease reflect congestion and imbalance in the body.** Reflexologists maintain that relieving areas of congestion in the reflex zones of the feet can relieve congestion in the organs, glands, and body parts that are associated with them.

TYPICAL SESSION

- **A reflexology session typically lasts thirty to sixty minutes.** The client sits comfortably in a chair or lies on a firm padded table. The client remains fully clothed except for socks and shoes. The reflexologist may apply a light, greaseless lotion or powder to the feet or may use no lubricant at all.

- The reflexologist uses her hands, particularly the thumbs and fingers, to apply a series of manipulative strokes aimed to relax the foot and break up areas of tension.

- Treatment is particularly noninvasive. The reflexologist works only on the feet—the more sensitive, vital areas of the body, near the torso, are left undisturbed.

- Expect to pay $30 to $120 for an hour session.

BENEFITS

- **Reflexology achieves its healing effects by improving circulation and increasing relaxation.** It is particularly recommended for stress-related disorders, such as low back pain, chronic indigestion, headaches, and high blood pressure. Practitioners also use it for emotional disorders, such as addictive behavior, sexual dysfunction, and overeating.

- Recipients often report feeling more alert, creative, and vital.

CONTRAINDICATIONS

- Reflexology is contraindicated in the case of serious systemic illnesses, where increased circulation might spread infection, and in the case of injuries to the feet.
- Because reflexology manipulates only the feet in order to affect the rest of the body, it can be used to treat traumatized or diseased body parts where direct manipulation might be contraindicated.
- In the event of injury to the feet, reflexologists can manipulate reflex zones in the hands to achieve the same effect as working the feet.

BACKGROUND AND TRAINING OF PRACTITIONERS

- **The background and training of reflexologists vary.** There is no national licensure for reflexology. However, a voluntary national certification procedure for reflexologists does exist.
- A number of massage therapists, doctors, chiropractors, podiatrists, and nurses learn reflexology to incorporate into their practices. Many laypeople study reflexology in a one-day to two-week workshop format to use on themselves or their loved ones.
- The International Institute of Reflexology, which offers the oldest course of instruction, has taught more than seventy thousand students worldwide.

CHAPTER 10

REFLEXOLOGY: BARING YOUR SOLE

Where congestion exists disease will result. . . . No one can deny the well-known fact that circulation is life; stagnation is death.[1]

—EUNICE INGHAM

WHAT IS REFLEXOLOGY?

Reflexology is a technique of manipulating the feet in order to improve circulation, ease pain, and increase relaxation in the body. Reflexology is based on the theory that all body parts, organs, and glands are associated with specific areas, called reflex zones, in the feet, hands, ears, and surface of the skin. By manipulating the associated zone, changes can be effected in the corresponding body part. For this reason, reflexology is sometimes called zone therapy. The feet have a large concentration of nerve endings and are, therefore, particularly sensitive; in addition, they are easier to grasp for firm focused manipulation. Consequently, reflexology treatments generally concentrate on the feet.

THE ORIGINS OF REFLEXOLOGY

Because it maintains that particular zones of one part of the body are related energetically to other parts of the body and the energy of the total body can be affected by manipulating the feet, reflexology calls to mind shiatsu. Indeed, manipulating the feet to restore balance to the body is a time-honored healing technique, which was practiced in ancient Egypt, China, Africa, India, Russia, and Japan. Some experts report its early use in Asia, where finger pressure rather than acupuncture needles was used on the feet due to the heightened sensitivity of the feet.[2] An ancient Egyptian wall painting more than four thousand years old from the tomb of Ankhmahor, known as the physician's tomb, depicts the practice of reflexology.[3] Native Americans were also extremely aware of the powerful role the feet play in maintaining the crucial connection to the life-giving energy of the earth.

While its origins are ancient, the techniques of reflexology as practiced today represent a more recent development. The individual who is generally considered the discoverer of zone therapy is Dr. William Fitzgerald, a physician from Hartford, Connecticut. In 1902, while working at the Central London Ears, Nose, and Throat Hospital, Fitzgerald became acquainted with zone theory. This approach used manipulations based on the premise that various body parts have referral areas associated with them throughout the body (for instance, on the surface of the skin of the back, hands, and feet).

This idea had been exciting interest in Europe since the 1800s. As early as 1834, Per Heinrik Ling, frequently called the father of Swedish massage, observed that pains originating in certain organs were associated with unrelated surface areas of the skin.[4] Later in the century, Sir Henry Head, a British neurologist, mapped areas of reflex zones on the back, which came to be known as Head Zones. And still to come, in the 1930s, Elizabeth Dicke in Germany would develop a technique of massage, known as connective tissue massage, based on a theory of reflex zones.

Dr. Fitzgerald returned to the United States, where, in 1917, he published a text on his work, entitled *Zone Therapy, or Relieving Pain at Home*. Dwight Byers, the author *of Better Health with Foot Reflexology*, recounts a particularly dramatic anecdote recording Dr. Fitzgerald's success with zone therapy. A famous concert singer, who was a guest at a 1934 dinner party that was also attended by Dr. Fitzgerald, had been having trouble reaching her high notes. Various medical specialists had been unable to diagnose or treat the problem. Upon examining her, Dr. Fitzgerald traced the problem to a callus on the singer's right big toe. He manipulated the affected toe for a few minutes, the singer regained her range, and according to a newspaper account of the time, "miraculously . . . reached two notes higher than she had ever sung before."[5]

In his clinical practice, Dr. Fitzgerald concentrated mainly on the reflex zones of the hand. Applying pressure to appropriate points on the hand enabled him to anesthetize patients successfully during minor surgery, thereby avoiding the use of cocaine and opium, which were commonly used for this purpose. In fact, in an early experiment, Fitzgerald's colleague, Dr. Edwin Bowers, was able to demonstrate that a needle could be inserted into a patient's face without pain if an appropriate spot were pressed on the hand.[6] In addition to using his fingers, Fitzgerald and the early zone therapists incorporated the use of various mechanical appliances to exert pressure, including aluminum combs and rubber bands. Some dentists of the time incorporated zone therapy into their practice to lessen the pain of their work.

In the United States, Dr. Fitzgerald's work was taken up by another American physician, Dr. Joseph Shelby Riley, but the individual credited as the founder of foot reflexology is Eunice Ingham (1889–1974), a physical therapist who was working in Dr. Riley's office and became intrigued by zone therapy.

Ingham developed her approach to reflexology through trial and error. Early in her practice, she taped cotton wads over tender spots on her client's feet, then had her clients walk about. Treating a variety of patients over a number of years, she kept notes on the correspondence between points she manipulated on the foot and associated dysfunctions in organs and glands. As a result of her clinical experience, she developed a detailed map of the foot, identifying each area of the foot with a corresponding organ, gland, and/or body part.

In 1938, Ingham published her findings in *Stories the Feet Can Tell*. She subsequently founded the International Institute of Reflexology to preserve and promote the Original Ingham Method of Reflexology. An unflagging advocate of reflexology, Ingham practiced and taught reflexology throughout the country until the age of eighty. The International Institute of Reflexology continues its educational function, headed by Dwight C. Byers, Eunice Ingham's nephew. Dwight Byers has brought the teachings of reflexology to ten foreign countries, establishing schools around the world.

Today, reflexology is one of the most popular and rapidly growing approaches to nontraditional healing. The Institute reports a fivefold growth in its membership (comprised of former students) from fourteen thousand in 1982 to a current roster of seventy thousand.

THE THEORY UNDERLYING REFLEXOLOGY

Zone therapy maintains that the body is divided into ten zones, just as we each have ten fingers and ten toes. These ten zones run longitudinally from the tip of the head to the toes, with five zones on each side of the body, right and left. By working any spot within a particular zone, a reflexologist can affect the energy in another part of the same zone.

Insofar as they represent pathways of energy flowing through the body, reflex zones can be compared to the meridians of the body. However, while there appear to be many similarities between meridians and reflex zones, the two stem from different systems. Experts have cited visual similarities between maps of the body outlining meridian flows and the ten zones of zone therapy. Research study conducted by Ralph Alan Dale, Ph.D., of the Acupuncture Education Center in North Miami Beach, Florida, demonstrated that manipulating the reflex zones of reflexology has the effect of stimulating the same energy balancing that is accomplished using traditional acupuncture points.[7] However, the mechanism by which each system works is not fully understood, and any comparison of the two systems at this point is more conjecture than solid scientific evidence.

In reflexology, the foot is considered a microcosm, or mini map, of the whole body. The five zones of each side of the body traverse each foot from toe to heel, so that the energy anywhere in the body can be affected by working the zones of the feet. In addition, the foot is like a homunculus, or "little man," in its appearance: Reflexologists maintain that it represents the appearance of the body of a human being, with the toes being the head; the balls of the feet the shoulders; the indentation where the foot becomes narrowest the waist; the beginning of the heel the pelvis; and the bottom of the heels the feet. Within this map, all the limbs, organs, and glands of the body can be located. For instance, the area in the middle of the foot represents the middle of the body, and it is there that you would find reflex zones for the stomach, liver, spleen, and other organs that lie in the abdominal cavity.

Reflexologists believe that problems relating to places anywhere in the body can be helped by manipulating the associated reflex zones in the feet. Treating the outside edge of the balls of the feet, just below the base of the toes, can unknot a tensed shoulder, while working the big toe can help relieve a headache.

Reflex zones exist throughout the body, not just in the feet. The hands are also a mini map of the body, with referral areas interrelating all the major body parts to one another. Referral areas are also known as helper areas, because working on a referral area can help the functioning of the area with which it is associated. For example, the elbow and knee mirror one another, so that working on the elbow can help a knee that is in a cast. Similar correspondences exist for the rest of the body: The ankle, wrist, and neck correspond (yes, according to reflexology, you can ease a stiff neck by stroking your wrist) as do the shoulder and the hip; the palms of the hands and the soles of the feet; the calf and the fleshy part of the forearm; and the shin and the bony part of the forearm. You may be able to appreciate these correspondences more fully when you consider that earlier in our evolutionary development, we walked on all fours, so that our arms were truly mirror images of our legs.

The feet, however, are especially important to reflexologists. As Dwight Byers points out, almost one-fourth of all our bones are located in our feet.[8] Twenty-six bones, 33 joints, 19 muscles, 107 ligaments, and more than 7,000 nerve endings in each foot support and balance the human structure. The feet represent one of the most complex and richly innervated surface areas of the body. The nerve endings in both the feet and hands are particularly close to the surface of the skin and so more available to manipulation. However, the feet are generally protected by socks or shoes, so that their surfaces remain unexposed and sensitive, unlike the hands, which are unprotected and exposed by constant use. Because the feet bear a physical resemblance to the outline of the body, it is easier to remember and locate the various anatomical landmarks of the body when working on them. The feet are also easier for a practitioner to grasp with two hands, yet small and sensitive enough to provide a surface for focused treatment.

Due to their position at the bottom of the body, the feet represent the locus where the greatest amounts of toxins have a chance to accumulate: As the blood flows to the feet, it is aided in its downward journey by gravity, but the return of blood to the heart through the venous system is an uphill battle, as evidenced by the propensity of varicose veins to form in the legs, where blood tends to pool and stagnate. The feet are thus the depositories of various chemicals and toxins in the body, most notably crystalline deposits formed by uric acid, which is also a major component in the formation of other crystalline deposits, including kidney stones and the trouble spots in the feet associated with gout. Reflexologists claim that by breaking up these crystalline deposits, they are ridding the body of toxins and improving overall circulation.

For all of these reasons, reflexologists generally work on the feet. They can, however, work on other parts of the body, most notably the hands, if there are any problems in the feet, such as a broken toe, inflammation, or a swollen ankle. Working the hands can be an effective form of self-treatment that is sometimes suggested as a homework exercise to promote self-healing.

Reflexologists also point to the importance of all those nerve endings in the feet. If deposits impinge upon a nerve ending, this could cause referred pain, dysfunction, or discomfort to the organ or gland that is innervated by the same nerve. Since the nervous system represents a complex system of interweaving nerves in large clusters known as plexuses, resembling the configuration of a computer switchboard, this could have ramifications throughout the body.

Finally, many reflexologists consider reflex zones to be energy zones, like the meridians of shiatsu, with vital life energy, or ki, flowing through them. If this flow of energy becomes congested, as reflected in tension and the formation of mineral deposits in the feet, it will throw the whole organism out of balance. Reflexology aims to restore homeostasis, or the natural balancing of all the body's systems. As in traditional Chinese medicine, disease is viewed as a disharmony of energy.

The truth is that all explanations of why reflexology works are speculation. Reflexologists claim that their work is neither medicine nor massage. They refer to it as a science and an art, but most research into reflexology is empirical rather than clinical. Practitioners by and large are satisfied with the fact that this methodology appears to work, without being able to answer why.

THE TYPICAL FORMAT OF A REFLEXOLOGY SESSION

A typical reflexology session lasts thirty minutes to an hour. Out of respect for the practitioner, it is recommended that you wash your feet before a reflexology session. Some reflexologists apply a nongreasy cream to the feet to make the work smoother while others use baby powder or cornstarch or nothing at all. During the session only the feet are exposed, which is reassuring to those who feel uncomfortable about exposing the rest of the body. In this respect, reflexology is particularly noninvasive.

A reflexology session usually begins with a repertoire of relaxing strokes and manipulations to prepare the feet for deeper work, which is applied with the sides of the thumbs or fingers in movements that creep up the sole of the foot. These strokes are known as thumb walking or finger walking. As a general rule, if an area is tender, it needs to be worked on. Most reflexologists today do not use mechanical appliances because the practitioner has more difficulty assessing the depth of pressure when touch is not involved.

After introductory relaxation strokes, a reflexologist applies pressure to areas of congestion. This pressure is firm, but should not feel painful. Reflexologists keep their fingernails cut especially short since they apply direct deep pressure with the fingernail border of the thumb and fingers to very sensitive areas of the foot. As with any type of bodywork, let a practitioner know if anything feels uncomfortable. Often areas of tenderness will relate to what is considered congestion in the associated organs and glands of the body, although tenderness may also be due simply to areas of local inflammation or adhesions from scar tissue in the foot itself. A reflexology session usually ends with a few minutes of relaxing and calming strokes.

When reflexologists discover an area of tenderness, they are usually reluctant to say that it relates to a particular organ or system. First, this might cause undue alarm on the part of the client. Second, and more important, many of the organs and glands overlap one another. When you consider that every body part, organ, gland, and bodily system is represented on the relatively small surface of the foot, you can understand better how it can be difficult to determine with pinpoint accuracy which organ or gland is being treated at a given spot. Again, tenderness may relate to local inflammation or trauma unrelated to other body parts.

Reflexologists often recommend that in the case of a specific complaint, an individual begin treatment with sessions spaced one to three times a week for several weeks. In cases of general maintenance or preventive care, a session once every two to four weeks is sufficient. As to how long it may take to help clear up a problem, that depends on the severity of the problem and the length of time it has been present, as well as the client's overall level of health and vitality.

THE EXPERIENCE: FEET FIRST

What do Regis Philbin and I have in common? We've both bared our soles to Laura Norman, the high priestess of feet. Laura Norman is a preeminent practitioner, a teacher, and the author of *Feet First: A Guide to Foot Reflexology*. After studying at the International Institute of Reflexology, she continued to develop her own program of foot reflexology, founding Laura Norman & Associates, a leader in the field of reflexology training.

Regis Philbin became a believer in the power of the feet when he first encountered Laura Norman. Philbin was scheduled for surgery to remove a kidney stone that his doctors said was too large for him to pass by himself. The night before surgery, Philbin's wife called Norman, who worked on his feet in the hospital. By morning he had passed the stone; no surgery was necessary.

"This woman gave me the rub of my life. She saved my life, and I don't forget things like that," Philbin swears.[9] Another time, Norman was a guest on his television talk show when he was suffering from painful enlarged glands in his neck. Norman worked on him that morning, and by the time of the next show, the swelling had disappeared.

Deciding that this recommendation was good enough for me, I contacted Laura and arranged an appointment to experience a session of reflexology. The timing of my session with her could not have been better for me. Having had a grueling schedule of writing and massaging, I'd gone for several weeks without having time to receive bodywork. The psychological stress of work (which included frequent, intense treatments of a terminally ill client) as well as the occupational stress of bending over a massage table for hours at a time left me with a nearly debilitating aching back and shoulder and neck tension—the kind of pain that made me wish someone would come and pry my shoulder blades off my back and crack my neck in twenty different directions.

Laura greets me warmly when I arrive at her cozily decorated apartment in midtown Manhattan. Laura is a tall, trim, vivacious woman who exudes enthusiasm for reflexology. She is a frequent consultant on professional books on healing and bodywork and an eloquent spokesperson for the benefits of reflexology.

Laura begins our meeting by asking me if I have any question about reflexology and by taking the time to answer any concerns. She asks me to complete a short intake form, requesting information regarding medical history, previous experience with reflexology, and any particular areas of my body where I'm experiencing problems.

Like many bodywork practitioners, Laura works out of her home. "I've worked in a variety of professional spaces, including doctors' and chiropractors' offices," she explains, "but my clients keep telling me they prefer the intimacy of working in my apartment. They say it's so much more welcoming."

I must say I agree with Laura's clients. I've removed only my shoes and socks, otherwise remaining in my street clothes, and am lying on my back on a standard padded treatment table. It's covered with a sheet, and Laura has placed a pillow under my head for support. A towel lies under my feet. Soft music is playing in the background, Laura dims the lights, and a candle flickers gentle waves across the room. I close my eyes. Am I in heaven?

Laura asks me to take a moment to relax. "This session is for you, just to relax," she cajoles. "You've been busy writing, taking care of other people. Now it's time to let you be taken care of." Her soft, soothing voice lulls me into relaxing as effectively as a hypnotherapist's. "Forget all your cares. Forget your writing, your journalistic brain. Just relax. Trust that whatever you need will come to you during this session."

Boy, does she have my number.

I gratefully accept her invitation. I allow myself to relax and just be, as her knowing hands respectfully salute my feet. She applies lotion simultaneously with her two hands to my two feet. She spreads the lotion in a gentle, relaxing gliding stroke that covers each foot, starting from above the ankle bone and moving down to the tips of my toes. These broadly flowing strokes are punctuated by some more specific applications of pressure, where Laura applies her thumbs to points in the balls of my feet and alongside my ankles, holding for a few seconds. The pressure is deeper, but comfortable. I find myself beginning to waft.

Having greeted both my feet, Laura gently covers my left foot as she prepares to focus her full attention on my right foot. She is careful throughout to maintain some contact between one of her hands and one of my feet so that the flow of communication between us remains unbroken. She knows from my intake form that my back pain is more severe on the right side and that I am taking a homeopathic preparation to tone my liver. Both of these are indications for some focused work on my right foot. (Because the liver is located more on the right side of the body than the left, the reflex zone associated with the liver lies more on the right foot than the left.)

Laura's work on my right foot begins with some additional introductory relaxing strokes. Then she exerts greater pressure with her thumb and fingers in specific areas along my toes, the ball of my foot, the fleshy part of the sole of my foot, my heel, and the areas along the inside and outside of the ankle bone.

One of the first things that strikes me about this session is how odd it seems at first to have someone work only on my feet. I'm used to receiving, and giving, full-body treatments, where head, neck, shoulders, back, arms, and legs are all touched and treated. (Laura later explains that she and her associates often incorporate some gentle neck, shoulder, and face massage into their treatments. She also has available a treatment program that incorporates aromatherapy, having clients soak their feet in aromatic waters before treatment, and providing skin scrub supplies and aromatherapy lotions to apply to the feet at home.)

The initial strangeness of this situation gives way to a sense of deep relaxation as I feel my whole body responding to the ministrations to my feet. Laura's touch is gentle, warm, nurturing. It progresses from light to deep, bordering on pain, but a pain that feels oh so good. As Laura works my big toe, I can feel my neck lengthening and relaxing. I even feel my jaw releasing, accompanied by a kind of high, vibratory buzzing sensation that spreads around my teeth as the tension there melts. As she works on my little toe, I feel a tingling in my right ear and move my hand to scratch it. Is this a reflex reaction to the ear, which is associated with the reflex zone of the little toe? As Laura works on the balls of my feet, I feel a releasing of my back, which now feels as though it is melding with the table.

As my back releases, my mind seems to relax as well. My consciousness feels as though it's floating somewhere above the table. Even though this is my first reflexology treatment, I'm a believer: I'm in a state of deep relaxation, somewhere between sleep and conscious awareness, which permits me to wallow in the luxury of total peace, fulfillment, and relaxation.

Laura completes the treatment of my right foot by working the lower part of my foot and heel. I can feel my pelvis sinking into the table, my waist widening and relaxing. I experience a wonderful feeling that combines letting go of holding with wholeness and expansiveness. When Laura completes treatment of my right foot, I notice a marked difference between the feeling of my back on the right side versus the left side: The right side is soft, loose, relaxed; the left is still taut as a steel cable.

Laura covers my right foot and proceeds to treat my left foot. Her sequence of movements parallels that to the right foot. She concludes the session by uncovering my right foot and administering a few relaxing strokes to both feet, followed by some bracing tapping strokes to the fleshy soles of both feet. Her brisk taps seem to encourage circulation while helping to rouse me from the state of deep relaxation, bordering on sleep, that I entered during the session.

Laura disengages from my feet as she gives a few nerve strokes, or light, brushing strokes using the tips of all her fingers, passing gently down from the shins of both legs and out past my toes. She urges me to rest and relax for a few moments.

Following treatment, I chat with Laura. She offers me a glass of water. "It's important to drink lots of fluids today and tomorrow," she counsels, "because you'll be flushing out a lot of toxins that we released during today's treatment."

"Pay attention to how you feel over the next couple of days," she suggests. "Some people sleep really well after a session; some people feel really energized; others feel tired from the release of all the toxins, almost the way you do when you're really tired and have gotten too much sleep. You may have a particularly good elimination, because we worked a lot on the digestive organs."

I ask Laura what other areas in particular she worked on.

"We also focused specifically on the areas relating to the pain you're experiencing in your back as well as the liver, since you're taking something for that. I think it's important to do a good intake interview and find out as much as possible about what's going on with a client. That allows me to understand better what I'm feeling with my hands, to distinguish an area of local inflammation, for instance, from some complaint that might be related to an organ system. As you know, reflexologists don't diagnose, and I can't tell from an area of tenderness whether there is a medical problem or not."

Skeptic that I am, I cannot help but ask Laura, "Can working on the feet really help a neuromuscular problem like back pain? I know that's the theory, but it's hard to believe that working on the feet can unknot muscles located so far away."

"Sure it can help." Laura explains, "The muscle pain is caused by tension, and by inducing such a deep state of relaxation, the muscles can relax and relieve the pain. I'm a licensed massage therapist and I've studied Swedish massage, shiatsu, the Trager Approach, and many other modalities. But in my experience, nothing can induce such a deep state of relaxation as reflexology. Clients fall asleep on my table when I touch their feet, and their relaxation is deeper than with other forms of bodywork with which I'm familiar."

Following my session with Laura, I float out of her apartment. I'm feeling relaxed, indeed, a little spacey. I feel slightly washed out, the way you feel after you've been working really hard and finally let your guard down and the fatigue catches up with you. I feel energized and fatigued at the same time. My back feels looser, more relaxed, although I still feel some of the pain I felt before.

That evening, I feel so tired I barely want to move. I drink plenty of fluids and go to bed a little earlier than usual. I sleep incredibly soundly and remember a dream where I go into the bathroom and clean out my medicine cabinet, which is full of old bottles of various oils and preparations that have been sitting there for years. I realize it's finally time to get rid of this unused, outdated stuff. I can't help but wonder if this dream is mirroring my releasing of old toxins in my body.

The next morning, I feel terrific. I am surprised to find that even though my bowel movements are regular, I have an especially large and satisfying one. It feels as though this is the physical manifestation of the dream image of cleaning out the medicine cabinet. How could Laura be so sure this would happen? My back feels 100 percent better. The tightness I'd been suffering for days is gone—just a memory. I give four massage treatments in rapid succession without a twinge of pain or fatigue. I feel energized and ready to take on the world.

THE BENEFITS OF REFLEXOLOGY

Laura Norman points to a variety of benefits of reflexology. Chief among these is relaxation and the release of stress. Reflexology induces the relaxation response, which counters stress and activates the release of endorphins into the bloodstream. It also improves circulation, most notably from the feet. By improving circulation, reflexology helps to cleanse the body of toxins. It also aids the exchange of oxygen, nutrients, and essential chemical metabolites among the cells of the body. This helps the body to maintain homeostasis, or a balance of dynamic equilibrium within its ever-changing internal environment. By inducing relaxation and improving circulation, reflexology supports the optimum functioning of the immune system and therefore can be an important part of a preventive healthcare program.

In addition to increased relaxation, individuals who have received reflexology report greater alertness, vitality, and creativity. Practitioners claim reflexology has helped individuals suffering from disorders ranging from asthma to sciatica, and even provided support in overcoming addictions, morning sickness, weight disorders, sexual dysfunction, and infertility. Reflexology is particularly recommended for stress-induced disorders, such as high blood pressure, chronic indigestion, headaches, and backaches. One of the most powerful yet intangible benefits of reflexology is the sense of trust and nurturing it can help foster.

CONTRAINDICATIONS TO REFLEXOLOGY

Reflexology is seldom contraindicated. Because it manipulates the feet in order to effect change in problem areas of the body, it can often be used when massage or other forms of bodywork directly on a site of inflammation, trauma, or disease would be contraindicated. In fact, reflexology claims to affect internal organs deep within the body's core that traditional massage cannot reach.

Anyone suffering injuries to the feet or serious systemic illnesses where increased circulation might spread infection should refrain from reflexology treatments. As with other types of bodywork, treatment for the very young, elderly, or sick should be administered in shorter, more frequent sessions, with the use of less pressure. Individuals on medication should consult with their doctor when undergoing reflexology treatment because improved circulation may help the medication to be absorbed more efficiently, thus warranting a lowering of dosage.

While reflexology has not been known to do any serious harm, overworking may cause some minor side effects, such as a runny nose or diarrhea.

For those readers who are concerned that reflexology may feel ticklish, Laura Norman explains that ticklishness can result from nervousness and that a reflexology session begins with a series of relaxing strokes to allay nervousness. Additionally, ticklishness can be caused by sluggish blood circulation, and reflexology assists circulation. Finally, ticklishness can be induced by light rubbing or scratching of the surface of the skin, and reflexology uses firm, directed pressure.

BACKGROUND AND TRAINING OF PRACTITIONERS

While there is currently no nationally recognized license for reflexologists, a voluntary national certification program is administered by the American Reflexology Certification Board (ARCB). The ARCB was legally formed in 1991, and administered its first test in 1992. ARCB is an independent, non-profit organization whose primary aim is to certify the competency of those reflexologists who practice on a professional basis and wish to be recognized as meeting national standards. In order to be certified, candidates must have 110 hours of hands-on, in-class instruction in reflexology, including 90 hours of practical sessions. ARCB certificants must obtain twelve hours of continuing education every two years.

The International Institute of Reflexology claims more than seventy thousand members around the globe who have taken its course. Some licensed massage therapists as well as podiatrists, doctors, chiropractors, and nurses learn reflexology to incorporate into their practices. Many laypeople study reflexology in a one-day to two-week workshop format, to use either for personal fulfillment with family or friends or professionally. In fact, reflexology is one form of bodywork that you can easily learn in a weekend workshop to share with a loved one. However, in seeking professional treatment, you are advised to check the background of any practitioner.

FOR FURTHER INFORMATION

The International Institute of Reflexology offers seminars in major cities throughout the world and training in the theory, demonstration, and practical use of the Original Ingham Method of Reflexology. For further information on its certification program, books and charts on reflexology, as well as local referrals, contact:

The International Institute of Reflexology
P.O. Box 12642
St. Petersburg, FL 33733-2642
Tel: (727) 343-4811
Fax: (727) 381-2807
Website: www.reflexology-usa.net
E-mail: iir@tampabay.rr.com

Laura Norman and her personally trained staff of instructors offer courses ranging from one-day workshops to a six-day basic certification course and a twelve-day advanced certification course in the Laura Norman Method of Reflexology, which is billed as the most comprehensive training and certification program in the field. Norman also offers a course specifically designed for health professionals in both New York and Delray Beach, Florida. For further information on training, books, visual aids, and Norman's accessory line of reflexology and aromatherapy products, contact:

Laura Norman & Associates
41 Park Avenue, Suite 8A
New York, NY 10016
Tel: (800) FEET FIRST (800-333-8347) or (212) 532-4404
Fax: (212) 532-4504
Website: www.800feetfirst.com
E-mail: info@800feetfirst.com

In Florida, contact:

Laura Norman Enterprises, Inc.
Delray Beach, FL
Tel: (561) 272-1220

For information on reflexology certification procedures as well as the name of a certified reflexologist near you, contact:

American Reflexology Certification Board
P.O. Box 740879
Arvada, CO 80006-0879
Tel: (303) 933-6921
Fax: (303) 904-0460
Website: www.arcb.net
E-mail: arcbnet@aol.com

SUGGESTED FURTHER READING

Dwight C. Byers, *Better Health with Foot Reflexology* (St. Petersburg, FL: Ingham Publishing, Inc., Revised 2001). This book presents the Original Ingham Method of Reflexology as updated by the author. It includes a brief section on hand reflexology, with related charts of the reflex areas in the hands as well as the feet.

Eunice D. Ingham, *The Original Works of Eunice D. Ingham: Stories the Feet Can Tell Thru Reflexology and Stories the Feet Have Told Thru Reflexology* (St. Petersburg, FL: Ingham Publishing, Inc., 1984). This is Eunice Ingham's inspirational account of her pioneering work, as revised by Dwight C. Byers.

Laura Norman with Thomas Cowan, *Feet First: A Guide to Foot Reflexology* (New York: Simon & Schuster, 1988). This is a how-to book that provides a clear, readable introduction to the theory of reflexology as well as detailed information on how to perform reflexology. Easy-to-follow drawings, suggested visualizations, and case histories are provided to supplement technical descriptions.

AROMATHERAPY MASSAGE AT A GLANCE

BASIC FACTS

- **Aromatherapy uses essential oils extracted from plants and flowers to heal.** Essential oils, which contain vitamins, plant hormones, antibiotics, and antiseptics, are used to fortify the function of internal organs and boost the body's defense system.

- **The use of plants and oils for healing dates back thousands of years.** The individuals who most influenced aromatherapy massage as practiced today were both French: René-Maurice Gattefossé, a chemist, and Marguerite Maury, a biochemist.

THEORY

- **Essential oils are reputed to have unique, specific attributes.** For instance, lavender is relaxing while peppermint is stimulating. Essential oils can be used to imbue their qualities in individuals. Aromatherapists maintain that essential oils are antiseptic and promote efficient functioning of the immune system.

- **Essential oils can be absorbed through the skin.** While they can also be ingested orally or inhaled, the most pleasurable form of administering aromatherapy is through massage. Once absorbed by the skin, essential oils can be carried to the whole body via the circulatory system. The beneficial effects of aromatherapy continue to be felt by the body for several hours following a massage.

TYPICAL SESSION

- **Aromatherapy can be incorporated into nearly any type of massage.** Frequently, aromatherapists use strokes and techniques drawn from Swedish massage and shiatsu.

BENEFITS

- **Essential oils contain vitamins, hormones, antibiotics, and antiseptics.** Once absorbed by the skin, they are transported through the body's blood and lymphatic systems to diverse organs, glands, nerves, and soft tissue.

- In addition to promoting proper body functioning, aromatherapy enhances massage's therapeutic and uplifting benefits because essential oils are so pleasant-smelling.

CONTRAINDICATIONS

- Because aromatherapy is incorporated into specific massage and bodywork methods, see the contraindications for individual bodywork listings.

- **Essential oils should not be taken internally without the supervision of a physician.** They can have damaging side effects if misused. Essential oils should not be placed undiluted on the skin as they can be irritating.

BACKGROUND AND TRAINING OF PRACTITIONERS

- **The background and training of aromatherapists vary.** There is no national licensing or certification in aromatherapy. Anyone interested in aromatherapy massage should explore the background of practitioners for training in both the use of essential oils and the specific bodywork modality to which they are applied.

CHAPTER 11

AROMATHERAPY MASSAGE: APPEALING TO THE "SCENTSES"

Essences are like the blood of a person. . . . They are like the personality, or spirit, of the plant.[1]

—ROBERT TISSERAND

WHAT IS AROMATHERAPY?

Aromatherapy uses essential oils extracted from plants and flowers to heal. Essential oils, which represent the "essence" of plants, are a highly concentrated volatile mixture of potent chemicals; they are found in the flowers, roots, leaves, bark, wood, resins, and, in the case of citrus fruits, rinds of plants. Essential oils are extracted from plants by a variety of methods, the most common of which is distillation. While essential oils may be used in any number of ways, including diffusion into the air, aromatic baths, the application of scented waters, and even ingestion, they are most frequently mixed with oil and applied to the skin in the form of an aromatherapy massage. While this branch of bodywork was comparatively unknown until recently, it is now attracting widespread interest.

THE ORIGINS OF AROMATHERAPY

The use of plants and oils for healing dates back thousands of years. Cave paintings in Lascaux, France, dating from 18,000 B.C. portray the healing use of plants. Cleopatra is said to have charmed by using perfumed potions, Mary Magdalen washed the feet of Christ in precious oils, and Hippocrates fumigated Athens with aromatic plants to combat the plague. The first recorded uses of essential oils for healing occurred in ancient Egypt, Babylon, and India, which is why aromatherapy is included in this section on bodywork therapies that trace their origins to Asian roots.

191

More than six thousand years ago, the ancient Egyptians were adepts in aromatherapy. Aware of the antiseptic properties of plants, they used essential oils to preserve the bodies of their dead. To the amazement of modern scientists, the tissues of these embalmed mummies have survived remarkably intact. From Egypt and the Middle East knowledge of the art of essential oils traveled to Greece, Rome, Constantinople, and the Arab world. The ancient term for massage was "anointing," reflecting the prominent role that unguents have played throughout the history of massage. During the Middle Ages, alchemists experimented with the healing, energetic properties of essential oils, which they considered to represent the quintessential spirit of a plant. Their knowledge of essential oils was expanded by the Crusaders, who brought exotic aromatic preparations back from their travels to the East. Essential oils continued to be a major remedy in the pharmacopoeia of eighteenth- and nineteenth-century physicians until they were replaced by synthetic drugs.

Current interest in aromatherapy is a more modern development, however. The father of aromatherapy as we know it today is René-Maurice Gattefossé, a chemist who was born in Grasse, France, at the turn of the twentieth century. Grasse, which is in the sunny southern part of France, was, and still is, the center for the cultivation and extraction of essential oils for use in cosmetics. Gattefossé was born into a family whose business was the extraction of essential oils. When his hand was badly burned during an explosion in his laboratory, he immersed it immediately in lavender oil. His hand healed rapidly, without infection and without leaving a scar. This confirmed Gattefossé's belief in the healing properties of essential oils; he dedicated the rest of his life to scientific research in this field. Gattefossé, who is credited with coining the term "aromatherapy," published his findings in a book by that name in 1928.

Research in aromatherapy waned until World War II. At that time, Jean Valnet, a French medical doctor, recognizing the antibiotic and healing properties of essential oils, used them to treat soldiers wounded during the war. In 1964, through the publication of his landmark book, *Aromathérapie*, Dr. Valnet was responsible for focusing medical attention on this exciting field. While aromatherapy began to make major inroads in the United States only in the late 1980s, it has been a respected therapy for many years in France, where it is taught in medical schools. As a sign of its acceptance, French pharmacies routinely dispense essential oils for medicinal use. Aromatherapy is also widely popular in other European countries, most notably England, Germany, Switzerland, and Italy.

Maintaining the French connection in aromatherapy, the individual who did the most to introduce aromatherapy into massage was Madame Marguerite Maury. Trained as a biochemist, Mme. Maury was not qualified to prescribe essential oils for internal consumption. She therefore sought a method of using them externally for both therapeutic and cosmetic benefits. Her work confirmed that massage is ideally suited to aromatherapy because essential oils combined in a carrier oil are easily absorbed through the skin during treatment—a convenient and pleasurable way of introducing essential oils into the body while compounding the beneficial effects of massage.

THE THEORY UNDERLYING AROMATHERAPY

Research into essential oils has shown that the extracts of certain plants have specific, unique qualities. For instance, lavender is considered to be relaxing to both the nervous system and the muscles; clove is a powerful antiseptic; peppermint is stimulating; and ylang-ylang ("flower of flowers") is reputed to be an aphrodisiac. Some oils can be either relaxing or energizing, depending upon the dosage. An aromatherapist can custom tailor a blend of essential oils to meet a particular individual's emotional and physical makeup. While the chemical ingredients of essential oils can be synthesized in the test tube, proponents of aromatherapy say it is not only the primary chemical ingredient of an essential oil but the trace elements and their unique combination that give the natural essential oil greater efficacy over its synthetic counterpart. In addition, since essential oils are natural, they are more easily assimilated by the body without the toxic side effects of synthetic substances. In fact, essential oils actually stimulate the body's natural defense mechanism. Renewed interest in the healing properties of plants is reflected in growing research into the pharmaceutical properties of a variety of plants, including those growing in the rapidly dwindling tropical rain forests.

Aromatherapy is directed at our sense of smell, which is extremely refined. We can distinguish 1 part of aromatic matter in up to 10,000 billion parts, enabling us to distinguish up to 4,000 different scents. Much of what we consider our sense of taste is actually smell, as evidenced by our inability to taste food when we have a stuffed-up nose. While we now tend to rely heavily on vision, at one time the sense of smell played a crucial role in our survival and evolution as a species, enabling us to smell our predators and track our prey. The olfactory nerves that register the sensation of odor lead directly into the oldest and most primitive part of the brain, the limbic system, which controls our basic emotional, visceral, and muscular responses. The sense of smell can subconsciously influence our emotions, sexual urges, and certain involuntary physiological responses as well as bring back old memories in a flash. Anyone familiar with the vividly sensuous novel *Remembrance of Things Past* is familiar with how the taste and smell of a pastry reawakened a lost world of childhood memories for the novelist Marcel Proust. Recent studies have shown that sexual attraction is caused in part by the release of pheromones, subtle sexual odors, that act as signals to attract members of the opposite sex.[2] Perfume makers have capitalized on this finding to develop perfumes to enhance sex appeal. There is evidence that these same pheromones play a role in the well-documented synchronization of menstrual cycles that takes place among women living together in college dormitories. So influential is our sense of smell that many people refuse to check into a hotel if it has odors in the lobby.[3] Companies are using aromatherapy to relax employees and clients, while airlines have used it to help passengers beat jet lag.[4] Negative odors, such as smog molecules and some man-made chemicals, can cause stress.[5]

Aromatherapy is distinct from what is known as herbal medicine, and it is studied as a separate discipline. While approximately one-third of plants used in herbal medicine are also used in aromatherapy, herbal medicine uses the whole plant to heal. Aromatherapy uses only essential oils, which Robert Tisserand, author of *The Art of Aromatherapy,* has described as the personality or distilled essence of a plant. In the case of roses, for instance, it may take as much as a ton of rose petals to produce two pounds of essential oil. Tisserand explains that essential oils (which account for anywhere from .01 percent to 10 percent of the total plant) represent the subtlest, most refined energy of the plant; consequently, they heal on a more etheric plane than the whole plant. Their effect is often as much psychological as physiological due to their pleasant smell (anyone who has taken medicinal herbal teas knows that by contrast their taste can be bitter and decidedly unpleasant).

Aromatherapy also differs from the Bach Flower Remedies developed beginning in the 1920s by Dr. Edward Bach (1886–1936), a British physician. The Bach remedies represent the extraction of one or a combination of flower essences, which are ingested orally in small doses. Dr. Bach believed that illness is caused by negative emotions, and the Bach Flower Remedies aim to overcome negative emotions to restore mental and physical balance.

THE TYPICAL FORMAT OF AROMATHERAPY MASSAGE

Aromatherapy massage incorporates essential oils in the ministration of massage strokes drawn from virtually any massage or bodywork practice. The long, deep, flowing strokes of Swedish massage, for example, can be used to apply essential oils and aid their penetration and circulation in the body. Massage deep into body tissues can allow the aromatherapist to work locally on areas of congestion and tension in the body. Working with acupressure points, a shiatsu practitioner can apply essential oils to important energetic points and reflex zones in the body.

Tisserand explains that massage with essential oils usually takes one of three forms: a massage to the back; a full-body massage; or a facial massage, which may also include the neck and shoulders. In the case of an acute, or local, problem area, aromatherapy massage would pay particular attention to that area. The back is of special importance because the spinal nerves that innervate the whole body below the head exit the spinal column between the vertebrae. Therefore, any massage done along the spine has the potential of affecting every muscle and organ influenced by these nerves. In addition, in shiatsu, each meridian has a point associated with it along the spine, so that working on the back has the potential of impacting every meridian in the body. Massage to the back, therefore, could affect both the local areas of congestion—through massage to the corresponding area of spinal nerve or acupoint association—and the full body. In cases where there is no particular local problem, the aromatherapist will most likely perform a facial or a full-body massage.

THE EXPERIENCE: MASSAGE AS A "SCENTSUAL" EXPERIENCE

My experience with aromatherapy massage takes place in a very special setting. I've decided to treat myself to some luxurious relaxation and have just spent a week at Spa'Deus, one of the world's premier fitness spas, located in Chianciano Terme, Italy. While enjoying the beauty of the Tuscan hills, I've been experiencing pampering bodywork treatments, healthy eating, and fitness training in an atmosphere designed to help me destress from my day-to-day worries.

Founded by Christina Newburgh, whose lifelong commitment to health and well-being sent her searching the globe for the best in health and beauty treatments, Spa'Deus offers a wide range of treatments based on the use of natural plants, herbs, and essential oils. I've had my body massaged with salt from the Dead Sea to scale off layers of dead skin; painted with honey to moisturize it; and baked in sea mud and algae to draw out toxins. The crowning moment of my stay, however, is an aromatherapy massage session with a talented and sensitive therapist named Greta.

I visit Greta in her treatment room, where she greets me at the door. She is a young, attractive Italian woman in her mid-twenties, with long straight black hair. Her glasses give her a certain studied look, and the white lab coat she wears enhances her air of professionalism. Her manner is gracious and friendly.

Her massage area is a quiet, intimate, wood-paneled room with a raised padded table in the center. Shelves filled with essential oils and lotions line its walls as well as some high-tech–looking beauty treatment equipment. The lights are low. Soft music by Kitaro, a New-Age composer, plays from a small portable tape deck. The delicately fragrant scent of jasmine incense lingers in the air.

For my experience of aromatherapy I've selected a massage focusing on my face and neck; treatment will be administered using a massage technique based on Dr. Vodder's lymph drainage. This method of massage was developed in the 1930s by a Danish couple, Dr. Emil Vodder and his wife, Estrid, while they worked as massage therapists on the French Riviera. It uses light, slow, deliberate strokes, repeated numerous times, to aid the circulation of lymph in the body, which in turn facilitates removal of excess water, wastes, toxins, and foreign substances from body tissues. It is a routine form of therapeutic treatment in many parts of Europe and has been gaining popularity in the United States since it was introduced in the 1980s.

Greta gently applies a blend of massage oil to my face. Her touch is soft, sensuous, gently relaxing. Next, she applies a light cream, which she works into my skin. She picks up a small glass vial, and a few drops of clear liquid fall like a soft fragrant rain of apple blossom on my face. This blend contains the specific essential oils that Greta has selected to use for my treatment session in a carrier oil.

Greta and I communicate with one another by intuition as much as words: My Italian is limited to the vocabulary of northern Italian cuisine, and Greta's knowledge of English seems no larger. However, when I ask her which oils she is using I recognize the words "chamomile" and "juniper." I know that these oils are frequently used in aromatherapy. Chamomile has been prized for centuries for the calming effect it has on both the mind and the body. It is also helpful for allergies and sinus problems, from which I suffer. Juniper relaxes while at the same time it energizes. It is said to stimulate the circulation as well as being a diuretic. As part of my treatment at the spa, I'm drinking lots of water to detoxify my body; the juniper should aid in the elimination of toxins. Both chamomile and juniper have antiseptic and astringent qualities, which make them good for various skin disorders, such as dermatitis, acne, and dry skin.

Greta's fingers gently trace the outlines of my eyebrows, bridge of my nose, my chin, my temples—over and over again until I feel my face is melting into her hands. Her strokes lengthen, and she continues these motions all down my neck, encouraging the flow of lymph through the important constellation of lymph nodes and glands in the neck. (These are the areas that become enlarged when you're fighting off an infection.) Greta is not only making me feel good; she's also bolstering the functioning of my immune system.

Greta's fingers make circles around the orbits of my eyes, figure-eighting back and forth. Her circles lengthen as she outlines ovals around the circumference of my whole face, from temples to chin to forehead. Round and round, again and again. These movements are interspersed with the figure eights around my eyes. Greta strokes my neck again. The delicate aroma of essential oils brushes my nostrils, calms my mind.

I am putty in Greta's hands, floating, flying, at peace. No need for language here: Greta is reminding me in a very concrete way that massage is indeed all about touch communication.

My sensuous journey with Greta comes slowly to an end. She has been massaging me for about a half hour. As she bids me adieu, I review myself mentally. I feel nurtured, calmed, relaxed, yet full of vitality. These sensations seem to come not only from the soothing massage strokes, but also from the delightfully calming scent of the essential oils Greta incorporated into the treatment. I float down the stairs from Greta's treatment room for lunch at the spa. I feel a lightness and ease from this treatment, which somehow seems to have penetrated my entire being, beyond my skin, and into my core. It is different from the sensations of any of the other treatments I've experienced. A fellow American guest at the spa is the first to greet me in the dining room. She takes one look at me and tells me that my face, which is usually oily, looks clear and clean. "You look as though you had a *very* relaxing treatment," she adds. And indeed I have.

THE BENEFITS OF AROMATHERAPY MASSAGE

Essential oils contain vitamins, plant hormones, antibiotics, and antiseptics. They act to fortify the function of internal organs and to boost the efficiency of the body's defense system. Once absorbed by the skin, essential oils can be carried through the body's blood and lymphatic transport systems to diverse organs, glands, nerves, and soft tissue. In addition to promoting proper body functioning, aromatherapy enhances massage's therapeutic and uplifting benefits because essential oils are so pleasant-smelling. (Religious rites have capitalized on the uplifting nature of aroma by using incense to raise the spirit.) Essential oils are absorbed into the skin within about an hour or two, and their pleasurable effects can often be felt for several hours following aromatherapy massage.

CONTRAINDICATIONS TO AROMATHERAPY MASSAGE

Since aromatherapy uses essential oils in the performance of specific massage techniques, contraindications correspond to the contraindications for the particular bodywork practice with which they are employed. Individuals interested in pursuing aromatherapy massage should check for contraindications in the individual chapters on bodywork.

A word of caution: While essential oils are sometimes taken internally, you should not ingest any oils without a physician's supervision. Essential oils are extremely potent substances. If misused, they can have profound, potentially damaging side effects. (For instance, nutmeg, if taken in large doses, can cause delirium and loss of memory.) Essential oils should always be diluted with a carrier oil before they are applied to the skin. They are potent chemicals that can be irritating if applied directly.

BACKGROUND AND TRAINING OF PRACTITIONERS

Finding a qualified aromatherapist may require some investigation. There is no national license for aromatherapists. Anyone interested in aromatherapy massage should explore the background of therapists to ascertain their credentials in their respective bodywork disciplines as well as specific training in aromatherapy.

FOR FURTHER INFORMATION

For information on essential oils and aromatherapy products, contact:

Aroma Vera
5310 Beethoven Street
Los Angeles, CA 90066
Tel: (800) 669-9514 or (310) 574-6920
Fax: (310) 306-5873
Website: www.aromavera.com
E-mail: cservice@aromavera.com

SUGGESTED FURTHER READING

I am indebted to the following books, which served as the basis for much of the information presented in this chapter:

Marcel Lavabre, *Aromatherapy Workbook* (Rochester, VT: Healing Arts Press, 1990). This book offers a concise easy-to-read introduction to the history and theory of aromatherapy, with practical information on the healing properties of various plants and recipes for blending your own oils.

Robert B. Tisserand, *The Art of Aromatherapy: The Healing and Beautifying Properties of the Essential Oils of Flowers and Herbs* (Rochester, VT: Healing Arts Press, 1977). This is one of the principal works on aromatherapy since it was first published in 1977. It contains a separate chapter on the principles of aromatherapy massage, including do-it-yourself tips.

PART V

ENERGETIC BODYWORK:
HEALING WITH THE HUMAN ENERGY FIELD

Up to the Twentieth Century, reality was everything humans
could touch, smell, see, and hear. Since the initial publication
of the chart of the electromagnetic spectrum, humans have
learned that what they can touch, smell, see, and hear is less
than one-millionth of reality.[1]

—ALBERT EINSTEIN

What is essential is invisible to the naked eye.[2]

—THE LITTLE PRINCE, THE FOX TO THE PRINCE

Energetic bodywork is on the cutting edge of modern thought,
where scientist, mystic, and sage meet. Practices grouped under this
heading have a common goal of influencing a subtle, invisible electromagnetic flow of energy that surrounds and infuses the body
and that is referred to as the human energy field. This life energy is
known variously as ch'i or qi (Chinese), ki (Japanese), prana (Sanskrit),
orgone (Reichian theory), and bioplasm (Soviet research). Energetic
bodywork approaches represent contemporary interpretations and
syntheses of age-old practices that are descended from a variety of

healing traditions, including traditional Chinese medicine, Indian Ayurveda, Tibetan Buddhism, and Western metaphysics. They are complemented by contemporary insights gleaned from quantum physics, the burgeoning field of psychoneuroimmunology (PNI), depth psychology, Western medical practice, and modern consciousness research.

THERAPEUTIC TOUCH (TT) AT A GLANCE

BASIC FACTS

- **Therapeutic Touch (TT) is a healing modality that modulates the energy field which surrounds and penetrates the human body.** Practitioners assess and balance this field to support an individual's own powers for self-healing.

- **TT is a contemporary interpretation of several ancient healing practices.** It was developed collaboratively by Dolores Krieger, Ph.D., R.N., and Dora Kunz, a spiritual healer.

THEORY

- **TT works with the human energy field,** which is an open energy system and is bilaterally symmetric.

- **Disease reflects imbalance in the energy field.** A TT practitioner assesses a receiver's, or healee's, energy field to determine areas of imbalance. (In TT, practitioners often refer to their clients or receivers as healees.) Treatment is directed toward rebalancing the energy field. This enables the client's own recuperative powers to reassert themselves.

- **The process of centering is key to the practice of TT.** During treatment, the practitioner enters a state of stillness where her own inner wisdom connects to that of the client.

TYPICAL SESSION

- **TT treatments typically last twenty to thirty minutes.** The client remains fully dressed in street clothes. Generally, he sits on a stool or straight-backed chair, sideways, so the back is exposed for treatment.

- The practitioner assesses the client's field by feeling for cues given by temperature differences, areas of pressure and tingling, or other sensations perceived through the palms of the hands.

- The practitioner's hands are usually held several inches away from the receiver's body, although the practitioner may sometimes apply gentle touch to the body.

- Fees for a TT session are usually based on a client's ability to pay. In case of need, TT is most frequently offered gratis.

BENEFITS

- TT facilitates healing by mobilizing the patient's own inner healing capabilities.
- TT has been the subject of much scientific research. Studies have shown that TT induces the relaxation response, usually within two to four minutes of the start of treatment. TT alleviates pain, even in some patients for whom medication has proven ineffective. TT can accelerate the healing process.

CONTRAINDICATIONS

- Because TT is gentle and is performed at a slight distance from the body, it has proven to be a very safe form of intervention.
- TT treatments for the elderly, the young, the weak, or individuals with head injuries should be particularly gentle and short.

BACKGROUND AND TRAINING OF PRACTITIONERS

- Dr. Krieger is a research scientist and professor emerita at New York University's Division of Nursing, where she instituted the teaching of TT. TT has since been taught at more than eighty colleges in the United States and in seventy foreign countries.
- Dr. Krieger has focused on teaching fellow nurses and members of the healthcare profession. She estimates that she has taught more than forty-one thousand practitioners herself. A growing number of massage therapists incorporate TT into their practice.
- Dr. Krieger maintains that TT is a natural human potential. It can be learned by anyone demonstrating compassion, dedication, and the intention to heal. The foundational techniques of TT can be taught in one day to groups. Many laypeople have studied TT to use on loved ones.

CHAPTER 12

THERAPEUTIC TOUCH (TT): MODULATING THE HUMAN ENERGY FIELD

Healing is a natural potential that can be actualized under the appropriate circumstances.[1]

—DOLORES KRIEGER, PH.D., R.N.

WHAT IS THERAPEUTIC TOUCH?

Therapeutic Touch (TT) is a contemporary interpretation of several ancient health practices, one of which is the laying on of hands. A practitioner assesses subtle, invisible energy fields that surround and permeate the physical body in order to detect areas of unbalance. She then restores balance by clearing the field and transferring energy to the receiver, or healee. (In TT, practitioners often refer to their clients or receivers as healees. As a massage therapist, I am most comfortable using the terms "client" and "receiver.") The name Therapeutic Touch is in a way misleading: Most often, the practitioner does not even physically touch the receiver's body but instead places her hands several inches away from the body.

Therapeutic Touch was developed collaboratively by Dora Kunz, a noted metaphysician, and Dolores Krieger, Ph.D., R.N., professor emerita of nursing at New York University's prestigious Division of Nursing. A gifted spiritual healer trained by C. W. Leadbeater, a legendary clairvoyant, Dora Kunz studied diverse healers at work to determine what, if any, principles form a common basis for healing. The techniques we now associate with Therapeutic Touch grew from these investigations.

Dolores Krieger is the person most often associated with Therapeutic Touch. With Dora Kunz, she refined this approach to healing and coined the term "Therapeutic Touch." Significantly, as a teacher and researcher at the nation's largest private university, she approached the subjective practice of Therapeutic Touch with the intellectual rigor of a scientist.

THE ORIGINS OF THERAPEUTIC TOUCH

Like many people involved in the healing arts, Dolores Krieger is a seeker. Her quest for spiritual truth led her to study the religions of the world and even, for a time, to live in a monastery.

Dr. Krieger's historical research has revealed that the therapeutic use of the hands for healing dates back at least fifteen thousand years; cave paintings in northern Spain depict its practice. Laying on of hands was prevalent throughout the early Christian era, with both clergy and royalty performing it. In Ireland, St. Patrick healed the blind with his hands while St. Bertrand cured the lame and deaf in France. In the twelfth century, Pope Alexander III banned the clergy from exercising the laying on of hands. Its practice persisted sporadically and furtively, however. In the seventeenth century, Valentine Greatrakes, a well-known Irish landowner and veteran of Oliver Cromwell's army, made a celebrated healing tour of London, curing people of paralysis, deafness, headaches, swelling of tumors, and arthritis.[2]

Dr. Krieger's contribution to study in this field is particularly exciting because her unique background empowered her to analyze the assumptions of ancient healing practices in the light of contemporary developments in the life sciences. As an academically trained health professional, Dr. Krieger subjected the effects of Therapeutic Touch to intellectually rigorous academic research. Her work has proven that Therapeutic Touch will elicit dependable beneficial responses in subjects who are treated with it. Therapeutic Touch was the first healing modality of its kind to be taught within a fully accredited master's degree program.

As a result, Therapeutic Touch serves as a bridge between Western bodywork practices (traditionally based largely on the scientific principles of anatomy and physiology) and more esoteric approaches to energetic bodywork (like Reiki and Polarity Therapy, which are presented in following chapters).

One of the most celebrated healers studied by Kunz and Krieger was a colorful elderly Hungarian military colonel who had retired to Montreal. Oskar Estebany, known simply as Mr. E, came to public attention for his ability to heal both animals and humans through the simple laying on of hands. He first realized his healing ability when he was serving in the Hungarian cavalry and his beloved horse fell ill. Mr. E stayed up all night massaging and caressing it. To everyone's surprise, the horse was well the next day. As Mr. E's reputation spread, he was soon healing scores of humans as well as family pets.

In the 1970s, Mr. E's healing abilities were the subject of scientific curiosity, when they were studied by a seemingly odd collaborator, Dr. Sister M. Justa Smith, a Franciscan nun, biochemist, and enzymologist. In 1974, *Esquire* magazine featured the laboratory experiments that Dr. Sister and Dr. Bernard Grad, a biochemist at McGill University, had performed with Mr. E. The article reported Dr. Grad's original findings—that merely by placing his hands around test materials, Mr. E was able to accelerate the healing time of wounded mice, improve the growth and development of plants that were watered with harmful salt water, and increase the activity of enzymes needed for proper body metabolism. Subsequent studies showed that other healers were able to replicate these results.[3]

THE THEORY UNDERLYING THERAPEUTIC TOUCH

The theory underlying Therapeutic Touch has developed from an impressive array of research findings. At least twenty-two doctoral dissertations on the subject have been formally accepted. Additionally, at least twelve postdoctoral studies have been completed.

Dolores Krieger took the time to explain to me the basic assumptions that are fundamental to Therapeutic Touch. She is a short, rotund woman with a doll-like face and short gray hair. She has a sense of humor, and she exudes compassion, experience, and groundedness, as well as charisma. An individual with eclectic and wide-ranging interests, she represents a synthesis of cultural vantage points. Her choice of clothing reinforces her original style: She was dressed in black ski pants, a tie-dyed printed T-shirt, and moccasins.

TT, as Dr. Krieger affectionately calls her life's work, is a natural human potential. It can be actualized by anyone showing compassion, a focused intention to help others, and the discipline to learn the practice. Of the more than forty-one thousand people she estimates that she has taught in classes, workshops, and professional conferences over the course of her career, she can recall only six individuals who were not able to master TT.

Therapeutic Touch is based on two fundamental principles. The first is that each human being is an open energy system in dynamic interface with the environment. Energy enters this system, circulates throughout, then exits. This principle is founded on the ancient Hindu concept of prana (the vital energy that is the Indian equivalent of ki) and the chakra ("wheel") system. According to the ancient teachings of India, everyone is endowed with a set of seven major chakras, which are nonphysical energy centers. Each chakra is positioned at a strategic, vital area of the human energy field. Chakras take in and transform prana for use by the body. Prana enters the body through the spleen chakra, located where the physical spleen lies, in the upper left quadrant of the abdomen, just beneath the rib cage. It then travels systematically through the remaining chakras in the body, along the way passing through a vast network of interconnecting channels, called nadis (similar in many respects to the meridians of traditional Chinese medicine). Prana leaves the body by traveling through the shoulders, down the arms, then out the center of the palms. The palms are secondary chakras; they make the hands important energy centers that are powerful instruments for healing.

The second principle of TT is that each individual is bilaterally symmetrical, with the right and left sides of the body mirroring each other. Because of this bilateral symmetry, a practitioner can detect imbalances from one side of a client's body to the other based on cues in the energy field. Pinpointing areas of imbalance is fundamental to administering a Therapeutic Touch treatment. TT, like shiatsu, views disease as an imbalance in the human energy system. Each individual has a unique configuration and supply of energy. The energy of ill people is depleted and disorganized while healthy people have excess energy that is better integrated. (Other examples of individuals with excess energy include charismatic personalities, such as actors, performers, and public speakers who, Dr. Krieger observes, often make excellent healers.)

The role of the healer in Therapeutic Touch is to be a vehicle for the transfer of energy to the weak or ill person, thereby being a support mechanism in the healing process. All living organisms have an innate tendency to wholeness and order. In TT, the practitioner works to modulate the subtle flow of energy in the fields that surround and intersect the receiver. In fact, the energy fields of healer and receiver intermesh during treatment, which allows the healer to impact on the receiver. The healer uses her own energy system as a pattern of wholeness to subtly influence the client's system to reorganize itself in a more balanced and unified way.

According to Dr. Krieger, we do not stop at our skins: We are surrounded by subtle, invisible electromagnetic fields of energy that infuse every individual. While the human energy field may sound like scientific hocus-pocus to some, skeptics should be reminded that science accepts the fact that up to 99 percent of the universe exists in an invisible and unknowable fashion (in the form of the dark matter), and speculates that subatomic particles from the Big Bang may be speeding through us even now. The study of energy fields is closely tied to advanced findings in the area of quantum physics and associated with the ideas of such respected scientists as Albert Einstein, Niels Bohr, and Max Planck, the founder of quantum physics. Quantum physics holds that the majority of what we call the universe is actually space rather than matter. Einstein, through his celebrated equation $E = mC^2$, postulated that energy can be transformed to matter and matter to energy. The electromagnetic fields that surround us contain energy that is on the verge of becoming matter.

Challenging the traditional Newtonian view of the world—which described the universe as one gigantic machine operating within a prescribed linear fashion with one cause leading to one effect—the new science views the universe as one interactive dynamic dance of energetic relationships, with all its components "participating" to make the whole. It is alive and ever-changing.[4]

As an analogy, you might consider a television set. We are accustomed to watching the visual images that are displayed on its screen, yet the wavelengths of energy by which the signals are transmitted are invisible to the human eye. They travel through space (in fact, countless radio and TV signals are passing through us at this very moment) and materialize as images or sounds coming from our TV sets. Another model that illustrates the dynamic interplay of energy is the hologram, which is a three-dimensional image created by the intersecting play of waves of energy in the form of light.[5]

Beginning in the 1940s, a Russian photographer, Kirlian, developed a technique for photographing the energy fields surrounding objects. By capturing their emanations on film, he was able to provide pictorial evidence that these fields continue to exist even when the physical material to which they relate is gone. When a leaf was cut in half, for example, his photographs captured the energetic field that continued to surround the *whole* leaf, even though the original form of the leaf was no longer visible to the unaided eye. Other Kirlian photographs have captured emanations of energy from the human body.

I've had several rather startling demonstrations of the existence of these subtle energy fields. Once, I was treating a friend whose left leg had been amputated decades before as a complication of cancer. I held my hands around the empty space of what would have been her leg. I was astonished to find I could feel the energy of her phantom limb pulsating. My friend could also feel a tingling, even though she had no leg. In another instance, I was performing TT on a colleague whose dog was in the room. As I held my hands around my colleague's energy field, her dog jumped up and ran to my hands, slurping away at my palms. In classical mythology, dogs were considered the guides to the underworld. This dog certainly seemed knowledgeable about some unseen world.

THE TYPICAL FORMAT OF A THERAPEUTIC TOUCH TREATMENT

A typical TT treatment lasts from twenty minutes to a half hour. The client remains fully clothed and either sits in a chair or lies on a padded table. During most of a TT session, the practitioner holds her hands two to five inches away from the body. She works with subtle fields of energy that encircle the body. TT deals with human energy, not with the material body. The energy field surrounding the outside of the body is continuous with the energy field inside the body. By balancing and clearing the energy that surrounds the body, the healer enables the client's own natural healing abilities to assert themselves. The physical body responds as well.

The process of performing Therapeutic Touch involves four steps or stages:

Centering In order to help another, the healer must be focused and centered before beginning a Therapeutic Touch session. The practitioner centers in a variety of ways: by breathing slowly, deeply, rhythmically; recalling a peaceful image or feeling; visualizing a tranquil light or symbol; or silently repeating a calming sound. At the same time that the healer centers, the receiver should center, too. The art of centering is important in TT because in order to perceive and understand what is happening in a client's energy field, the healer must enter a state of stillness in which she can listen and be attuned to the receiver. Otherwise, she is distracted by external chatter. Centering helps the healer connect with her own deeper resources, so that her inner wisdom can connect with the inner wisdom of the receiver. Healing occurs at this level, through reaching deeper recesses of the self. The healer's focused intention to help the receiver is the most important factor in this process.

Assessing The second step in Therapeutic Touch is assessing the field of the receiver. The practitioner stands, then generally kneels, in front of the client and rapidly, yet gently and rhythmically, passes her hands, palms toward the receiver, about four to six inches away from the client's body. The practitioner then repeats this pass through the space behind the client's body.

The healer is feeling for any cues of imbalance in the client's energy field. This imbalance can manifest in a number of ways, but most frequently is felt as a variation in temperature (a hot or a cold spot); pressure; pulsation; static buildup; or as a tingling sensation. Some healers may experience the field as colors, sounds, or intuitive hunches about the receiver's emotional state. These sensations differ from practitioner to practitioner and seem to reflect a subtle quality, a feeling-tone of energy that eludes words. Each practitioner may describe the same energy field in a unique way, depending upon her own inner workings, just as some artists are drawn to expressing themselves through music and others through visual images.

The reason the practitioner's hands are positioned off the body in TT is that they are actually able to register more precise information than if they were placed on the body, where they would pick up such distracting interference as the feel of the client's clothing, skin sensations, muscle movements, and other body rhythms. The hands are not held farther than a few inches from the body because the energy field becomes fainter. The assessment is a quick pass through the receiver's energy field, taking generally less than a minute to do. Its purpose is to gain a fast, snapshot understanding of the receiver's energy field.

Unruffling This unscientific yet highly descriptive term describes the effort of the TT practitioner to clear the receiver's energy field. When passing through a client's energy field, the practitioner will have noticed areas of pressure or static buildup, where energy has congested. The purpose of unruffling is to release this blocked energy with a gentle downward motion of the hands, from the top of the client's head to his feet. It is as though the healer were ironing out a wrinkled piece of cloth. Unruffling the field makes the receiver's energy feel free and flowing.

Transferring Energy Once the client's energy field has been cleared, the practitioner transfers energy to him. The assessment will have revealed certain deficient areas in a client's field, places that seemed to want to suck in energy. The practitioner positions her hands near those spots, directing and modulating the flow of energy to them. In addition, the practitioner works according to the law of opposites. Since her intention is to rebalance the receiver's field, she will direct warmth to areas that feel cold, fullness to areas that feel empty.

In transferring energy, the practitioner does not draw upon her own store of energy. Anyone who has ever tried sending energy to others for healing might have found himself exhausted from the effort. This usually results from trying to send personal energy, which can quickly become depleted. The Therapeutic Touch practitioner taps into a greater universal energy, the cosmic source of prana, and directs this energy without using her own personal store. A helpful analogy is the relation of a vacuum cleaner's hose to the vacuum cleaner: The power for doing the cleaning comes from the vacuum itself; the hose is just the vehicle through which it acts to effect its work. In performing Therapeutic Touch, the practitioner is like the hose and the vacuum cleaner is like the universal power source of prana.

In TT, the practitioner does not deplete herself; in fact, she generally becomes vitalized because the energy passing through her gives her an energy boost. Once when preparing for an interview on *Today*, the morning television talk show, Dr. Krieger discovered a line of production crew members forming outside her dressing room. Having heard she was a guest on the program, they were all coming for TT to heal a host of aches and pains. She worked on one after another and, rather than feeling tired, was rejuvenated for her appearance before the cameras.

An important concept to recall is that our energy systems are integrated. The place where the TT practitioner detects a deficit may not correspond precisely with an area where an individual reports pain. The pain may be the result of an energy imbalance elsewhere in the body. The practitioner is intuitively moved to replenish an energy deficit wherever she feels it. The TT practitioner does not attempt to diagnose from a medical point of view what the client's condition is. Instead, she feels for the subtle energy cues. A practitioner can sometimes feel disturbances in the field surrounding the body before they manifest as physical symptoms.

It is difficult to predict how long an energy transfer will take. A practitioner knows when it is time to stop transferring energy—she can tell by the feel of an area that it has taken in all the energy it needs. This may require only a few seconds or perhaps minutes.

Most experts on Therapeutic Touch report—and many other healers acting in a variety of modalities would agree—that both the healer's and the receiver's perception of time during a treatment period differs from their perception of time during ordinary day-to-day reality. Significant changes, which we might think would take a long time to accomplish, can take place in just a few seconds or a few minutes. Additionally, our sense of time changes, so that a session that lasts a half hour may seem to have taken only a few seconds. It is as though we entered into a deep recess of our unconscious where time ceased to have meaning in the way in which we normally perceive it.

These are the elements that form the protocol for a Therapeutic Touch session. These stages are part of a process and do not necessarily need to follow one another in a linear progression, but may occur in a different sequence or simultaneously. A TT treatment is a dynamic interchange; the receiver's energy field is in constant movement, and the practitioner frequently reassesses it to know how best to encourage the free flow of energy.

Some practitioners incorporate other healing modalities, such as shiatsu or guided visualizations, into their work. Many practitioners weave hands-on contact into their work, particularly early in the session, when a gentle back or shoulder rub might help a receiver to relax. In certain cases, a practitioner may refer a receiver to another allied health professional (for instance, in cases where emotional issues are raised, the individual might be referred to counseling).

A typical TT session lasts no longer than a half hour. Often treatment will take only fifteen or twenty minutes. Two practitioners can even work on one client at the same time, synchronizing their work in a rhythmic pattern. This treatment can be even more powerful than a session performed by a solo practitioner.

THE EXPERIENCE: I GET ENERGIZED

It is a cool, damp, crisp, spring afternoon. I arrive at the office of Dr. Janet Macrae, Ph.D., R.N., for a Therapeutic Touch treatment.

Janet, the author of the simple yet sophisticated book *Therapeutic Touch: A Practical Guide*, lives the Therapeutic Touch as a practitioner and teacher of TT and meditation (she is on the faculty of New York University's Division of Nursing). A registered nurse with a Ph.D. in nursing, Janet has studied and practiced Therapeutic Touch since 1976, and its practice has affected her deeply. She also writes about healing and the spiritual quest. Tall and thin, her posture erect, she exudes a firm yet caring, nurturing presence. When I meet her, I am reminded of pictures I've seen of Florence Nightingale, whose writings she has helped to edit.

In preparation for treatment, Janet politely asks me to remove my shoes. "Most people are relieved that's all they have to take off," she jokes, putting me at ease immediately.

She motions me toward a straight-backed wooden chair in the center of her treatment room, an open, airy, well-lighted meditation room situated in the heart of bustling midtown Manhattan. The room is peaceful; no music or outside noise disturbs, except for the faint hum of passing cars occasionally wafting through an open window.

Janet asks me to sit sideways on the chair, so that both my back and abdomen are exposed. "That way I can pass my hands around both your front and your back," she explains.

"The treatment will take only about twenty minutes to thirty minutes," she adds, "which is good because sitting without back support can become uncomfortable. We've experimented with other positions (for instance, with clients lying on the floor) but it just isn't comfortable for the practitioner, and it's hard to reach both front and back of the client's body. If you do become uncomfortable, please feel free to get up, walk around a bit, and stretch."

She then moves behind me and begins to massage my shoulders and back lightly. This helps me to relax and allows our energies to become synchronized. "This is important," Janet tells me, "because some people have such low energy that they start to draw in your energy the moment you start to work with them."

Centered and synchronized, Janet moves to my side and makes passes with her hands—one held in front of my body, the other in back—beginning at my head and progressing down to my feet. Shortly thereafter, she reports her findings: "Your energy in general is full. I feel a slight tightness around your chest and an indentation as the energy comes down to the area of your stomach." Considering that I've been suffering from allergies for the past two days, with congestion in my chest and lungs (which I hadn't mentioned to Janet), her remarks sound on target.

"I'm going to begin with your kidneys." Janet kneels behind me and places her hands gently halfway down my back, at the level of the bottom border of the rib cage, where the kidneys are located. These organs are considered a particularly vital storehouse of energy in TT. I can feel this area filling up with energy, as though Janet were charging my batteries.

She then moves up to my chest area, one hand several inches in front of my chest and the other several inches behind my back. I'm not watching her as she works. My eyes are closed. I could have kept them open, but I prefer to close them in order to aid me in my own centering. I can sense the subtle movements of her hands in my energy field. I can feel the congestion in my chest releasing. I breathe more fully; even my nostrils feel clearer.

As she works, I see a blue wave washing across my mind's eye. I often see this color myself when I'm performing energetic bodywork on clients. I connect it to what is known as the blue of Therapeutic Touch. Colors are in fact emanations of vibrational frequencies whose wavelengths are ranked on the familiar scale of the color spectrum. Certain colors are associated with certain emotional states or vibrations and are used by many healers in their work. In TT, green is considered healing; yellow is considered energizing; and blue is considered to be especially calming and soothing. When all other techniques fail, Therapeutic Touch practitioners visualize sending a deep royal blue light to help their clients heal. Whenever I see this color, I associate it with a deep level of relaxation and a sense of inner balance.

Janet moves down to my solar plexus, one hand on my abdomen, the other on my lower back. She is weaving hands-on with hands-off-the-body touch. My solar plexus feels as though it is expanding. The blue wave feels as though it is sinking, coming down to my abdomen from my chest. I am filling up like a balloon. I feel waves of energy pulsing between Janet's two hands, rhythmically, front and back, through me, like the murmur of a beating heart, growing ever fuller. My energy is radiating out into the cosmos. Am I leaving my body?

As if in response to my unspoken question, Janet moves down to my feet, holding the arch of each foot securely in her hand. She is helping to stabilize my energy. When a TT practitioner works on people, especially in the area of the head, neck, and upper body, it is possible for receivers to become light-headed and dizzy—the energy is literally floating upward, and they may feel as though they are having an out-of-body experience. By holding my feet, Janet is guiding energy into the lower half of my body, making certain I stay fully balanced. I feel a reattachment to the earth, a sense of connectedness. I feel a flow of energy all the way from the tip of my head to my feet. Janet's act of unruffling my field enabled my energy to circulate freely. I feel as though my pelvis is a faucet, with water flowing through the pipe of my legs to the ground at my feet.

Janet holds my feet for what seems a long time. I appreciate this grounding. I'm a very mental person, living much of the time in my head. I allow myself to give up thinking for now and sink into this feeling of flowing into the earth.

As she holds my feet, Janet moves her hands to stimulate various areas of my feet—the arches, the fleshy pads under the balls of my feet. This helps release my upper body. She later explains that she incorporates reflexology in her work, pressing the reflex zones in the feet to help balance the energy in the corresponding organs. This is a good illustration of how many healers today integrate techniques from various modalities in their practice.

Janet rises and passes her hands through my energy field. She lingers to feel the area around my chest and abdomen again. "You feel much fuller, more balanced now," she says. "I don't think you need much more today."

With that she concludes the treatment and suggests I take it easy for a half hour or so. "A lot of people rush out into hectic activity because they feel so vitalized by the treatment. But then they crash. Better to take it slowly."

I appreciate her concern. I do feel energized, balanced. My chest expands fully and I breathe deeply. My nostrils and airways feel clear and dry. They will continue to feel this way for several days afterward, and I will continue to feel increasingly more energized.

"Keep in touch," Janet quips as we part.

THE BENEFITS OF THERAPEUTIC TOUCH

TT has been shown to produce a number of highly reliable effects. First and foremost, it has been shown to induce the relaxation response, which is helpful in alleviating stress-related disorders. Second, TT has been shown to reduce pain. Third, it can accelerate the healing process. In the case of fractured bones, TT can decrease to two and a half weeks from the customary six-week period the time it takes for split bone ends to reunite. Fourth, it can alleviate certain psychosomatic illnesses, such as restlessness, anxiety, and hypertension. No one claims that Therapeutic Touch can cure anyone. Rather, TT practitioners believe that they are helping to clear, stabilize, and shore up the receiver's energy field. They create a window of opportunity for the individual's own self-healing powers to reassert themselves. Any healing that is accomplished is performed by the receiver himself.

Therapeutic Touch is especially recommended for acute conditions, such as infections (like the common cold), wounds, and sprains. It has not proven as effective in chronic conditions or life-threatening diseases, such as cancer. TT is administered to people receiving chemotherapy, both about a week before and then frequently following chemotherapy treatment, to lessen the side effects of nausea and headaches. While it is not so effective in relieving the underlying factors involved in life-threatening illnesses, TT is helpful in inducing the relaxation response and alleviating pain, even where medication has not been effective. It has also assisted the terminally ill to experience a state of calm and serenity that has made their transition to death much more peaceful. In fact, some TT practitioners have developed specialties in helping the dying prepare for transition.

One of Dr. Krieger's first experiments involved observing the effect of Therapeutic Touch on the components of blood, particularly levels of hemoglobin. She reported that subjects who received TT exhibited significant increases in blood hemoglobin levels versus subjects who did not receive Therapeutic Touch.[6] Hemoglobin has the important function of binding oxygen molecules within red blood cells, so that oxygen can be delivered most efficiently to the other cells and tissues in the body that need it. Oxygen is the fuel our bodies use for most of their metabolic reactions. It is essential to the proper functioning of a body in general and specifically to the repair and healing process. Dr. Krieger reasoned that if Therapeutic Touch could increase hemoglobin levels, our systems could deliver more oxygen to our bodies' cells, and this would facilitate more rapid healing. Her experiments proved that Therapeutic Touch does indeed raise hemoglobin levels.

Later studies concluded that within two to four minutes of beginning treatment, Therapeutic Touch induces the relaxation response, as evidenced by a lowering of subjects' voice levels by several decibels; slower and deeper breathing; an audible sign of relaxation (such as involuntary sighing); and a rosy flush to the skin, attesting to an increase in circulation of blood to the extremities of the body.[7] Other studies of hospitalized patients and female college students have shown that Therapeutic Touch reduces anxiety. Additionally, TT can alleviate or eradicate the pain associated with premenstrual syndrome and tension headaches.

No one really knows why Therapeutic Touch works. While Dr. Krieger is the first to admit this, she speculates that it is connected to the concept of prana: There is a vital energy in the air that we take in through the breath. The practitioner taps into this and transfers it during TT. Ashley Montagu, the noted scholar of touch, has speculated that Therapeutic Touch may trigger some complex chemical reactions in the body—with touch receptors on the skin relaying information to the central nervous system, which then causes chemicals to be released that activate other systems in the body.[8]

Some skeptics may argue that Therapeutic Touch works solely through the placebo effect, or the power of suggestion. It is conceivable that an individual who believes he will get better may in fact have a better chance of getting better. For example, have you ever known anyone who has been in terrible pain, made an emergency appointment with a doctor, then arrived at the doctor's office only to discover the pain gone? Visiting someone in the hospital can help them feel better (and for this reason, some argue that we have an obligation to visit the sick).

However, controlled studies have shown that a receiver's belief or lack of belief in Therapeutic Touch has no correlation to the outcome of treatment. Believers in Therapeutic Touch do not respond differently from those who do not believe with one exception: TT does not seem to be effective for those people who are adamantly opposed to treatment. Studies where some nurses merely mimicked the hand movements of TT showed that only those who were actually performing Therapeutic Touch achieved effective results. In a particularly elegant and groundbreaking double-blind controlled study, subjects received wounds to their arms by skin incision. They then put their wounded arms through a partition with a hole cut in it. TT was administered to some of the subjects while others received sham exposure. The study found superior wound healing in an accelerated period of time for those treated with TT versus those who were not.[9] The studies done with Mr. E showed that his healing touch could affect mice, seedlings, and enzymes, which would not have been affected by placebo effects. Additionally, TT has proven effective when used on premature infants and comatose or catatonic subjects. Even paraplegics have reported feeling sensations in the areas around which TT is being performed, even though these people had no sense receptors because the nerves supplying them had been severed. Finally, Dr. Krieger queries, *even if* Therapeutic Touch worked because of the placebo effect, so what? Be grateful that it makes people feel better. "TT is not a miracle cure," she quips. "The miracle is that it works at all."

Dr. Krieger has often expressed her conviction that once you begin to engage in a healing practice, such as TT, your life is changed. This belief is based upon her own experience and that of her students, who over the years have kept journals as part of the process of learning TT. Practitioners of Therapeutic Touch note significant changes in their awareness of themselves and others, often opening up to greater dimensions of spirituality. Their sense of unity with other people, animals, and objects in the world increases; they develop a sense of greater purposefulness; and often their sense of intuition, or telepathy, grows. Dr. Krieger reports that typically people who engage in a healing lifestyle start to feel these shifts happening within two and a half weeks of beginning the practice of Therapeutic Touch. While many other healers reiterate this, Dr.

Krieger has been noteworthy in focusing on this important aspect of healing. Her book *Living the Therapeutic Touch* specifically deals with the changes that healers undergo in their own lives as they begin to engage in a healing lifestyle.

CONTRAINDICATIONS TO THERAPEUTIC TOUCH

Since Therapeutic Touch is performed gently and usually without even touching the body, it has proven to be a safe and effective form of intervention. There are, however, cases when caution should be exercised. Treatments should be gentler and shorter but more frequent for the elderly, young, weak, near-term pregnant women, and individuals with head injuries. Therapeutic Touch should be administered to infants and newborns for only a few minutes at a time. In general, a TT practitioner should underdo rather than overdo. It is possible to overdose from too much TT. Signs of excess energy transfer include irritability, anxiety, restlessness, hostility, and sometimes pain.

BACKGROUND AND TRAINING OF PRACTITIONERS

Of all the therapies presented in this book, Therapeutic Touch is probably one of the most widely studied and practiced today. Because the ability to heal is a natural human potential, anyone can learn to do TT. Its widespread acceptance has largely to do with the untiring enthusiasm of Dr. Krieger. As a nurse-educator, Dr. Krieger has purposely taught her method to the healthcare community, most especially nurses but also doctors, psychiatrists, chiropractors, and dentists, because she feels these professionals are in the best position to impact the greatest number of people in need of TT. A growing number of massage therapists incorporate Therapeutic Touch into their work. Therapeutic Touch has been taught at more than eighty colleges in the United States and in some seventy foreign countries from Austria to Zimbabwe. Dr. Krieger estimates that she has taught Therapeutic Touch to more than forty-one thousand healthcare professionals and that Dora Kunz has taught nearly an equal number of practitioners. Taking into account Dr. Krieger's students—she calls them Krieger's Krazies—who have in turn taught other practitioners, the number of individuals trained in Therapeutic Touch could be as high as a hundred thousand.

The foundational techniques of Therapeutic Touch can be taught in one day (six contact hours) to groups. Laypersons can learn TT for home healing purposes: For instance, expectant parents learn it to ease pain during and after childbirth while senior citizens use it to alleviate the pain of arthritis and other aches and pains. Dr. Krieger encourages the teaching of TT in peer therapeutic groups, where individuals with similar medical problems, such as cancer or AIDS, learn TT to use on one another. This provides the powerful benefits of support and empowerment to those whose lives often seem out of control.

Dr. Krieger is an unflagging spokesperson for Therapeutic Touch. She has made presentations at numerous international scientific conferences, has appeared frequently on television and radio, and has been interviewed regularly by the press. She is particularly proud of having been cover girl for the *American Journal of Nursing.*

FOR FURTHER INFORMATION

Nurse Healers-Professional Associates International, Inc., is the only national group to which Dr. Krieger has given all her original TT materials regarding teaching, clinical practice, and the policies and procedures regarding the use of TT in hospitals and other formal health agencies. If you would like to find out more about Therapeutic Touch or learn the name of a practitioner in your area, contact:

Nurse Healers–Professional Associates International, Inc.
P.O. Box 158
Wanerville, NY 12187-0158
Fax: (509) 693-3537
Website: www.therapeutic-touch.org
E-mail: nhpai@therapeutic-touch.org

Pumpkin Hollow Farm is the only year-round setting where a spectrum of Therapeutic Touch, from beginning classes through advanced practices, is taught:

Pumpkin Hollow Farm
1184 Route 11
Craryville, NY 12521
Tel: (877) 325-3583 or (518) 325-3583
Fax: (518) 325-5633
Website: www.pumpkinhollow.org
E-mail: pumpkin@taconic.net

For information on TT in Canada, contact:

The Therapeutic Touch Network of Ontario
P.O. Box 156, Station U
Etobicoke, Ontario
Canada M8Z 5P1
Tel: (416) 65-TOUCH (658-6824)

Website: www.therapeutictouchnetwk.com
E-mail: cookes4@lks.net

Suggested Further Reading

Dolores Krieger, Ph.D., R.N., *Accepting Your Power to Heal: The Personal Practice of Therapeutic Touch* (Santa Fe, NM: Bear & Co., 1993). In this book, Dr. Krieger lays out the theory and practice of Therapeutic Touch in light of her insights into the mechanism of healing.

_____. *Living the Therapeutic Touch: Healing as a Lifestyle* (New York: Dodd, Mead, 1987). This is a provocative analysis of the personal transformation that individuals begin to experience once they engage in a healing lifestyle.

_____. *The Therapeutic Touch: How to Use Your Hands to Help or to Heal* (New York: Prentice Hall, 1979). This is Dr. Krieger's first groundbreaking introduction to Therapeutic Touch.

Dora Kunz with Dolores Krieger, Ph.D., R.N., *The Spiritual Dimensions of Therapeutic Touch* (Rochester, VT: Bear & Co., 2004). Based on transcribed audiotapes of lectures by medical intuitive Dora Kunz, this book explores the relationship between expanded levels of consciousness and the healing process, and contains healing exercises for common complaints and managing stress.

Janet Macrae, Ph.D., R.N., *Therapeutic Touch: A Practical Guide* (New York: Knopf, 1987). This is a simple, clear, concise introduction on how to do Therapeutic Touch.

CRANIOSACRAL THERAPY AT A GLANCE

BASIC FACTS

- CranioSacral Therapy is a recently developed hands-on approach to healing that applies gentle noninvasive pressure. Its goal is to restore harmony by balancing the craniosacral system.

- Craniosacral osteopathy originated in the early nineteenth century from a branch of the medical practice of osteopathy. Since the 1970s, its practice has grown substantially through the innovative research and teaching efforts of John E. Upledger, D.O., O.M.M., who modified it significantly and called it CranioSacral Therapy.

THEORY

- CranioSacral Therapy is aimed at the craniosacral system. This system is composed of the three-layered meningeal membranes (of which the dura mater is the tough outer waterproof layer) that surround and protect the brain and spinal cord; the clear, colorless cerebrospinal fluid (CSF) that circulates within these membranes; and the structures that control CSF input and outflow.

- The craniosacral rhythm points to areas of abnormality in the body. The CranioSacral Therapist evaluates the rate, symmetry, quality, and amplitude of the craniosacral rhythm to detect areas of holding in the body.

- A practitioner uses the bones and soft tissue of the skull and pelvis as handles to release areas of tension. This permits the inner wisdom of the client to self-correct imbalances and leads to improved functioning of the body.

TYPICAL SESSION

- A typical CranioSacral treatment lasts forty-five minutes to an hour. The client remains fully clothed and lies on a comfortable padded table.

- The practitioner begins a session by palpating the craniosacral rhythm to determine areas of restriction. He then applies gentle touch with the fingers, palm, or whole hand to restricted areas or to areas of maximum motion to facilitate release. The pressure used is very light—only 5 grams (the weight of a nickel).

- Expect to pay $40 to $150 per treatment, depending on the credentials of the therapist.

BENEFITS

- **CranioSacral Therapy is used to alleviate pain and stress.** It is especially effective in treating problems related to the head, such as chronic and migraine headaches; TMJ disorder; sinus problems; dizziness; tinnitus; eye strain and vision problems; Bell's palsy; and insomnia.

- **CranioSacral Therapy has proven effective in dealing with problems related to brain and spinal cord injury.** Examples include cerebral palsy and other forms of paralysis, nervous disorders, chronic back pain, and even some cases of depression.

- **CranioSacral Therapy is used widely with children.** It has proven helpful in treating the hyperactive, dyslexic, and learning disabled.

CONTRAINDICATIONS

- Because CranioSacral Therapy is gentle and nonintrusive, there is little danger of adverse reaction.

- Since it affects the pressure of the fluid in the brain, its use is contraindicated in recent acute conditions of stroke, cerebral aneurysm, brain stem tumor, head injury, or bleeding within the head.

- In treatments for infants, be sure to find a highly trained practitioner: An infant's craniosacral system is much more delicate than an adult's.

BACKGROUND AND TRAINING OF PRACTITIONERS

The Upledger Institute is the most comprehensive source of training. It offers a series of courses and programs in CranioSacral Therapy. Its graduates are generally credentialed in a related healthcare profession. They include massage therapists, osteopaths, chiropractors, physical and occupational therapists, M.D.s, dentists, and psychotherapists, among others.

- The Upledger Institute has trained tens of thousands of healthcare professionals in CranioSacral Therapy.

CHAPTER 13

CRANIOSACRAL THERAPY: THE SKULL SPEAKS

My belief is that somewhere inside of you is the answer to every question that can be asked about you. My concern, as your health care practitioner, is that we make a connection with that part of you that knows the answers, and that those answers be shared with us and used for the good of the total you.[1]

—JOHN E. UPLEDGER, D.O., O.M.M.

WHAT IS CRANIOSACRAL THERAPY?

CranioSacral Therapy is a recently developed hands-on approach to healing that applies gentle, noninvasive pressure to balance what is known as the craniosacral system. This system extends from the skull, face, and mouth (the cranium) down and within the spinal column to the sacrum and coccyx, the bones that form the tail end of the spine. At the center of this network is a system of cerebrospinal fluid (CSF), which circulates throughout the system within an envelope of meninges, bathing, nourishing, and protecting the brain, the spinal cord, and the nerve roots. CSF is constantly being made from, and reabsorbed into, the blood supply. It is enclosed in a watertight, semiclosed hydraulic system formed by the connective tissue lining the skull, spinal column, and sacrum. Practitioners of CranioSacral Therapy maintain that by working with the rhythm and flow of CSF through the bones and soft tissue that encase it, they can provide relief for a variety of acute and chronic neuromuscular and musculoskeletal complaints.

THE ORIGINS OF CRANIOSACRAL THERAPY

CranioSacral Therapy evolved from a branch of medical science known as osteopathy. The individual who has done the most to foster the study of this method and develop it into a widely practiced healing modality is John E. Upledger, D.O., O.M.M. An osteopath, he founded the Upledger Institute, an educational and clinical research center located in Palm Beach Gardens, Florida.

Osteopathy was founded in the nineteenth century by Andrew Taylor Still, M.D. Dr. Still, who was a Civil War surgeon and country doctor in Missouri, became disillusioned with orthodox medicine when his three children died during a meningitis epidemic in 1864. Rebelling against the unsanitary surgical conditions of his time, as well as the crude pharmaceutical remedies available, Dr. Still developed osteopathy. His approach to healing eschewed surgery and drugs except as a last resort. He relied primarily on body manipulation, advice on lifestyle, and exercises. (The word "osteopathy" is in fact a misnomer. Literally, it means "bone disease," and Dr. Still's system addressed the entire structure of the body, not just bones.)

In its early days, osteopathy was rejected by the orthodox medical establishment as quackery. Osteopathy has evolved from Dr. Still's original ideas; today, it is widely accepted as a legitimate medical discipline. Osteopaths undergo a seven-year training program (not unlike doctors) and are licensed to practice in all fifty states. They are designated by the initials "D.O." (doctor of osteopathy) after their name, and have many of the privileges associated with medical doctors.

In the 1900s, William G. Sutherland, a pioneering osteopath, began to explore the bones of the skull. He designed a helmetlike device (especially constructed to exert controlled and varied pressure on different cranial bones), which he wore around his head. Dr. Sutherland recorded the effects he felt as a result of the pressure on different parts of his head. These included motor dysfunction, depression, and various mood changes. Because of his concern for the skeptical reaction of the medical establishment to his work, Dr. Sutherland published his first research articles under the pseudonym "Blunt Bone Bill." He summarized the results of his research in 1939 in a book entitled *The Cranial Bowl*. (His wife also noted her husband's strange behavior during this period and recorded her views of his experiments in a book of her own.) From his research, Dr. Sutherland developed a subspecialty of osteopathy called cranial osteopathy, based on the manipulation of the cranial bones.

Cranial osteopathy was generally ignored by the medical establishment at large, and even by other osteopaths, until the 1970s. (In fact, currently only a small number of osteopaths follow Dr. Sutherland's principles.) At that time,

Dr. Upledger had a transformative revelation, the kind of "Aha" experience that spurs scientists to breakthrough discoveries. In 1970, as a young osteopathic surgeon freshly out of medical school, he was assisting a neurosurgeon during an operation on a patient's spinal cord. It was Dr. Upledger's function to hold back the flap of the thick connective tissue membrane that surrounds the spinal cord so that the neurosurgeon could remove a layer of deposit below it. To Dr. Upledger's amazement, he couldn't hold the membrane still. The tissue continued to pulsate rhythmically, at a rate independent of the patient's heart rate or breathing. Awestruck by his experience, Upledger set out to investigate cranial osteopathy.

In 1975, Upledger was invited to join Michigan State University's (MSU) College of Osteopathy as a professor of biomechanics. He formed part of a multidisciplinary research team investigating what he later named the craniosacral system—either to prove its existence once and for all or to debunk the myths surrounding it. Examining fresh laboratory specimens (rather than dried ones whose bones had hardened), this team proved that the tissue between the bones in the head is alive and moving. They were further able to quantify the rhythm of the craniosacral system and demonstrate that it could be used to evaluate and treat a variety of health problems.

While at MSU, Dr. Upledger participated in a number of research experiments, some of them sponsored by the Michigan Board of Education and the National Institute for Mental Health, designed to analyze and evaluate the craniosacral system. Among his landmark findings was a close correlation between children with motor coordination and developmental problems (those classified by such designations as "hyperactive," "not normal," "behavioral problems," and "learning disabled" by school authorities) and restrictions in the movement of the craniosacral system.[2] Dr. Upledger realized that CranioSacral Therapy had tremendous potential to help such children as well as others suffering from such diverse complaints as headaches and cerebral palsy. (At the time of these studies, one out of every twenty children in Michigan suffered from some form of neurological dysfunction.) Unfortunately, there were only three osteopaths trained in his brand of CranioSacral Therapy in the entire state of Michigan. So Dr. Upledger began to teach CranioSacral Therapy to nonphysicians, such as physical therapists and nurses, in the Michigan area under the auspices of the Meninger Foundation. Dr. Upledger found himself running up against the orthodox medical establishment, which considered him a heretic for teaching his techniques to nonphysicians and, later on, to parents of brain dysfunctioning children. In 1985, Dr. Upledger established his own teaching institute and nonprofit foundation in Florida to provide CranioSacral Therapy to those in need.

THE THEORY UNDERLYING CRANIOSACRAL THERAPY

CranioSacral Therapy is new because until recently very little was known about the craniosacral system. The key elements that comprise this system are the three-layered meningeal membranes that line the bones of the head, spinal column, and sacrum; the cerebrospinal fluid (CSF) that circulates within these membranes; and the structures that control CSF input and outflow. The outermost meningeal membrane, which is formed of tough connective tissue, is called the dura mater ("tough mother") and is an impermeable membrane that protects the brain and spinal cord and contains the CSF within a closed system. The portion of the dura mater that encases the spinal cord is called the dural tube. The whole craniosacral system resembles a tadpole in shape, with the cranium being the head of the tadpole, the spinal column the long skinny body, and the sacrum the tail.

CSF is a clear, colorless liquid that normally contains no red or white blood cells. It has a watery consistency, which is thinner than blood plasma. CSF is extracted from fluid in the blood through a network of capillary beds, called choroid plexuses, that are located in the ventricles, or cavities, in the brain. CSF acts as a shock absorber for the brain and spinal cord, bathing them in a protective liquid that also permits the brain to "float" (the brain has so little tensile strength that it would probably collapse unless supported in this way). CSF is formed in the brain, flows down the back of the spinal column to the sacrum, then upward in front of the spinal column to the head, where it drains back into the bloodstream via a network of veins. The average person has 125 milliliters (about 4 ounces) of CSF in circulation at any given moment. There is a complete turnover of CSF about six times per day, so that a total of about 800 milliliters of CSF is formed and reabsorbed into the bloodstream during a twenty four-hour period. While the amount of CSF circulating at any given moment may seem small, anyone who has had a spinal tap in which even a little CSF fluid has seeped out of this closed system knows the excruciating pain that can result from a disruption to this delicate system.

The craniosacral system pulsates with a unique rhythm created by expansion and contraction of CSF fluid volume. Dr. Upledger has theorized that this system is a semiclosed hydraulic system: When the volume of CSF created exceeds the amount that is reabsorbed, this causes fluid pressure to build up within the system, causing expansion. When the pressure reaches its high level, fluid production shuts off and pressure is relieved as the CSF is absorbed and the system contracts. When pressure reaches a low point, production resumes and once again pressure begins to build up and the system expands. The movement of expansion and contraction produces a distinct rhythm in the body, which CranioSacral Therapists can palpate. Called the craniosacral rhythm, this pulse serves as a basic evaluative tool in determining proper functioning of the system.

A key assumption in CranioSacral Therapy is that the pulsating rhythm of CSF causes the bones of the skull to move in accommodation of the changing CSF pressure and volume within the system. Because this impacts the brain and central nervous system, the accommodation or lack thereof of these bones has far-reaching effects. Movement restrictions of any part of the craniosacral system can result in dysfunction at virtually any place in the body. The bones of the head can and often do retain the impact of the traumas an individual has experienced, both sharp and subtle, not infrequently as far back as injuries sustained in utero or during the birth process. (For instance, the use of forceps during delivery can have a seriously traumatic effect on the bones of the head.) This can lead to restriction in movement of the cranial bones.

While these concepts may seem noncontroversial, indeed simplistic, this theory was considered heresy by the orthodox medical establishment until recently. That's because anatomy as taught in the United States, based on British anatomical tradition, had always maintained that the bones of the skull are immovable. Most of us are probably not even aware of all the bones we have in our skull. Anyone who feels his head is likely to feel what seems to be just one big oval-shaped hard bone, and a casual glance at the skulls of skeletons would seem to confirm this. Actually, however, there are eight different cranial bones (plus three small bones in each of our ears). Anyone who has felt what is called the fontanel, or soft spot, on the head of an infant knows how pliable it is. That's because at birth an infant's skull bones are not completely formed. This permits its head the resilience to be compressed through the birth canal without being crushed. Slowly, over time, the soft tissue in the head calcifies into bones that are joined by a type of joint known as a suture, which is formed of connective tissue. The word "suture" means "seam" and is related to the act of stitching. Some sutures even look like stitches: They interlock the bones of the head in a zigzag formation that resembles a zipper.

Traditional medicine looked at the cranial bones of dead bodies—in whom the sutures had hardened—and assumed that the bones were immovable. Upledger and others, however, examined live humans and other primates and demonstrated that the sutures are living connective tissue that allow a slight degree of flexibility among the bones of the head. The discipline of CranioSacral Therapy required this initial finding. (By the way, anatomists of other countries, such as Italy and Israel, have long taught that cranial bones are movable.)

Through assessing the rhythm and flow of CSF, the CranioSacral Therapist is able to identify areas of restriction and holding in the bones of the skull and vertebral column. Through gentle manipulation, he is able to release areas of constriction, thereby restoring homeostatic functioning to the craniosacral system.

THE TYPICAL FORMAT OF A CRANIOSACRAL THERAPY SESSION

Robert Harris, trained as an instructor of CranioSacral Therapy at the Upledger Institute, explains the format of a typical CranioSacral Therapy session. Like many practitioners of CranioSacral Therapy, he is also a massage therapist: His training in hands-on skills makes him particularly sensitive to working with the craniosacral rhythm. As a registered massage therapist in Ontario, Canada, he has undergone an especially rigorous training of 2,200 classroom hours. With his wife, Alix McLaughlin, Robert operates a clinic in Ontario where he has provided CranioSacral Therapy to such celebrities as Steve Podorski, the world-cup downhill ski champ, stars of the National Ballet of Canada, and the heads of some of the world's largest multinational corporations. He and Alix were first attracted to CranioSacral Therapy when his wife underwent knee surgery. After receiving little help in recovery from traditional physical therapy, she obtained dramatic and significant results from a single CranioSacral treatment.

A typical CranioSacral session lasts forty-five minutes to an hour. The client lies fully clothed on a comfortable padded table, sometimes further cushioned by an inflatable air mattress. No oil or lotion is used.

The CranioSacral Therapist begins a session by assessing the rate, symmetry, quality, and amplitude of the craniosacral rhythm in order to evaluate any areas of abnormality or holding in the body. He carefully palpates the rhythm at any of a variety of "listening" stations—the head, feet, knees, hips, virtually anywhere on the client's body. Robert notes that palpation, often equated with the vague word "touch," has a specific connotation in CranioSacral Therapy. The touch used in CranioSacral Therapy is as gentle and light as a caress. But exactly how light is that? Generally, a therapist applies no more than 5 grams of pressure wherever he is working. A nickel weighs approximately 5 grams (so you might picture placing a nickel on your forehead)—that is approximately the amount of force used in CranioSacral touch. (If you are skeptical that such light weight can affect the body, consider how even the slightest of breezes can send ripples across a vast body of water as far as the eye can see. This analogy is not random: Two-thirds of our body is water.)

The therapist measures the craniosacral rhythm in cycles, with each cycle consisting of one complete contraction followed by one complete expansion of CSF within the craniosacral system. On average, this rhythm consists of six to twelve cycles per minute. A rhythm either faster or slower than this points to a potential imbalance in the craniosacral system. Hyperactive children and individuals suffering acute illnesses with high fever have, for example, characteristically rapid craniosacral rhythms while brain-damaged patients may have slow rhythms.[3]

The craniosacral pulse is akin to, but different from, the pulses caused by the heart beating and the lungs breathing. While the craniosacral pulse can be felt at any point on the body, it is palpated most commonly at the head or sacrum, where it is particularly pronounced. When first beginning to palpate, the therapist is noninvasive, just making contact with the client to become acquainted with the nature of her particular craniosacral system. The therapist's eyes are often closed so that he can focus on what his hands are experiencing. He engages in a quiet, nonintrusive melding with the patient, using his hands as exquisite listening devices. Laced with more sensory receptors than almost any other body part, the hands act as amplifiers of what they are feeling. "Patients can tell you anything they want about their symptoms but their bodies don't lie," Robert counsels. "In some cases, you can even pick up disturbances in the body, such as headaches, that are not revealed to even the most sophisticated of magnetic resonance imaging [MRI] equipment." In an evocative analogy, Dr. Upledger compares the hands in this attitude of listening to a dry sponge resting in a pool of water, waiting to absorb information about the client.[4]

CranioSacral Therapy focuses largely on the fascia, or soft connective tissue, that is attached to the bones that form the craniosacral system and that extends throughout the body. When the fascia becomes distorted, it pulls on the skin, muscles, connective tissue, and bones beneath it, causing pain and discomfort. (There are certain places in the body where the fascia is more likely to become twisted: areas where longitudinal fibers of fascia cross vertical fibers. This occurs in places like the chest, where constrictions can inhibit full, deep breathing, and at joints, giving way to such problems as shoulder pain.)

Once the therapist has assessed the craniosacral pulse, he proceeds to release various parts of the body, from the feet to the head. Like releasing a snag in a sock, if a therapist unwinds or unlatches distorted fascia, underlying body tension will be relieved. A successful release is signaled by a softening and relaxation of the contracted tissue and restoration of normal function.

Like Rolfing, which also developed from osteopathy, CranioSacral Therapy emphasizes the important role of fascia and focuses on realigning lines of pull within this network of connective tissue. However, CranioSacral Therapists achieve this through delicate, noninvasive touch while Rolfers generally manipulate the muscles and connective tissue that form the fascia much more deeply. Like chiropractic, CranioSacral Therapy seeks to release restrictions in the spinal column. CranioSacral Therapists achieve this by freeing the fascia and dura mater that surround the craniosacral system rather than by adjusting the bones of the vertebrae as do chiropractors.

A distinguishing characteristic of CranioSacral Therapy is the gentleness of the approach. A manipulation in CranioSacral Therapy is more an invitation to the body to relax than an aggressive movement. If the therapist's pressure is too hard, treatment becomes a contest between the practitioner and the client's tissue, which guards against the intrusion. In this case, neither therapist nor client wins.

CranioSacral releases may take seconds to minutes to complete. They are necessary in order to relax the body for more active work. Following these releases, the therapist applies gentle, nonintrusive pressure to coax the soft tissue covering the bones in the craniosacral system to relax and separate. In performing these manipulations, he uses the bones of the skull, neck, vertebrae, and base of the spine as handles to evaluate and effect change in the circulation of CSF and thereby release soft tissue. These gentle movements reestablish a strong, healthy craniosacral rhythm, which in turn assists the body to self-correct for optimal functioning.

CranioSacral Therapy also uses techniques to achieve still points, which are defined as periods of time when the craniosacral pulse ceases altogether. This is a powerful technique used in enabling the craniosacral rhythm to reestablish itself. It also helps our autonomic nervous system to enter the parasympathetic, or relaxation, mode. Quite frequently during CranioSacral treatment a client will experience what is known as a therapeutic pulse—a sensation of strong pulsation that is an indication that a powerful healing mechanism is at work. While a client is experiencing a therapeutic pulse, the therapist always remains still in order to allow natural healing to occur.

CranioSacral practitioners sometimes incorporate a technique called the V spread, initially developed by Dr. Sutherland. The practitioner holds his hands on either side of a restriction and aims energy toward that restriction through his intention to send energy in whatever way is most healing for the patient. The V spread resembles techniques used for transferring energy used in other types of energetic bodywork, such as Therapeutic Touch.

THE EXPERIENCE: MY SKULL SPEAKS

I arrive at the offices of Ken Frey, a physical therapist, to experience CranioSacral Therapy firsthand. Ken's office forms an adjunct to a health club.

I obtained Ken's name and background, along with references to a number of other practitioners in my area, from the Upledger Institute. Ken is a physical therapist who has not only taken a number of courses at the Upledger Institute, but has also assisted in its training program. After contacting several CranioSacral practitioners, I selected Ken because of favorable referrals from other practitioners, his breadth of experience, and the positive reaction I had toward him during our exploratory phone conversations. I had to plan my appointment several weeks in advance: Because Ken has a strong reputation, the demand for his work is great and he has a long waiting list.

At the time I visited Ken, my primary-care physician had recently diagnosed me as suffering from fibromyositis. Fibromyositis is doctorese for inflammation of muscle and the fibrous connective tissue attaching to it. In laymen's terms, it means stiff, tender, painful muscles. In my particular case, it means the nagging pain I get in my back, on the right hand side right below the shoulder blade, the kind I get from sitting hunched over a desk writing all day or stooping hunched over a massage table. You may get it by sitting at a desk in an office or hunching over a computer terminal. It involves those tender areas of tension that one of my colleagues unscientifically yet evocatively calls "crunchies," that, by the end of the workday, you wish you could break up with a sledgehammer.

I enter Ken's office and meet him for the first time. He is young and robust and exudes energy and concern. Observing us today is Debbie, a student who is completing her training in physical therapy and who is eager to find out what CranioSacral Therapy is about. I am lucky to have her present because I get double the attention; in addition, I learn not only from Ken's hands, but also from his verbal explanations directed to Debbie.

Ken asks me some preliminary questions, taking a brief medical history to explore my complaint, as well as gather other pertinent medical information. Ken asks me how long I've experienced my pain, and I realize probably all my life, at least as long as I can remember.

The preliminaries over, Ken begins the bodywork. I lie fully clothed on my back, on a comfortable padded massage table. Ken positions himself at my feet, his hands placed over the tops of my ankles. He is "listening" for my craniosacral pulse. "You have a beautiful pulse," he tells me. "The rate is good. It is even, nice and full, and the expansion is fuller than the contraction."

Then he reports, "There seems to be some restriction in the right hip." On the surface, this seems surprising, because I'd told Ken that not too long ago I'd had surgery to repair a hernia in my left groin, and you might suspect that would be the side of the restriction. But Ken is interested in finding the ultimate cause of my imbalance, not just the symptoms. He feels that because of the restriction in the right hip, my left side has had to work extra hard.

Ken is like a detective. "The chase is on!" he exclaims. The chase he is referring to is actually a subtle listening to my body as it directs his hands to its most deep-seated areas of restriction so that his hands may guide them to release.

Ken moves to my head and positions his hands under the base of my skull to feel the pulse there. I try to experience this rhythm along with him. I feel like I have just stepped into the ocean, in between waves, and am waiting to catch the crest of the next wave that's coming. That is my clue to the movement of the craniosacral rhythm. I feel my skull expand and contract in measured beat. The contraction feels almost like my brain and skull are sinking in on themselves— I picture a walnut with its shell collapsing onto the nut within.

"You've received some fine bodywork," Ken reports. "I can feel the traces of some very fine signatures in your body. Your energy is very clear and easy to work with." Ah, yes, the "signatures." Each practitioner who works on a body leaves a kind of imprint of his energy, like a painter who signs his painting. And because the body is an energetic field, it retains that imprint, almost like the traces of light found on a photographic negative or the fingerprint that a discerning detective uncovers.

"You're very easy to work with because your body possesses the ability to respond to deep work as well as to light energetic work." Yes, this is something I have been realizing myself; this is why I am in a unique position to write this book—because I can respond to the full spectrum of bodywork, from deep tissue work to gentle energetic work.

"Many people cannot be sensitive across the full range of bodywork. For instance, Rolfing would be agonizing pain to some people, who would armor themselves and not respond to treatment. On the other hand, some people are not capable of responding to the gentle cues of more subtle energy work."

Ken begins to appraise my body, tracking the trail of imbalance from one area to another. The holding in my right hip resulted in overtaxing my left hip. The holding in my right side seems to come from a lack of mobility in my viscera, the liver and gall bladder in particular. Because of this lack of mobility, a couple of my midribs are compressed, inhibiting breathing on my right side; this imbalance is caught in the fascia, which is twisted and distorted all the way up through my body so that it pulls and holds my neck bent over to the left in compensation. "Many practitioners might have seen the imbalance in your neck and worked on that," Ken adds, "but that's not the source of the problem."

Ken believes that the soreness in my shoulder is also related to the lack of mobility in the fascia surrounding or attached to my visceral organs. To remedy this, he releases those structures associated with the liver and gall bladder by placing his hands lightly under my low back and rib cage, exploring for areas of tension and holding. I feel a dull ache. "This may hurt a little," he warns me. "The liver is frequently associated with anger, so if you get angry, please don't blame me." He's preparing me for the fact that the physical release may be accompanied by a psychological release in the form of an emotional outburst.

I am familiar with anger. I've spent a lifetime holding it in, so it's unlikely I'll break into a string of expletives right now. I've also learned that we can experience deep inner changes without necessarily having to act them out in ways that are observable in the external world. I can feel the profound impact Ken's releasing is having on me, and I feel freer. In addition to moving slightly with the restriction to release it, Ken is transmitting energy to the area through his intention to help and to heal. As the restriction passes, I feel for an instant as though I've passed a stool. Not that I have physically, but as though there has been the sweet kind of release that comes from passage from an area of greater restriction to wide openness. I breathe more deeply. I can feel my neck beginning to unhitch itself from its locked position. I can feel it more evenly centered above my torso.

Having released the fascia associated with the area of my liver and gall bladder, Ken moves to release the restriction in my ribs, which have become compressed. His releases consist of holding his hands, lightly, one in front of me, one in back, while at first I lie on my back, then sit up, gently supported by him. As he releases my ribs, my breathing opens up even more. I feel as though Ken has taken a broom and swept out all the cobwebs and dust that have accumulated in my chest and lungs over the years. My lungs are becoming open and free, pristine and clean. I also have flashbacks to early traumas: Several times as a child I fell while racing about the yard, landing flat on my back, my breath knocked out of me. Yes, I remember whacking those ribs that are meshed together now. Somehow in the stillness and clarity of this moment of knowing, my body remembers the position it was in when I experienced those traumas. They involved hurt, sadness, and pain in addition to physical shock. I can understand how the restrictions began. And knowing this, I am free to let them go, slowly, in an atmosphere of trust.

As I am thinking this, Ken says to Debbie, "There has been a lot of holding in here. We're undoing some of it. There's still more to do, but Thomas can feel it. There's an emotional component here, too. Thomas knows this and knows what has to be done." Yes, within the memories deep in the tissues of my body, Ken's inner physician is consulting with my inner physician, and both somehow know, in a way that surpasses conscious understanding, what needs to be done.

As my chest is released, I can feel my shoulder opening up, too. Ken thinks only so much can be done in one day. He also knows that whatever restrictions exist in my body have been built up over years, and gentle unwinding over time is better than an aggressive, invasive approach to treatment.

Ken completes the session by returning to my head and creating a still point, which provides a final therapeutic release to the session. A CranioSacral Therapy session nearly always ends with a still point, a final gesture designed to appease the inner gods and make right whatever may have been left undone during the session.

I sit up, refreshed and invigorated. The pain that was in my right shoulder seems much less pronounced now. I breathe freely, deeply, ready to meet the day. In addition to a deep sense of calm and relaxation, I feel energetic, alive, vibrant.

THE BENEFITS OF CRANIOSACRAL THERAPY

CranioSacral Therapy aims to facilitate one's own self-healing process. Dr. Upledger believes that we each have an inner physician who has the answer to any question we might ever ask. The role of a CranioSacral Therapist is to ease making the connection with that inner physician or inner self. The patient "knows a lot more about how to fix herself than I do. So I'm here to help her, not to decide what needs to be done," Dr. Upledger explains.

CranioSacral Therapy has achieved promising success with a variety of ailments throughout the body. It may seem hard to believe that such gentle work on the head, neck, and torso can impact the entire body. It can, though, because these body parts contain and protect the all-important central nervous system, which is responsible for receiving sensory input, registering pain, and effecting movement throughout the whole body. It also houses the autonomic nervous system, which controls involuntary functions, such as digestion and respiration, as well as the glands of the endocrine system. Because they release hormones into the bloodstream, the endocrine glands have a system-wide effect on the whole body. Nerve roots exit the spinal column between the vertebrae. Any pressure on the spinal nerve roots can cause tension throughout the body. Additionally, fascia forms one continuous web in the body: A distortion in the fascia attaching to the bones of the craniosacral system could pull fascia, and hence muscles, bones, and neural structures, out of alignment to the rest of the body.

The fact that CranioSacral Therapy applies gentle pressure is seen as facilitating release. More aggressive pressure would cause the soft tissue of the body to armor itself against invasive touch and that would cause more tightening. The light pressure coaxes the body gently, patiently, to relinquish any holding in a safe embrace. CranioSacral Therapy is performed with the client fully clothed, in part because the absence of direct skin-to-skin contact lessens the amount of guarding.

Proponents believe that CranioSacral Therapy can be used to alleviate pain and stress; calm down the autonomic nervous system; lower high blood pressure and fever; remove transient and minor restrictions; improve fluid exchange and blood flow; lengthen the spine; and promote general relaxation.

CranioSacral Therapy has proven particularly effective in relieving complaints related to the head—chronic and migraine headaches (Dr. Upledger reports an 80 to 90 percent success rate in treating headache conditions), sinus problems, whiplash, torticollis (stiff neck, or wryneck), dizziness, tinnitus, eye strain and vision problems (such as lazy and crossed eyes), Bell's palsy (facial paralysis), and even insomnia. Because it has proven particularly helpful in relieving TMJ disorder, a growing number of dentists incorporate CranioSacral Therapy into their work. CranioSacral Therapy has proven helpful in treatment of some cases of endogenous depression (a type of depression not attributable to any known cause), where such depression results from overlapping and constriction of cranial bones.

In many of Dr. Upledger's early studies, performed on elementary school-children, CranioSacral Therapy was shown to help slow, hyperactive, dyslexic, spastic, and cerebral palsied children. Robert Harris, whose practice includes a large number of children, has reported instances of success in helping dyslexic children achieve better grades in school after only four or five CranioSacral treatments. Sharon Weiselfish, a physical therapist, has incorporated CranioSacral Therapy into her treatment of paralyzed children. She has reported a 100 percent success rate in treating children with Erb's palsy (a paralysis of the arm often sustained in breeched births and once considered incurable) using CranioSacral Therapy in conjunction with manual and neurodevelopmental therapies.[5] She has also reported success in treating children with cerebral palsy using cranial with neurodevelopmental therapy.[6] Studies performed in hospitals in Canada have shown that newborns treated with CranioSacral Therapy within the first few days of life die less frequently from sudden infant death syndrome (SIDS) and have fewer respiratory problems.

CranioSacral Therapy is also helpful for problems related to chronic back pain, especially in cases such as ruptured disks, where abnormal tension is exerted upon the dura mater. Dr. Upledger maintains that 50 percent of brain dysfunction problems could be helped by CranioSacral Therapy. CranioSacral Therapy has also provided relief for people with paralysis, cerebral seizures, and other spinal cord and nervous disorders where no other treatment has helped. In fact, the Brain and Spinal Cord Dysfunction Center at the Upledger Institute is dedicated to treating individuals with these conditions.

Other problem areas that CranioSacral Therapy helps are acute systemic infectious conditions; localized infections resulting from sprains, strains, bumps, and bruises; chronic pain syndrome; arthritis; emotional disorders; and scoliosis.

CONTRAINDICATIONS TO CRANIOSACRAL THERAPY

CranioSacral Therapy involves very gentle movement, so there is little danger of an adverse reaction. Because it affects the pressure within the cranium, however, it is clearly contraindicated in the case of recent, acute conditions of stroke, cerebral aneurysm, brain stem tumor, head injury, or bleeding within the head. You should wait at least two weeks after these occurrences before seeking CranioSacral Therapy and obtain a physician's note authorizing treatment. On the other hand, CranioSacral Therapy can benefit people suffering from what are known as transient ischemic attacks (TIAs), or ministrokes. Individuals who are on medication for such disorders as high blood pressure may wish to consult with their doctors after several weeks of treatment: Cranio-Sacral Therapy can bring blood pressure down to the point where less medication might be required. CranioSacral Therapy is safe for infants and children, but treatment should be performed by a very experienced practitioner due to the delicacy of an infant's system.

BACKGROUND AND TRAINING OF PRACTITIONERS

Dr. Upledger has done much to expand the accessibility of CranioSacral Therapy. The Upledger Institute seeks to train practitioners who are already licensed in other healthcare disciplines. It views CranioSacral Therapy as a postgraduate discipline and assumes a thorough knowledge of anatomy and physiology among the practitioners who attend its trainings.

The Upledger Institute offers a progressive series of advanced workshops and certification programs at convenient sites throughout the world. Those who have attended its courses include osteopathic physicians, allopathic physicians, doctors of chiropractic, doctors of Oriental medicine, naturopathic physicians, nurses, psychiatric specialists, psychologists, dentists, massage therapists, physical therapists, occupational therapists, speech and language pathologists, acupuncturists, and other professional bodyworkers. Dentists find CranioSacral Therapy particularly effective in treating TMJ disorder, which has reached epidemic proportions in the United States. Interestingly enough, in the state of Colorado, dentists had to sue in court for the right to incorporate CranioSacral Therapy into their practice: The orthodox medical establishment did not believe that dentists should be manipulating cranial and sacral bones. The dentists proved their point and won the suit. In other states, some dentists have sought additional accreditation as licensed massage therapists to gain the right to practice CranioSacral Therapy on their patients.

FOR FURTHER INFORMATION

The Upledger Institute is the most comprehensive source of information on

CranioSacral Therapy. For lists of its publications, course schedules, and alumni, contact:

The Upledger Institute
11211 Prosperity Farms Road, Suite D-325
Palm Beach Gardens, FL 33410
Tel: (800) 233-5880 or (561) 622-4334
Fax: (561) 622-4771
Website: www.upledger.com
E-mail: upledger@upledger.com

SUGGESTED FURTHER READING

The following books by Dr. Upledger are highly recommended:

John E. Upledger, D.O., O.M.M., *CranioSacral Therapy, SomatoEmotional Release, Your Inner Physician and You* (Berkeley, CA: North Atlantic Books and Palm Beach Gardens, FL: The Upledger Institute, 1991). This is a highly readable book that explains Dr. Upledger's findings and techniques to the layperson.

_____. and Jon D. Vredegvoogd, M.F.A., *CranioSacral Therapy* (Seattle, WA: Eastland Press, 1988). This is the essential text on CranioSacral Therapy and is geared to the professional.

Also recommended is:

Harold Ives Magoun, A.B., D.O., O.M.M., *Osteopathy in the Cranial Field*, Third Edition (Kirksville, MD: Journal Printing Co., 1976).

OTHER PRACTICES ASSOCIATED WITH CRANIOSACRAL THERAPY

While Dr. Upledger's work was at first considered unorthodox, it is rapidly becoming accepted within mainstream medicine. Tens of thousands of health-care professionals around the world have taken courses offered by the Upledger Institute. The Upledger Institute HealthPlex Clinical Services in Palm Beach Gardens, Florida, offers private sessions as well as innovative intensive programs that address concerns such as brain and spinal cord dysfunction, learning disabilities, autism, therapist rejuvenation, post-traumatic stress disorder, and numerous other conditions. In 2004, the Upledger Institute HealthPlex added Dolphin-Assisted Therapy Intensive Programs, which are held in the Bahamas. Dr. Upledger, who was one of the original twenty-five-member advisory board of NIH's Office of Alternative Medicine, was surprised to learn at the board's first official meeting that three other board members had studied CranioSacral Therapy. One even remarked, "Gee, I thought your work was mainstream by now, not alternative!"

Dr. Upledger has continued to expand the frontiers of his work. In addition to offering courses in CranioSacral Therapy, he has also developed a type of work known as **SomatoEmotional Release** (SER). SomatoEmotional Release is based on the belief that our bodies hold the energy of past traumas, both physical and emotional, in the form of memories in the physical tissues of the body. He has coined the expression "energy cysts" for these areas of congestion, which disrupt the normal functioning of the body. SomatoEmotional Release seeks to find and discharge the energy that has become embedded in these cysts.

Visceral Manipulation is a hands-on therapy that seeks to encourage normal movement and tone in the viscera, or internal organs, of the body. If these organs do not function harmoniously with one another, irritation and disease can ensue. Visceral Manipulation was developed by Dr. Upledger's collaborator, Jean Pierre Barral, a French osteopath, and expanded by Barral's American protégé, Frank Lowen.

Another adjunct modality within the umbrella of the Upledger Institute is **Zero Balancing** (ZB). This hands-on technique was developed by Fritz Smith, M.D. It draws on Smith's training as an osteopathic medical physician and acupuncturist and integrates Western manipulative techniques with the Eastern energy system. Zero Balancing uses hands-on touch to balance the body's deep energy currents with the structural components of bone, muscle, and joints.

FOR FURTHER INFORMATION

For further information on Zero Balancing, contact:

Zero Balancing Health Association
Kings Contrivance Village Center
8640 Guilford Road, Suite 240
Columbia, MD 21046
Tel: (410) 381-8956
Fax: (410) 381-9634
Website: www.zerobalancing.com
E-mail: zbaoffice@zerobalancing.com

Also recommended is Fritz Smith's book, *Inner Bridges: A Guide to Energy Movement and Body Structure* (Atlanta, GA: Humanics New Age, 1986).

REIKI AT A GLANCE

BASIC FACTS

- **Reiki is an energetic healing practice that utilizes hands-on touch and focused visualization.** It aims to balance and amplify energy on the physical, mental, emotional, and spiritual planes.

- **Reiki (pronounced "ray-key") is a Japanese word meaning "universal life energy."** According to popular legend, it is reportedly based on ancient Tibetan Buddhist teachings rediscovered in the mid-1800s by Dr. Mikao Usui, a professor of theology at a Christian seminary in Kyoto, Japan.

THEORY

- **Reiki is based on a universal life force energy.** This energy, which surrounds and animates all of creation, is available for use in healing.

- **The Reiki practitioner acts as a channel for accessing the universal life energy.** While everyone has access to this energy, Reiki practitioners maintain that over the course of time the ability to access it has become blocked. Reiki practitioners undergo a series of initiations (called attunements) that enable them to tap into this energy.

- **Practitioners use Reiki energy to balance and amplify an individual's energy to promote healing.** Disharmony in the physical body or subtle energy fields that surround it can result in physical or emotional disease and dysfunction. During treatment, the practitioner draws on Reiki energy to restore balance. She does not use her own personal energy.

TYPICAL SESSION

- **A hands-on Reiki session typically lasts sixty to ninety minutes.** The practitioner holds the palm surface of both hands gently on a receiver's body. She moves her hands in a series of ten to twenty positions that cover the subtle energy centers known as chakras as well as the major physical organs and glands. The practitioner maintains each hand position for three to five minutes while the receiver draws in any required energy.

- Reiki practitioners also perform absentee healings, working from a photograph, at remote distances from the client. The techniques for such treatment are learned in advanced initiations.

- Expect to pay $30 to $100 for a Reiki treatment.

BENEFITS

- **Reiki practitioners view their work as a powerful tool in stress reduction and relaxation.** Advocates point to success in treating a variety of acute and chronic complaints ranging from asthma to arthritis.

- While not requiring belief in any religious system or dogma, many practitioners see Reiki as a form of self-discipline that can lead to spiritual transformation and insight.

- Reiki can be used not only to accelerate physical healing, but also to heal emotional and mental distress. Adherents maintain it can also be used to help animals, plants, and problem situations (such as war and famine).

CONTRAINDICATIONS

- Because it uses gentle touch and visualization, Reiki can be used in nearly any situation. Treatments should be abbreviated in the case of the elderly, the very young, or the seriously ill.

BACKGROUND AND TRAINING OF PRACTITIONERS

- Reiki is learned through initiation into various levels ranging from beginning practitioner to Master. Initiations often take place in weekend workshops, during which practitioners learn theory and technique.

- The background and training of Reiki practitioners vary. A number of massage therapists, doctors, dentists, chiropractors, podiatrists, nurses, and even veterinarians learn Reiki to incorporate into their practices. Many laypeople learn Reiki to use on themselves and their loved ones.

- There are thousands of Reiki Masters worldwide; in addition, many more practitioners have been initiated into other levels of practice.

CHAPTER 14

REIKI:
UNIVERSAL LIFE ENERGY

Just for today, do not worry.

Just for today, do not anger.

Honor your parents, teachers, and elders.

Earn your living honestly.

Show gratitude to every thing.[1]

—DR. MIKAO USUI,
THE FIVE ETHICAL PRINCIPLES OF REIKI

WHAT IS REIKI?

Reiki (pronounced "ray-key") is an ancient energetic healing technique utilizing the laying on of hands. Its practitioners assert that it brings balance and harmony to the body, mind, and spirit. Reiki is a Japanese word that means "universal life energy." *Rei* refers to the greater, universal spirit of energy that permeates the entire cosmos; *ki* refers to the vital life energy that animates every individual being and thing. Reiki aligns and balances universal with individual energy. Reiki practitioners have been trained and empowered to serve as channels to draw universal energy in order to transfer it to themselves and others for the purpose of healing.

Practitioners draw on two techniques: They can place their hands over key areas of a receiver's body, where the principal organs and glands are located (these areas correspond to the chakras, or subtle energy centers, of esoteric tradition), or they can visualize special symbols, enabling them to send healing energy, even at a distance. Hands-on touch can be combined with visualization in a bodywork session for a particularly powerful effect.

239

Reiki is considered a powerful tool in self-transformation, and proponents of Reiki claim universal life energy can be used to help not only individuals, but also animals, plants, emotional situations, and even machinery such as automobiles and appliances. (Yes, some Reiki practitioners believe a Reiki treatment might help to jump-start a stalled car.) Many practitioners perform Reiki on their food to increase its healing energy. Groups of Reiki practitioners gather to transmit Reiki energy for such purposes as healing the planet and ending wars.

If all of this sounds a little too much like hocus-pocus to you, Reiki practitioners would be quick to point out that their practice does not represent any religious dogma, nor does it require any particular set of beliefs on the part of the receiver. They maintain that their art is a science whose value has been demonstrated over an extended period of time in a growing body of anecdotal reports that attest to its efficacy.

Of all the healing modalities presented in this book, Reiki is the one that will probably strain your credibility the most. You may have to suspend your ordinary belief system to read about Reiki with an open mind to see if it holds genuine appeal for you.

THE ORIGINS OF REIKI

The origins of Reiki are recorded in legend, which contributes to its mystique. Reiki is unique among bodywork approaches because, by and large, Reiki practitioners adhere to a code of secrecy and are reluctant to disclose the details of their techniques to the uninitiated. They feel that Reiki energy is so powerful that only those who have been properly instructed should attempt its use. Instruction in Reiki is conferred from Master to student through a process of attunements. Reiki is the only bodywork system profiled in this book that requires an initiation, or attunement, to empower a practitioner to channel its energy.

According to a popularly recounted story, Reiki represents the rediscovery in the mid-1800s by Dr. Mikao Usui of ancient healing techniques developed in Tibet more than ten thousand years ago but lost to obscurity. According to some experts, the information regarding these healing techniques made its way to India, China, Japan, Egypt, and the Greco-Roman Empire, where it formed part of the training afforded initiates in the mystery schools of antiquity.

Dr. Usui was not a medical doctor but a doctor of philosophy. He was a Japanese convert to Christianity, professor, and dean of a Christian theological seminary in Kyoto, Japan. His students reminded Dr. Usui that Christ healed with his hands and admonished his disciples to do the same. "If this is so," they challenged, "show us how to heal."

Usui was stumped. Nothing in his training had prepared him to answer such a question. He felt honor-bound to answer his students' questions, so he set off on a journey around the world to discover the secret of healing.

Usui's teachers of Christian doctrine had been American, so he traveled first to the United States, where he spent seven years studying theology at the University of Chicago, trying to learn firsthand from Christians how to heal. No one there could help him, though. Usui then traveled to northern India to study ancient Hindu texts in the original Sanskrit. Again, he could find no answers to his questions. Ultimately, his quest brought him back to Japan to a Zen Buddhist monastery outside Kyoto. The head of this monastery believed some ancient Sanskrit Buddhist texts preserved there might hold the answer to Usui's question.

Dr. Usui studied these texts, then went on a kind of vision quest to the top of a holy mountain, Kuriyama, near Kyoto. There he fasted and meditated for twenty-one days in search of the key to healing. On the morning of the twenty-first day, in the midst of a black, moonless predawn, he saw a brilliant shining light racing toward him. It struck him in the center of his forehead, then erupted into countless tiny colored bubbles. A dazzling white light appeared, as did a number of Sanskrit characters in a radiant gold light. This represented Dr. Usui's initiation into the system of Reiki.[2]

Immediately following his transformative experience, Dr. Usui was able to effect a series of cures that were considered miracles. The Sanskrit characters from his vision formed the basis of his healing tools. Dr. Usui's reputation grew as he spent many years healing the sick in the beggars' quarter of Kyoto. Before his death, Usui appointed Dr. Chujiru Hayashi, a retired naval officer, Grand Master and successor to his legacy of Reiki healing. Hayashi in turn founded the first Reiki clinic, in Tokyo, to treat the severely ill around the clock.

The tradition of Reiki as practiced today was preserved largely through the efforts of Hawayo Takata. Born on the island of Hawaii to Japanese sugarcane farmers, Takata was widowed at a young age. Suffering a number of life-threatening illnesses, she went to Japan at the age of thirty-one to prepare for death. While in Tokyo, she received an inner message to seek treatment at Hayashi's clinic. Takata was healed after a series of Reiki treatments, and she became a devoted student. Hayashi initiated Takata as Reiki Master in 1938 to preserve the tradition of Reiki.

Takata returned to Hawaii, where she quietly practiced Reiki. Following Hayashi's death, she assumed the role of Grand Master. Aldous Huxley and Doris Duke, heiress to the Woolworth fortune, were among her early students. In the 1970s, Takata began to train other Reiki Masters. By the time of her death at the age of eighty in 1980, she had trained twenty-two other Reiki Masters. In recent years, evidence has been discovered to indicate that Reiki continued to be practiced in Japan as well as in Hawaii following Hayashi's death. Today, there are thousands of Reiki Masters practicing around the world, many of whom trace their lineage to Hawayo Takata.

THE THEORY UNDERLYING REIKI

Practitioners of Reiki maintain that everyone is born with the potential to access Reiki energy. However, over time, the human system has become blocked. A Master who has been empowered to grant initiations must open up this channel of energy flow before it can be accessed. The Sanskrit symbols recorded by Usui are a formulaic key that allow the Master to access Reiki energy. Once opened, the channel flows forever. The initiate develops a kind of antenna to draw in universal energy.

The Reiki Alliance, which supports its members as teachers of the Mikao Usui System of Reiki, as well as the American Reiki Master Association (ARMA), initiate individuals into three levels, called degrees, of Reiki practice. Each level is accompanied by a series of attunements, or initiations, that are meant to open up and amplify the channel of Reiki energy within the practitioner.

The first degree of Reiki initiation permits the practitioner to perform hands-on healing and is accompanied by an attunement process that opens up the higher energy centers. During second-degree Reiki initiation, the practitioner receives a further attunement and learns visual symbols that can be used to facilitate absentee treatment and healing emotional or mental distress. Second-degree attunement amplifies a practitioner's ability to perform hands-on treatment. Third-degree Reiki initiation imparts an additional symbol and empowers a practitioner to become a Master capable of teaching Reiki and initiating others while increasing the power of her own treatments.

First- and second-degree Reiki instruction usually takes place over a weekend or a series of several evenings. Preparation for initiation as a Master can require a practical demonstration and an apprenticeship over an extended period of time as well as substantial fees. This process is meant to screen aspirants for dedication and suitability.

Much is made of the attunement process, the initiations that are bestowed, and the role of the visual symbols employed in Reiki. Some people view them as magical power tools passed from one individual to another. Others see the initiations as occasions for heightening an individual's sense of self-awareness, helping to create an altered state of consciousness that permits the initiate to access deeper realms of the unconscious. ARMA founder Arthur Robertson described Reiki as consisting of "nothing more than keys to help you center and focus your consciousness."

No one is exactly sure how Reiki works. Proponents seem to be satisfied with the fact that they and the individuals with whom they work report physical and emotional benefits following its use. They point to the fact that healing by laying the hands on vital physical and subtle energy centers in the body participates in millennia-old traditions of healing that have spanned the world.

Reiki practitioners underscore the close, nearly one-to-one relationship between the chakras, which they cover with their hands, and the anatomical location of the glands that comprise the endocrine system. This vital system plays the important role of secreting hormones.

Many important physiological processes are regulated by hormones (the term literally means "to urge on"), including the rate of metabolism, growth and developmental processes, the functioning of the reproductive organs, the development of personality, and the ability of the body to cope with stress and resistance to disease. Consequently, a large number of pathological conditions are associated with malfunctioning of the endocrine system.[3] Reiki practitioners believe their work operates on the chakra system, which acts as a conduit of energy to the endocrine system. This accounts for the ability of Reiki to have such profound physical, emotional, and mental effects.

The ethical teachings of Reiki are encapsulated in the five principles that are inset as the epigraph to this chapter. These principles, which form an abbreviated guide to right living, are said to have evolved from Dr. Usui's personal experience. After having worked for seven years in the slums of Kyoto, Dr. Usui began to see some of his first patients, whom he had healed so that they might improve their lives, returning to him as beggars. When he asked why they still lived as beggars, they explained that it is easier to beg than to earn an honest living. Dr. Usui then realized he had overlooked an important consideration: He had failed to teach the beggars gratitude and responsibility. He realized he had mistakenly given his work away. Today, it is an important principle of Reiki that an individual must want to be healed, that he must take responsibility for himself and his own healing, and that he must compensate the healer in some way—otherwise he consumes energy without exchanging anything in return. All of life is a dynamic interchange of energy. It is important that every act reflect appropriate exchange.

THE TYPICAL FORMAT OF A REIKI SESSION

Reiki treatments can take various forms depending on the degree of Reiki energy the practitioner is using. Most typically, a Reiki treatment takes the form of a bodywork session following the protocol that is taught in first-degree Reiki.

A complete treatment can last from an hour to an hour and a half. The receiver lies on his back on a comfortable flat surface, such as a padded massage table. The receiver remains fully clothed: Reiki energy will pass through clothing; in fact, it will even penetrate plaster casts. No oils or lotions are used.

The practitioner positions her hands flat, fingers held closely together. The hands are generally placed so that one hand points toward the other as they cover the major surface areas of the body. The practitioner begins at the forehead and crown of the head and moves downward. Some practitioners stop at the pelvis while others continue to the feet.

After treating the front of the body, the practitioner asks the receiver to turn over onto his stomach. The practitioner then treats the back, starting with the shoulders and moving to the base of the spine. The practitioner may end the session by gently holding one hand at the top of the receiver's spine and the other at the base in a final balancing of energy. In all, anywhere from ten to twenty hand positions are used during treatment. This allows the practitioner to systematically treat all the major areas of the body.

During treatment, the practitioner holds her hands in each position with very light pressure for a relatively long period of time—three to five minutes. The hands are held in a stationary position and do not actively manipulate tissue. The beginning practitioner times the treatment and closely follows a prescribed course of hand positions. Advanced practitioners know by feel when an area has drawn in enough energy. They rely more heavily upon their intuition to know which parts of the body to treat and in what order. Advanced practitioners can also visualize the Reiki healing symbols to intensify the healing effect.

While a practitioner generally places her hands on the body during a Reiki session, it's also possible to administer a Reiki treatment with the hands held a few inches off the body, as in Therapeutic Touch. This approach might be used, for example, over the site of a traumatic injury, such as a burn or fracture. Abbreviated thirty-minute treatments can be administered, with the receiver typically seated in a chair. Healing treatments can also be administered from a distance, with the practitioner often using a photograph of the individual to be healed. Many Reiki practitioners incorporate other energetic healing techniques into their work, including the use of crystals, colors, and sound. Two or more Reiki practitioners sometimes work simultaneously on a receiver to intensify the effect of treatment. Reiki practitioners maintain that just the amount of energy that is needed is transmitted: Receivers cannot "overload" on energy.

One of the unique advantages of Reiki is the ease of administering self-treatments. While it is possible with most types of bodywork to do some self-treating, Reiki permits an individual to perform a complete self-treatment.

Indeed, in Reiki, individuals are encouraged to give themselves regular Reiki treatments, preferably daily, in order to further their own physical, mental, emotional, and spiritual well-being.

Reiki practitioners recommend that first-time recipients of Reiki receive three or four Reiki treatments over a period of about a week. Such a series enables an initial cleansing and attunement process to begin. As response to treatment frequently lags the treatment itself by up to three days, benefits may not be apparent until the end of this series. Frequency of treatments after the initial series depends upon the individual and the condition being treated. Acute conditions generally require fewer treatments than chronically ingrained ones.

THE EXPERIENCE: TAPPING INTO UNIVERSAL LIFE ENERGY

The following account, written by Richard Kaplan, describes his experience of a Reiki treatment I administered to him. Richard is an accomplished screenwriter, who approaches bodywork with a respectful yet critical attitude. I thought it would be helpful to share his perspective on a Reiki session.

When I enter Thomas Claire's Greenwich Village apartment, I am greeted with a fresh, clean aroma, soft lights, and a warm but respectful hug. He wears a white cotton tunic, loose-fitting white pants, and white *tabis*, Japanese mitten-like socks. Thomas explains that this attire is not an integral part of Reiki, but that he wears it for the effect of serenity it evokes. Subsequent to a mutual friend's recommending him, I have already enjoyed one shiatsu, one Swedish, and two Reiki sessions with him this past year. I always sense that Thomas thoughtfully prepares everything in advance, so that the session will flow as easily and be as calm and productive as possible. He has already set up the massage table, draped with a white sheet, and neatly centered it on an Oriental rug in a large open area of the white-walled, book-lined living room. He has drawn the shades; subdued the lights; and lit fragrant incense and several candles, heedfully positioned at pleasing intervals. Gregorian chants that remind me of Native American music play softly in continuous mode to avoid interruption. The answering machine is on, with the volume set all the way down. Thomas creates the impression of a sacred healing environment, like a Greek Orthodox church or a yoga ashram.

We sit on a couch to talk. He inquires as to how I'm feeling physically and emotionally and what I'd like to work on with him. I have already given Thomas a hypochondriac's detailed medical history that makes me wonder how, even though I'm in my mid-thirties and quite healthy, I'm still walking and talking. I tell Thomas that three things are bothering me. Starting at the top and working my way down: My neck and jaw are tense, a chronic problem. I grind my teeth at night. When I wake up, I feel tired from doing battle all night. The chronic TMJ problem can even cause occasional dizziness as the jaw affects the balance in my inner ear. Second, I have felt a tension in my solar plexus that has left me somewhat breathless and feeling rushed for the last few weeks—like I can never get done all the things I have to do. Third, eleven months ago, I tore ligaments in my ankle that were diagnosed as chronically torn. They are almost all healed, but not quite. Thomas states apologetically that Reiki won't repair the torn ligament in my ankle—that's a structural problem best left to my doctor to treat—but Reiki will encourage relaxation and blood circulation to the area, which will support the healing process. The jaw and solar plexus, however, he will definitely try to relax.

Thomas considers his work both spiritual and physical, balancing Eastern and Western interpretations and explanations. He explains, in esoteric and anatomical terms that even I, a layman who has forgotten all his biology, can understand, how the solar plexus is the locus of many emotions. . . . "the seat of security and feeling our place in the world—as if approaching the world with a 'here I am' attitude." He further clarifies how we instinctively tense the jaw in a fight-or-flight response to stress. I understand his points, rather than feeling "blinded with science" or befuddled with mysticism.

Thomas tells me I can leave my clothes on for the session. However, I take off my shoes, socks, belt, and watch and remove everything from my pockets. Although still dressed, I feel unencumbered, not having to worry about keys and coins falling during the session. Someone once told me not to have any metal on me during a massage as it could adversely affect the energy field. I don't really understand, but it's like being an agnostic instead of an atheist—better to hedge your bets.

I lie on my back on his massage table, placing my head on the folded white towel he has put there to support it. I assume the position yoga teachers call the relaxation pose—my eyes closed; arms and palms up, somewhat away from my body; legs spread slightly apart; feet relaxed. I try to breathe deeply into my belly and expand my chest in order to calm myself and focus on how Thomas will work. I remember that during our first session, he complimented me on my deep breathing. I thanked him but explained I'd been doing it all my life.

Ever solicitous, Thomas asks if I am warm enough and whether I would like him to drape a sheet over me. I tell him I am comfortable as is. He says I should inform him if I get cool at any time during the session. Sometimes Reiki can affect the body's thermostat, and I might get chilly. Thomas emphasizes that we do work on this together, but that I don't really have to *do* anything. I hear him rapidly rub his hands together. He announces that he will start by placing his fingers over my eyes, which he does, ever so gently touching his warm fingertips to my eyelids, eyebrows, and the area just below my eyes for several minutes. I am immediately calmed. Wordlessly, he moves his fingers to the crown of my head and again gently applies pressure—as he will throughout the session—with subtle variations. I feel his fingers quaver. I contemplate: Is he moving to produce a certain effect or is my energy causing his fingers to move? Is the ki or ch'i or life energy flowing from my head causing the movement? Or is it his subconscious impulses, like when holding a pendulum or Ouija board? I wonder as I drift into a meditative state. By the time his fingers move to the back of my head, I'm almost asleep, with the swirling colors of Jackson Pollock action paintings beneath my eyelids. I tranquilly resist sleep as I want to be aware of his process and to "work" with him. Various abstract ideas interchange with my daily must-dos. I breathe deeply trying to refocus on his seemingly hot fingertips, which are now resting lightly on the surface of my chest. I'm amazed at the heat generated. I feel my sinuses clear. Strange, I think. Why did they do that now and not when he was laying his hands on my face?

Thomas lifts his hands and stops them over my upper belly, then my lower belly. I notice that his movements from one zone to another are distinct discrete moves. In Reiki, I think, the practitioner's hands work on separate points with imaginary connecting lines rather than with the gliding lines that Swedish massage therapists utilize without lifting their hands while moving from one section to another.

Thomas walks to the foot of the table, where he gently holds my feet. I feel his thumbs press lightly into the center of my feet, which I imagine corresponds to my solar plexus or adrenals. (He later confirms that this is an energizing point for the adrenals.) His palms cradle the outside edge of my feet.

During some types of bodywork I like to ask what the practitioner is picking up from my body or which muscle he is working on. I find I learn a lot from this, even if it means I take myself out of a meditative and completely relaxed state. Thomas is very good at explaining his work, but today I don't feel like talking.

The first words spoken in a half hour or so are when he asks me to turn over on my belly. I don't feel nearly as sleepy as I did in the beginning. Nor, I realize, do I have to make such a concerted effort to turn over as I do during more physical deep tissue–style massages.

Thomas continues subtly touching my back. My attention, softly focused on his hands, begins to drift. I think of bodywork as I do of chicken soup: It may not cure the ailment, but it can't hurt. Maybe chicken soup helps colds because it tastes so good and eating it reminds one of being taken care of as a child. Or maybe the warm liquid opens up the chest and sinuses. Or perhaps it contains some healing chemical property that more research will bear out. Similarly, I remember an article I read about heart patients' responding positively to doctors and nurses who methodically touched them while treating them, frequently holding their hands, arms, and shoulders, and hugging them. This makes sense. If we relax, feel good about ourselves and others, chances are we'll feel better.

Getting a massage is a time to be touched by someone in an atmosphere of trust. Yet a professional massage is as different from the sensuous touch of a lover as speaking with a psychotherapist is from talking with a confidant. Both are beneficial and highly pleasurable, but the professional's efforts need not be reciprocated. You are there to heal yourself, not maintain a relationship.

About this time, I notice that I take a very deep involuntary breath, much deeper than my initial forced inhalations. Thomas's hands are working on my middle back. I now concentrate on his hands and my breathing. Thomas positions his hands on my lower spine.

Soon after, he tells me that he has finished and that I should rest. When he leaves the room, I gather my energy and assess my state: I feel relaxed, but my belly is still a little tight. I stretch out on the table. I feel frustrated that I didn't get a deep body workout. Yet I really do feel calm and much more centered, instead of feeling rushed and scattered as I have the last few weeks. I sit up slowly and as I do, a series of delicate burps come up from my belly like a string of bubbles from down deep in the water. My belly relaxes. Gone is that tension in the gut. I no longer feel frustrated but rather relieved. I'm quietly energetic and alert in an interior mode, like after a good yoga workout and meditation. I realize how different an aftermath this is from deep tissue massage, when I feel exhausted and relaxed, perhaps even sore, like after playing a hard game of basketball.

Thomas reenters the room and offers me a glass of water. I am thirsty. When I put on my watch, I notice that about an hour has elapsed since he started. I ask Thomas for his impressions of me from the evening's session. Trying to be as tactful, nonjudgmental, and enlightening as possible, he informs me that while he was first working on my head, he felt a "closure, in a metaphorical sense." He adds, "There was a kind of visual darkness, as if a veil were surrounding you, cutting the energy off . . . blocking, pinching." Regrettably, all this sounds right. I press him to continue. As he worked on the crown, side, and back of my head, he says he could feel my jaw relax. The darkness got lighter. My head opened up and he "saw" (with his eyes closed) a "nice wash of lavender," which he associated with "relaxation and a filling up with energy." That's reassuring and it corroborates my own sense of relaxation.

He continues about the tightness he felt in my chest, around the breastbone, which is often associated with a sense of "grief, possibly a very old and deep mourning," not necessarily for "a death, but mourning for not feeling loved, possibly as a baby or child," he adds. Knowing that "the body retains the emotional hurt," he worked on opening up my heart, the seat of love, compassion, and understanding. "When we feel unloved, it's hard for us to let go," he explains. Concerned that he might be getting too personal, he reassures me: "I'm just sharing some associations. If they resonate with you, they're something to reflect on." I ask him to proceed.

He felt a little tightness in my hips, even in the buttocks. While he worked on my back, he felt a "relaxing of tension there." My stomach had been "caved in," but after some holding there, it became "full and round." At this point, he "saw" a "nice bright white light." The stomach, he explains, is the place of grounding. He riffs on a now-familiar theme: "We are often brought up with insecurity and there's insecurity in our daily lives. It could be that you're feeling insecure about money, getting food, shelter, and work." He's on target. Thomas affirms, "I tried to encourage a feeling of security. To nurture you." He has.

"I felt a balance and an amplifying of energy . . . some nice bright white light while working on your back," he says. He also sensed a "nice flow of energy from my sacrum to my head, moving rhythmically through my back, which I associate with a balancing and attunement of your intellectual, spiritual, and intuitive side." Uncomfortable with the flattery, I think, Is this like all horoscopes beginning with "You are sensitive and creative"?

I thank Thomas and he thanks me—which always amazes me about bodyworkers. They have just performed a great deed for me. Doctors should take note. We hug again and I head out to the potentially rude awakening of a New York City night. After my first Reiki session, I felt relaxed and centered, as I do now. After the second, however, a great anger welled up inside me, even as I left Thomas's apartment and strode to the subway. I felt like the characters in *Network*, Paddy Chayevsky's film, screaming out their windows, "I'm mad as hell and I'm not going to take it anymore!" That whole evening, I felt anger, which lasted through the following day. I recall that during the first Reiki session I had with Thomas, I sensed yellowish-white light radiating from my forehead. At another point, I "saw" bluish light emanating from my abdominal region. These were not usual experiences for me. During this third session, even though Thomas had described his vision of the light within me, mine inner eyes have not seen the glory of such light.

All evening, I feel energized and relaxed, able to work late into the night. The next morning, I wake very refreshed, a half hour before the alarm, ready to work. Often, I wake up groggy and stunned. I can still feel that small ball of nagging tension in my diaphragm, but can focus my attention to breathe through it as I do during my morning yoga salute to the sun. I can sensorially remember Thomas's hands on my belly or back and the relaxing sensations that induced. I am more aware of when I clench my jaw during the day. I take a deep breath and relax the offending muscles. The Reiki work, like any type of bodywork or yoga, is no miracle cure, but it has given me an insight into how to calm myself.

THE BENEFITS OF REIKI

Reiki practitioners maintain that physical disease begins with imbalance in the emotional and mental fields. Reiki helps prevent physical illness by restoring balance to these more subtle fields before illness manifests in the physical body. In the case of physical illness, adherents believe Reiki can accelerate the healing process as well as aid relaxation and stress reduction.

Practitioners report success in helping patients with both acute and chronic illnesses, ranging from asthma and arthritis to more serious life-threatening illnesses. Reiki is considered helpful for debilitating chronic diseases because of the energy boost it gives people with depleted energy systems. While some Reiki practitioners claim to have healed people of such serious conditions as tumors, AIDS, and multiple sclerosis, such claims should be regarded with prudent skepticism: Be wary of any healing practitioner who promises to cure you of any illness.

In one of the few clinical studies performed on Reiki, researchers in California reported that students enrolled in Reiki training classes demonstrated significant increases in levels of hemoglobin in the blood following their periods of instruction versus control subjects who received no training.[4] These results, which seem to point to improved circulation and oxygenation, recall Dolores Krieger's findings related to the effects of treatment with Therapeutic Touch.

While it is not affiliated with any religion, Reiki embraces the spiritual dimension of healing. Reiki energy flows from a superior consciousness or spirit through a vital life energy force that permeates everything in the universe. Healing can occur in many ways—not only physically but also emotionally and spiritually. Reiki can be a powerful tool in helping people who are dying to find a place of stillness and calm within, which can help make their transition much more peaceful. Reiki practitioners would say that this in itself is a major healing, even if the physical body is not cured.

During a Reiki treatment, clients often report sensations of heat and tingling. They may drift into a deeply meditative state, somewhere between waking and sleeping. Takata's granddaughter Phyllis Lei Furumoto shares her experience with Reiki: "Some people have described it as coming home; some say it is like being plugged in again. I have the sense that I knew this feeling in the past and now am fully in touch with the energy again, without efforting."[5]

The most common effects people feel after a Reiki treatment are a deep sense of relaxation and an increased sense of vitality and mental alertness. Sometimes, people may feel an aggravation of their physical condition or of their emotional problems before they get better. This can be a normal, healing crisis.

Additionally, some people experience a shift in their level of awareness about the world, which they associate with spiritual transformation and growth. In particular, they report an especially strong connection to the here-and-now quality of life. They may feel more aware of flow and continuity in their lives. Greater insight into the self and subconscious may follow treatment through such mechanisms as vivid dreams.

CONTRAINDICATIONS TO REIKI

Reiki touch is gentle and can be applied off the body if necessary, so there is little risk of harming body tissue. Because it uses gentle touch and visualization, Reiki can be used in nearly any situation. Treatments should be shorter for the elderly and the very young.

Reiki practitioners do not use their personal energy. They maintain that no negative personal energy can be transferred, either from practitioner to client or from client to practitioner since Reiki is universal, not personal, energy. In fact, by serving as the vehicle of energy transmission, the Reiki practitioner herself becomes energized during the process of a Reiki treatment.

BACKGROUND AND TRAINING OF PRACTITIONERS

There are currently thousands of Reiki Masters worldwide, and many more people have been initiated into beginning and intermediate degrees of Reiki practice. The background of Reiki practitioners varies widely. The only prerequisites to becoming a channel of Reiki energy are a desire to learn, a commitment to use Reiki, and the series of attunements provided by a Master during the initiation process.

Healthcare professionals, including massage therapists, physicians, dentists, chiropractors, psychotherapists, nurses, and even veterinarians, learn Reiki to incorporate into their work. Because Reiki attunements activate the flow of Reiki energy, practitioners transfer Reiki healing energy to their patients even when not specifically using the prescribed Reiki hand positions. Reiki complements conventional medicine as well as other holistic healing modalities, and so can be used as an adjunct to many types of healing.

Many laypersons learn Reiki to practice on themselves and their loved ones. Since Reiki is easy to learn, its practice appeals to a wide range of people. Reiki classes are often taught in nonprofit alternative holistic healing centers to help people with life-threatening illnesses cope better with their condition. Because

Reiki is so simple to administer to oneself or others, it is a very effective tool for empowering the seriously ill and the loved ones who care for them.

Contrary to the practice in most U.S. hospitals, medical facilities in some foreign countries routinely offer spiritual healing therapies, such as Reiki. For instance, there are more than two thousand clinics in Great Britain in which patients can request spirit healing.[6]

In some locations, massage licensing laws make it illegal for practitioners of any type of hands-on bodywork to charge a fee for their services without having a requisite license. In such situations, Reiki practitioners sometimes label their work relaxation or ask for donations rather than fees. Some practitioners obtain a religious minister's license and ask for contributions for their work.

Reiki is a particularly esoteric form of bodywork. Practitioners claim it works on the emotional and spiritual planes to effect physical healing. I personally believe that working on these subtle levels can indeed be powerful. While most Reiki practitioners are well meaning and compassionate, not all practitioners seem to possess the gift of inner discipline that somehow transforms Reiki from a well-intentioned caring form of communication into a subtle, powerful healing art. In this modality, be particularly open and sensitive: Follow your intuition in finding a practitioner with whom you feel you can work.

FOR FURTHER INFORMATION

Before her death, Hawayo Takata is reported to have initiated twenty-two Reiki Masters to preserve her legacy. Today, her work is carried on by a number of independent teachers and organizations:

The Reiki Alliance
204 North Chestnut Street
Kellogg, ID 83837
Tel: (208) 783-3535
Fax: (208) 783-4848
Website: www.reikialliance.com
E-mail: info@reikialliance.com

The Reiki Alliance is an alliance of Reiki Masters that supports its members as teachers of the Mikao Usui System of Reiki.

ARMA
P.O. Box 130
Lake City, FL 32056-0130

Tel: (386) 755-9638
Website: www.atlantic.net/~arma/
E-mail: american_reiki@yahoo.com

The American Reiki Master Association (ARMA) was established by Arthur Robertson. He was trained by one of Takata's students, Iris Ichikuro, who asked him on her deathbed to make Reiki more widely available by providing affordable training. His work is carried on today by his wife, Cheri.

The International Center for Reiki Training
21421 Hilltop Street, Unit #28
Southfield, MI 48034
Tel: (800) 332-8112 or (248) 948-8112
Fax: (248) 948-9534
Website: www.reiki.org
E-mail: center@reiki.org

The International Center for Reiki Training offers Reiki classes throughout the world and publishes a free online newsletter.

SUGGESTED FURTHER READING

I am indebted to the following books, which served as the basis for much of the information presented in this chapter:

Bodo J. Baginski and Shalila Sharamon, *Reiki: Universal Life Energy,* trans. Christopher Baker and Judith Harrison (Mendocino, CA: Life Rhythm, 1988). This is an excellent easy-to-read introduction to Reiki, complete with a handy reference guide correlating physical symptoms of disease to emotional and mental issues.

Fran Brown, *Living Reiki: Takata's Teachings* (Mendocino, CA: Life Rhythm, 1992). This is an inspirational memoir of the history and practice of Reiki as told by one of its most influential teachers.

Lawrence Ellyard, *Reiki Healer: A Complete Guide to the Path and Practice of Reiki* (Twin Lakes, WI: Lotus Press, 2004). This is a heartfelt introduction to Reiki, which includes a summary of the most recent information regarding the history or Reiki.

Paula Horan, *Empowerment Through Reiki. The Path to Personal and Global Transformation* (Wilmot, WI: Lotus Light Publications, 1992). This is another easy-to-read introduction, which also suggests how adjunct healing modalities can be used with Reiki.

HOLOTROPIC BREATHWORK AT A GLANCE

BASIC FACTS

- Holotropic Breathwork combines rapid deep breathing, accompanied by evocative music, with focused bodywork. It is a powerful method of self-exploration and healing that aims to unify mind and body.

- "Holotropic" means "moving toward wholeness." Holotropic Breathwork was developed in 1976 by Stanislav Grof, M.D., a Czech-born psychiatrist and explorer of consciousness, in collaboration with his wife, Christina.

THEORY

- Holotropic Breathwork is based on modern consciousness research, depth psychology (the psychology of unconscious behavior), and various spiritual practices. It uses accelerated breathing and evocative music played at high volume to induce a nonordinary state of consciousness. The Breathwork loosens psychological defenses and leads to a release of unconscious material. This can free blocked energies, resulting in spontaneous healing of old, forgotten psychological traumas.

- Holotropic Breathwork uses a map of the unconscious. Developed by Grof, this map helps understand the experiences encountered during the Breathwork.

- The release of emotions and physical tension is facilitated by focused bodywork that involves massage, pressure, and resistance to areas of accumulated tension in the body.

TYPICAL SESSION

- Holotropic Breathwork is typically offered in group sessions in workshops from one to six days long. Group size can range from just a few participants to 150 or more. Some practictioners also offer individual sessions.

- Attendees of the workshop team up in pairs. One does Holotropic Breathwork while a partner observes and provides support. Roles are subsequently reversed. Breathers lie on the floor and perform deep accelerated breathing while music is played at high volume. If desired, certified facilitators apply focused resistance to areas of tension.

- Drawing of mandalas and group processing of the Breathwork experience conclude each day's session.

- Fees for a two-day workshop average between $150 and $300.

BENEFITS

- **Holotropic Breathwork is deeply experiential.** Its goal is to enable the participant to come into contact with her inner self. It provides a unique opportunity for combining personal growth with group interaction.

- Holotropic Breathwork is especially beneficial for individuals seeking greater psychological unfoldment, or an expanded spiritual dimension in their lives. It is also recommended for those showing little change after long-term psychotherapy.

- Holotropic Breathwork may result in the healing of psychosomatic disorders by releasing blocked energy.

CONTRAINDICATIONS

- **Holotropic Breathwork can involve varying degrees of physical stress and can evoke intense emotional experiences.** It is not advised for pregnant women or individuals with serious cardiovascular problems, lung disease (emphysema, tuberculosis), systemic debilitating diseases, epilepsy, glaucoma, or a history of mental illness.

BACKGROUND AND TRAINING OF PRACTITIONERS

- Practitioners, called facilitators, complete a program with Grof Transpersonal Training that takes a minimum of two years. Requirements for certification consist of 150 credit hours of general experience accumulated in Holotropic Breath Workshops; 350 hours of course work in the theory and practice of Holotropic Breathwork and related topics; private consultations with approved practitioners; and satisfactory completion of a two-week seminar. Training is offered in various locations around the world.

- Many facilitators have previous professional experience in the healing arts, such as bodywork, medicine, psychiatry, psychology, psychotherapy, and social work.

- There are approximately eight hundred certified facilitators located throughout the world. About 350 are in the United States. There are certified facilitators in Canada, Mexico, South America, Australia, Western and Central Europe, Scandinavia, Russia, Japan, Fiji, New Zealand, India, United Arab Emirates, South Africa, and Thailand. An additional eight hundred practitioners are currently attending practitioner training.

CHAPTER 15

HOLOTROPIC BREATHWORK: THE MUSIC OF BREATH

"Music," according to the ancient Chinese sage Seu-ma-tsen, "is that which unifies."

"Breath," according to consciousness explorer Stanislav Grof, M.D., "is the gateway to the unconscious."

WHAT IS HOLOTROPIC BREATHWORK?

Holotropic Breathwork is a powerful experiential method of self-exploration and healing that aims to unify mind and body. It is based on a synthesis of modern consciousness research, depth psychology (the psychology of unconscious behavior), and various spiritual practices. "Holotropic" means "moving toward wholeness" (from the Greek "holos" = whole and "trepein" = to move in the direction of). Holotropic Breathwork is typically offered in group sessions in workshops from one to six days long. Highly evocative music played at high volume is coupled with deep and faster breathing, a kind of hyperventilation to promote transformation. Focused bodywork using massage, pressure, and resistance to areas of accumulated tension is offered as an adjunct in healing.

THE ORIGINS OF HOLOTROPIC BREATHWORK

Holotropic Breathwork was developed in 1976 by Stanislav Grof, a Czech-born psychiatrist. Grof practices and teaches this technique with his wife, Christina, in the San Francisco Bay area and in other locations. Grof was interested in exploring ways to induce nonordinary states of altered consciousness without the use of drugs. His research and experimentation led to the development of Holotropic Breathwork.

THE THEORY UNDERLYING HOLOTROPIC BREATHWORK

Holotropic Breathwork is deeply experiential: Its goal is to enable the individual to contact her deepest self. It is a powerful way to reexperience early memories, and this practice mediates access to painful, unresolved conflicts in such a way as to allow the body and the psyche to process them in a healing way.

Grof distinguishes between two modes of consciousness: hylotropic and holotropic. Hylotropic consciousness characterizes everyday linear reality—it's the consciousness of being in a particular place at a particular moment in time—here in the here and now. Holotropic consciousness is beyond the boundaries of space and time as normally perceived. It moves us toward wholeness and totality of existence. It is characteristic of certain altered states of consciousness, such as meditative, mystical, and psychedelic experiences. The holotropic mode of consciousness is especially rich because it enables an individual to gain access to the full range of her biological, psychological, social, racial, and spiritual history as well as the realms of reality described by the great mystical traditions of the world. This is the mode of consciousness that Holotropic Breathwork is designed to induce.

Holotropic Breathwork uses accelerated breathing and evocative music played at high volume to induce a nonordinary state of consciousness. These techniques loosen psychological defenses and lead to a release of unconscious material. The unconscious knows what it needs and acts accordingly. Breath is the vehicle that allows the unconscious to take over. Whatever happens in a breathing session is exactly what is supposed to happen during that time: There is no right or wrong way to experience Breathwork.

Grof believes that everyone has built-in radar. At any given moment this radar will pick up whatever information is important for an individual to receive to help her deal with whatever issues are uppermost in her mind. When doing Holotropic breathing, this radar is extremely active and picks up whatever emotionally charged material one needs to tune into without any effort. The unconscious unerringly controls and guides a breather's process.

Grof developed what he calls a cartography, or map, of the psyche. This cartography reflects his theory of the unconscious and the kinds of experience that occur during a Holotropic Breathwork session. Consciousness is classified into four different bands, or levels.

The sensory band of consciousness is usually the first level to appear early in the breathing. The breath activates an individual's sensory receptors so that she may experience vivid visual images (for instance, colors and geometric patterns; sounds; and, less frequently, smells and sensations of touch).

Deep healing resolutions of old, forgotten biographical material occur in the

second level, the biographical band of consciousness. Here the individual experiences the area of her own individual consciousness—the area that is explored
extensively by traditional Freudian-oriented psychoanalysis. Within this band,
an individual becomes aware of the events in her life from birth to the present,
including unresolved conflicts and repressed memories.

The third level is the perinatal band of consciousness. It is extremely rich,
and it is the gateway to the deeper unconscious, the door to what Carl Jung
called the collective unconscious. It is the band of consciousness that surrounds
an individual's physical birth, from conception to delivery. As the bridge
between the personal and the transpersonal, the birth process is extremely
important. Grof divides experiences within the perinatal band of consciousness
into four basic perinatal matrices (BPMs). These four BPMs correspond to the
chronological stages in the birth process, beginning with the initial floating in
the amniotic fluid in the womb, continuing with the onset of biological delivery
and with movement down the birth canal, and concluding in the clinical act of
delivery. During a Breathwork session, an individual can actually experience
the sensations and feelings of her own birth.

The reenactment of the birth process typically opens the gate to the fourth
level of consciousness—the transpersonal band. Here, the breather transcends
conscious boundaries of space and time. An individual can identify with her
earliest memories, with her ancestors, with past lives, and even with experiences that are yet to occur. She can become one with the entire planet and all
the peoples on it. This is an extremely exalted state in which words seem inadequate to express the depth and range of what is experienced.

An individual does not necessarily have any or all of the above experiences,
and the experiences do not necessarily progress in the order described. No
effort is made to force this schema upon anyone. An individual's experience of
Holotropic Breathwork is hers alone, which makes this practice particularly
empowering.

THE TYPICAL FORMAT OF A HOLOTROPIC BREATHWORK SESSION

Holotropic Breathwork is generally performed in group sessions in workshops
from one to six days long. Group size can range from just a few particpants to
150 or more. Some practitioners also offer individual sessions.

A common format is a two-day weekend workshop. Certified facilitators
lead the workshop, and they begin with an introduction to the history and theory of Holotropic Breathwork. Attendees then partner up in pairs. On the first
day, one person lies down on the floor to breathe while her partner serves as a
sitter to protect the breather's space by providing support. The sitter attends to
any needs the breather may have, such as getting water, providing a blanket in

case of chills, or helping the breather to the bathroom. Roles are reversed the following day.

Everyone establishes a verbal contract with her partner before beginning to breathe. This contract defines whether or not an individual wants her sitter and/or the facilitators to touch her, or remind her to resume breathing deeply if she should stop doing so.

Each breathing session begins with a gentle, guided relaxation. Then the music and deep rhythmic breathing start. The musical selections consist of little-known classical pieces and movie scores (to avoid preconceived associations to them), music from spiritual traditions (such as Sufi chants, Hindu ragas, Gregorian chants), aboriginal drumming rhythms, trance-inducing and ethnic music, and New-Age pieces. Music is played for as long as four hours in order to ensure adequate time for personal processing. If requested and/or required, the facilitators provide hands-on touch, applying pressure to areas of resistance and tension to aid in their release. Drawing of mandalas and group processing of the Breathwork experience conclude each day's session. In addition to this workshop format, some practitioners offer one-on-one individual sessions with clients.

THE EXPERIENCE: I BREATHE TO MUSIC

It's a Friday evening in the sweltering heat of a New York summer. I'm sitting in a large open space in Manhattan with fifteen other people. We represent a diversity of backgrounds, including business professionals, homemakers, computer technicians, writers, social workers, and artists. We've all forgone the pleasure of spending a midsummer weekend in the outdoors to engage in some inner exploration. We will be breathing together over the next two days in a Holotropic Breathwork weekend workshop appropriately entitled "The Healer Is the Self."

Four facilitators have converged in New York City to initiate us into this work. Karen and Gary have just arrived from Florida, Ruby from Maryland, and Noah from California. These are our guides. They have all been trained and certified in Holotropic Breathwork by Stanislav Grof. Their personalities differ markedly, yet they complement one another superbly. Like a fine-tuned string quartet, they are going to play the music that will guide our bodies and our lives for the next forty-eight hours.

The first step in the Breathwork experience is choosing a partner. I do this on Friday evening in preparation for the first breathing session, which will take place on Saturday. I pair up with Nancy, an attractive blond New Jersey homemaker who sat next to me during the evening's introductory lecture. I know very little about her except that she seems very nice and has been involved in a variety of self-transformation work through a program that includes reading, psychotherapy, and assorted healing workshops. Somehow we seem to hit it off and feel comfortable with each other.

That night, I dream about my sister, who lives in the same Midwestern city where we both grew up. She's in trouble and needs my help. I dream about things in doubles: an unidentified friend who hands me a pair of frames for his glasses that are exactly like my own; and another friend who lifts his blue denim jacket off the back of a chair in a restaurant where we've been dining, only to find an identical jacket underneath it.

On Saturday morning, I learn that Nancy was born in the same town where I grew up and that she is one of a set of identical twins. We are already beginning our movement toward wholeness as a subtle unconscious bond is forming between us. According to Grof, such synchronicities often occur during Holotropic Breathwork experiences.

That afternoon, I prepare to breathe. I lie comfortably on my back, arms and legs stretched out. My body is supported by a comfortable padded blanket. Nancy sits cross-legged at my side; she will be my sitter for the day. She preferred to breathe the following morning, when she felt she'd be fresher. That was fine with me: I preferred to breathe first, before seeing how other people did it. I was concerned their experiences might bias my own.

I establish my contract with Nancy. I opt for the standard contract, the one used most frequently by those who are breathing for the first time: Nancy is to remind me to come back to my faster breathing if I should wander from it by tapping me lightly on my right am. Otherwise, she is not to touch me unless I specifically ask her to.

"Inhale deeply. Now release. Imagine a gold wave washing across your forehead, then flowing down from your head to your toes, and then slowly up past each part of your body, back to your head." Karen is softly guiding us through a deep relaxation visualization, not unlike that common in many meditation and yoga classes.

The relaxation comes to an end. The music begins to play—loud, lush, stirring, evocative—from six sense-surround speakers strategically mounted. Not so loud as to be uncomfortable, but pulsating and omnipresent. Karen exhorts us to breathe fast and deep, demonstrating the rhythm of the breath herself as she makes an exaggerated whooshing sound to show us exactly what she means. She encourages us to let out our own sound, the vibrating hum of our own vocal cord, so that our sounds blend with the swelling strains of the music. The room reverberates. The effect is truly powerful.

My immediate sensation is one of exhilaration, happiness, and joy. Then I become aware of severe tension in my forearms, thighs, and calves. I am amazed by the physical intensity of the feeling. This is not just a tingling. I feel tremendous physical pressure, as though an incredible amount of blood and energy were engorged in my limbs.

Our facilitators had recommended that we try to stay with whatever physical tension might arise, to go into those areas with our breath. So I send my breath and energy to areas of constriction. They do release, but the feeling of tension moves up to my solar plexus and lower chest. And my hands. My hands, especially. I feel as though I cannot open them, as though there are thick, tough elastic bands holding my fingers tight in a fist. Words seem inadequate to capture the intensity of sensation, how palpably real this feeling of tightness is.

My hands are infant hands; my fingers those of an unborn infant, trying to poke through the amniotic membrane, which feels like a layered sheet of thick latex. And I remember how difficult it was to be born, to break through this substance, and how much work I had to do to make my way through the womb.

I marvel at the magnificence of my hands, at how my fingers knew even before I was born how to work their way through the womb. I am struck with wonder at how many marvelous things hands can do. Play hauntingly moving pieces on the piano and violin and other musical instruments. Move in the sinuous, sensuous, graceful rhythm of a dance. How they can heal. All of this ability surpasses my intellectual understanding. I am humbled before the mystery and magic of my own body. I feel enormous power and beauty. I realize that I possessed both before I was even born. I have brought them forth into the world. Beauty and power are my birthright!

I feel as though I am traveling down the birth canal, and I experience the moment of my birth. I feel a sense of haunting disappointment. I'm all alone. I've come into the world expecting to be loved and there is no one to greet me. The ultimate truth of life is revealed to me as I experience it firsthand—I am alone. I associate this feeling with the sense of loneliness and isolation I've carried with me for as long as I can remember—from even before I can recall having any memory.

I say to myself, *Wait a minute. I don't have to be alone. I'm not an infant who's helpless and at the mercy of those adults who surrounded me as a child. I'm an adult. I can make my needs known. I can ask Nancy to hug me and make me feel welcome and loved.* I motion to Nancy to come near. I ask her to hug me. She does so, like a mother cradling a newborn, and I feel totally content, blissful. This single, simple gesture of caring human touch has done more to make me feel loved and secure than all the many years I've talked about why I feel so alone in traditional talk psychotherapy. I am complete and at peace. Finally, I feel total release. I experience a sense of well-being and fulfillment a million times more profound than that following six-alarm sex. I have arrived.

I need to pause in my breathing—I am exhausted, spent. Someone is crouching at my side, a mouth is next to my ear. Ruby is breathing with an exaggerated hyperventilation. She is reminding me to resume my breathing.

The experience of being born has opened the gateway to the transpersonal for me. I take off. I soar. I feel one with the cosmos. My solar plexus and chest vibrate with tremendous energy. I have limitless power. I see waves of gold and orange. They swirl around and off me like sunspots from the sun. I fling them across the farthest expanses of the universe. Galaxies erupt. I am present at the creation of the world. I am the earth, and I see the first green jungle ferns growing from me, sprouting roots deep below my skin. I see exotic jungle birds and primeval wild animals. I hear their first piercing screams in the primal forests.

The sky above is azure, slowly drifting ever higher, until it becomes black as the night. It becomes a great void. In this void, I see the stars. The power and brilliance of these stars seem as nothing compared to the power of the void. I am the void. The stars draw their power from me. I feel healing, incredible healing power in that void. There is enough power there to heal not only myself but everyone in this room, in the entire world.

The experience fills me with joy, indescribable joy. A strain of lush orchestral music from the Romantic period is playing loudly. But in my mind's ear, I hear Beethoven's *Ode to Joy*. I am joy itself. I have so much power and joy that I could create music as majestic as Beethoven's exhilarating salute to life. With the healing that has taken place, I feel an incredible sense of creativity, unity, compassion, and love. Tears of gratitude flow down my cheeks.

I see images of past faces and places, qualities of energy I associate with past life experiences. I am a wounded warrior in the Middle Ages, lanced in the prime of life. A widow dressed in widow's weeds sits near me. I try to comfort her but she cannot hear. I am enclosed in a granite tomb.

I arrive at a point where I feel spent and exhausted. I cannot breathe any longer. I feel as though I've been outside my body, flying high, in another space and time. That sensation changes. I'm coming back. I'm reentering the here and now.

Noah kneels at my side. He asks me how I'm doing. Do I want to get up? He seems to know intuitively that my process has run its course.

I tell him I've been in a beautiful place. I don't want to leave yet. I want to rest a little, then see if I can go back to that space. He says, "Fine. Just rest quietly and see what happens." I lie peacefully for some time, but it is clear that whatever extraordinary process had been taking place is now concluded. I ask Nancy to help me up.

She tells me how beautiful it was to watch me breathe. Even when I was crying, there was great beauty and joy in my face. "You looked so beatific," she says, "just like a baby. It made me want to cry, too."

I'm amazed at how weak I feel after the breathing. I can barely walk. My legs feel numb. I have to lean on Nancy for support. I can't believe this—I'm in peak athletic shape. I can easily bench-press my own weight. I fly through difficult aerobics classes. Now I can barely crawl.

I look at the clock. It's 4:15 p.m. I started breathing at 1:45. So I've been in an altered state of consciousness for two and a half hours. I had absolutely no sense of the passage of time. There are still a number of people breathing around me. Some of them will continue for another hour and a half.

I draw my mandala and chat quietly with my fellow workshoppers while we wait for the rest of the breathers to finish. We then have a group discussion of all our experiences to help process them. We break and go home about 7:00 p.m.

I'm exhausted. I eat a slice of reheated pizza, then go to bed, fast asleep by 9:00 on a Saturday night. The next morning, Nancy tells me she was totally exhausted, too. We learn that breathing often induces fatigue in those whose mothers were anesthetized during delivery: Traces of the anesthetic remain in the body through life. My mother was heavily anesthetized for my delivery—a common practice until more recently, with the popularity of natural childbirth.

On Sunday morning, I sit while Nancy breathes. I feel extremely protective toward her and her space. I want to be sure to provide as much support as I can so that her experience will be as healing as possible.

Noah leads today's breathers through a guided relaxation, much as Karen had the previous afternoon. The music begins and Nancy starts her deep, fast breathing. Like me, she is a quiet breather. She does not make many overt physical movements with her body, but I sense a deep intensity of emotion below her still, calm face. It's as though I can feel that she is revisiting some intensely charged emotional experiences. In an emotion somewhere between sorrow and joy, I find myself breaking into quiet tears. A deep connection continues to grow between us.

Other people in the room are going wild. One 200-pound guy thrashes about; it takes all four facilitators plus his sitter to hold him down. They are pressing hard, offering as much resistance as possible, helping him go deep into his tension so as to reach a deeper level of release. Another man is experiencing severe nausea. He's vomiting into a brown paper bag. From the far side of the room, I hear the cry of a newborn infant. I look to see whence this baby has materialized—I see a grown man bawling with the exact sound of a newborn. It is uncanny.

The breathing continues for four hours. At the end of the session, the breathers complete their mandalas and share their experiences in a group discussion. Many of them radiate inner calm—a delicate and beatific look in their eyes, like the otherworldly angels of Botticelli. They show us the mandalas they have drawn: They're filled with beautiful pastel colors that induce a sense of bliss. Some look like the works of accomplished artists. One picture in particular is striking, the work of a middle-aged woman down on her luck. It is a bright and joyful rendering of a field of fanciful flowers.

Some breathers remember nothing; they are aware only of having spent two to three hours in a state of great peace with no conscious memories of any visual images or sounds of any kind. Others, like Nancy, remember vivid images and thoughts that came to them. Nancy revisited important emotional moments with the people who have been most important in her life—her mother, husband, and son. Some breathers visited fantasy lands of sunshine, warm comforting waters, and clear skies. Still others had memories of intense physical sensations.

The man who vomited shares the fact that all his life he has had a tremendous fear of vomiting. No matter how ill he might have been and *wanted* to throw up, he couldn't. Today, he was able to vomit and release that fear for the first time in his life. The 200-pound man who thrashed about tells us his experience was positive also. He was reliving some of the pain and agony of his own birth experience and found an emotional support he never received from his mother when the facilitators reached out to help him.

Sharing these experiences enhances the bonds we've been forming. Parting is difficult for us all—we feel connected in a very fundamental, powerful way. The man who experienced nausea comes up to me and tells me how he enjoyed my description of my experiences the preceding day—of my flight into the transpersonal realm. He tells me he sincerely hopes to have an experience like that some day. In equal sincerity, I share my hope to have an experience like his some day—to be able to purge myself totally on the physical level of some great fear I've been holding on to all my life. What power and release there would be in that!

It's clear from the variety of experiences that individuals report during Holotropic Breath Workshops that no matter how many times an individual might undertake Holotropic Breathwork, each session can be different. Since the needs of the unconscious continue to evolve, a new experience of healing and transformation is always waiting. And it's only a breath away.

THE BENEFITS OF HOLOTROPIC BREATHWORK

As it acts strongly on the psyche, Holotropic Breathwork is especially beneficial for individuals seeking greater psychological unfoldment or an expanded spiritual dimension in their lives. It may result in the healing of psychosomatic conditions through releasing blocked energy. Holotropic Breathwork is especially recommended for individuals who have shown little improvement from long-term psychotherapy. Because it is usually done in a group, it also provides a unique opportunity to combine personal growth with the benefits of group interaction.

CONTRAINDICATIONS TO HOLOTROPIC BREATHWORK

Holotropic Breathwork can involve varying degrees of physical stress and can evoke intense emotional experiences. It is not advised for pregnant women or individuals with hypertension or other serious cardiovascular problems, lung diseases (such as emphysema or tuberculosis), systemic debilitating diseases, epilepsy, glaucoma, or a history of mental illness. Because reactions during a session can be very powerful, Holotropic Breathwork should not be attempted without the supervision of qualified facilitators.

BACKGROUND AND TRAINING OF PRACTITIONERS

Holotropic Breathwork sessions are conducted by facilitators who are certified by Grof Transpersonal Training. Requirements for certification consist of 150 credit hours of general experience accumulated in the theory and practice of Holotropic Breathwork and related topics; private consultations with approved practitioners; 350 hours in training workshops; and satisfactory completion of a two-week certification seminar. Many, but not all, facilitators have previous professional training in the healing arts, including bodywork, medicine, psychiatry, psychology, psychotherapy, and social work. There are approximately eight hundred certified facilitators practicing throughout the world. An additional eight hundred individuals currently attend training workshops around the world.

FOR FURTHER INFORMATION

If you are interested in receiving more information on Grof Holotropic Breathwork and the training program as well as how to obtain a list of certified Holotropic Breathwork practitioners near you, you can contact:

Grof Transpersonal Training
38 Miller Avenue, PMB 516
Mill Valley, CA 94941
Tel: (415) 383-8779
Fax: (415) 383-0965
Website: www.holotropic.com
E-mail: gtt@holotropic.com

A prerequisite for applying for training is to have experienced at least five Holotropic Breathwork sessions in the workshops of certified facilitators.

The following member organization sponsors periodic conferences and publishes a quarterly newsletter, *The Inner Door*. For information, contact:

Association for Holotropic Breathwork International
P.O. Box 7169
Santa Cruz, CA 95061-7169
Website: www.breathwork.com
E-mail: info@breathwork.com

SUGGESTED FURTHER READING
The following books by Stanislav Grof describe the practice and theory of Holotropic Breathwork:

Stanislav Grof, M.D. *The Adventure of Self-Discovery: Dimensions of Consciousness and New Perspectives in Psychotherapy and Inner Exploration* (Albany, NY: State University of New York Press, 1984).

_____. with Hal Z. Bennett, *The Holotropic Mind: The Three Levels of Human Consciousness and How They Shape Our Lives* (San Francisco: Harper-Collins, 1993).

The following guidebooks to the breathwork experience are written by a Holotropic Breathwork practitioner:

Kylea Taylor, M.S., *The Breathwork Experience: Exploration and Healing in Nonordinary States of Consciousness* (Santa Cruz, CA: Hanford Mead Publishers, 1994).

_____. *The Holotropic Breathwork Workshop: A Manual for Trained Facilitators* (Santa Cruz, CA: Hanford Mead Publishers, 1991).

POLARITY THERAPY AT A GLANCE

BASIC FACTS

- Polarity Therapy is an approach to healing that aims to restore energetic balance to the mind and body. It uses gentle touch, counseling on diet and nutrition, exercise, and psychological counseling.

- Polarity Therapy was developed in the mid-twentieth century by Randolph Stone, D.C., D.O., N.D. (1890–1981). A chiropractor, osteopathic physician, and naturopath, Stone combined his knowledge of Western structural manipulative methods with insights into energetic aspects of healing gained firsthand through the study of healing practices around the world.

THEORY

- The theoretical framework of Polarity Therapy is derived largely from the ancient healing practices of India known as Ayurveda. Polarity Therapy recognizes a vital energy that surrounds and animates every being. Illness results from a restriction in the natural flow of this energy.

- Energy pulsates in bipolar currents. These currents are either positive and expansive or negative and contractive. They surround and interpenetrate the body in a dynamic three-dimensional dance.

- The Polarity Therapist rebalances the bipolar charge in a client's body. She uses the connection between her two hands as a transmitter to effect balance and recharge the overall level of energy.

TYPICAL SESSION

- A typical Polarity bodywork treatment lasts thirty to ninety minutes. The client lies on a comfortable, padded massage table and is dressed in underwear or additional clothing. No oils or lotions are used.

- The therapist uses direct pressure and rocking and shaking movements to balance and amplify the client's flow of energy. Touch is typically gentle.

- Following hands-on treatment, the therapist may counsel the client in proper diet and nutrition, based mainly on the vegetarian principles of Ayurveda. She may also recommend a set of Polarity yoga exercises to stretch and balance the body. Supportive counseling that emphasizes positive thinking may also be offered.

- Expect to pay $30 to $100 for a Polarity session, which can be from thirty to ninety minutes.

BENEFITS

- **Polarity Therapy aims to redress imbalances in the vital energy that animates the body, mind, and spirit.** Polarity Therapists believe that all are connected at a deep level of being. Balancing energy may help to prevent the onset of physical illness or accelerate healing if illness has already set in. Proponents report relief from the pain and discomfort associated with many acute and chronic conditions, ranging from low back pain, muscle cramps, migraine headaches, and digestive disorders to emotional problems related to stress and tension.

- **Clients of Polarity Therapy often report a sense of deep relaxation following a session.** They often feel better balanced emotionally and mentally. A heightened feeling of energy and vitality can last several days afterward.

CONTRAINDICATIONS

- Because practitioners use gentle touch and can draw upon nonmanipulative means of treatment, they should be able to offer support for nearly any condition. However, since Polarity Therapy can involve body manipulation, anyone with a serious medical condition should consult a physician before treatment.

BACKGROUND AND TRAINING OF PRACTITIONERS

- The background and training of Polarity practitioners vary. Many practitioners learn Polarity Therapy after having studied other types of bodywork with which they integrate Polarity.

- The American Polarity Therapy Association (APTA) has established a code of ethics and minimum standards of training for Polarity practitioners. These include 155 hours of training for the level of associate practitioner and 520 hours for registered practitioner, 675 hours in total. The APTA maintains a registry of practitioners.

- There are more than one thousand practitioners registered by the APTA. In addition, many people have studied Polarity Therapy in weekend workshops or minicourses.

CHAPTER 16

POLARITY THERAPY: BALANCING CURRENTS OF ENERGY

Polarity is the law of opposites in their finer attraction from centre to centre. Unity is the merging of these currents into one Essence. Creation brings forth opposites by its centrifugal force, like a fountain spray of manifestation flowing out to the limits of the cosmos and of each pattern unit.[1]

—RANDOLPH STONE, D.C., D.O., N.D.

WHAT IS POLARITY THERAPY?

Polarity Therapy is a healing approach to restoring energetic balance to the mind and body. Like other practices that heal with energy, it is based on the principle that a life force surrounds and permeates the physical body. Illness is a sign of imbalance in this flow of energy. Polarity Therapy aims to restore harmony through four interrelated therapeutic methods: gentle hands-on bodywork; counseling on diet and nutrition; guidance in a series of exercises called Polarity yoga; and psychological counseling that emphasizes the importance of positive thinking.

If Polarity Therapy seems eclectic in both its goals and the resources it uses to achieve them, that's because it is. John Beaulieu, director of the Polarity Wellness Center in New York City, explains: "Polarity Therapy is the great integrator, drawing many healing modes together within an energetic framework."

THE ORIGINS OF POLARITY THERAPY

Polarity Therapy was developed in the mid-1900s by Randolph Stone, D.C., D.O., N.D. (1890–1981). Born in Vienna, at the age of eleven Dr. Stone immigrated with his family to the United States. He became a chiropractor, osteopathic physician, and naturopath. Dr. Stone held a deep interest in the healing traditions of all cultures, and he traveled the world to discover what elements these traditions held in common. This led him to study traditional Chinese medicine and herbal remedies, the Hindu Ayurvedic healing tradition, and Middle Eastern medicine and spiritualism, including Egyptian and hermetic cabalistic teachings. The results of Dr. Stone's studies are embodied in the theory and techniques of Polarity Therapy. This represents a rich blend of the Western tradition of structural body manipulation that Dr. Stone had mastered as a chiropractor and osteopath and the Eastern tradition of energetic work, particularly Chinese and East Indian, that he learned through his many travels and further study. It is fitting to conclude the presentation of bodywork practices with Polarity Therapy as it represents a synthesis of Western, Eastern, structural, and energetic approaches to healing.

Polarity Therapy is at its core an energetic healing modality. At the heart of diverse traditions throughout the world, Dr. Stone discovered, certain universal healing principles were at work: Every individual is animated by a universal life force energy. Blockages in the circulation of this energy lead to disease and illness. Movement is life; stagnation is death. Our degree of health is determined by the relative freedom in the movement of vital energy.

While Dr. Stone was deeply influenced by the Chinese concepts of ch'i and yin and yang, the theory upon which his work is based is derived more directly from the Hindu tradition of healing known as Ayurveda. Meaning "the science of life," Ayurveda stems from the teachings contained in the *Vedas,* the ancient holy books of India. Dating back some five thousand years, Ayurvedic medicine is considered the earliest system of health care based upon scientific principles. With Eastern theory, Dr. Stone integrated his knowledge of Western anatomy, physiology, and structural manipulation to develop the bodywork techniques used in a Polarity session. Drawing upon his background as a naturopath and natural healer, he offered dietary and exercise recommendations. The principles for these are derived mainly from Vedic literature and the Indian tradition of yoga postures. The bulk of Dr. Stone's extensive writings, which form the basis for Polarity Therapy, were written between 1948 and 1970.

When Dr. Stone retired in 1973, he appointed Pierre Pannetier (1914–1984) as his successor. As the leader of Polarity Therapy, Pannetier taught seminars all over the United States and Canada and treated a wide variety of clients in his own Polarity Therapy center in California. Since Pannetier's death, Polarity Therapy has been taught by a number of his students, who in 1985 formed the American Polarity Therapy Association (APTA).

Dr. Stone left behind an extensive body of writings. Even the greatest teachers and advocates of his work are quick to admit that these can be dense and at times downright contradictory and confusing. This has left his work open to broad interpretation, with the result that practitioners of Polarity Therapy may vary widely in their implementation of Dr. Stone's work as well as in the principles that they tend to emphasize. For instance, some practitioners use gentle touch while others use deeper pressure; some emphasize diet and psychological counseling while others focus primarily on bodywork.

THE THEORY UNDERLYING POLARITY THERAPY

The Ayurvedic tradition views all life as emanating from one single source of energy known as Brahman. Energy flows outward in a positive movement from a neutral source and back inward, in a negative contraction. (Quantum physicists have corroborated this dynamic at the subatomic level with an atom consisting of positively charged protons, negatively charged electrons, and neutral neutrons.) All nature manifests a polarity between positive and negative charges with an intermediate neutral area. All energy, whether positive or negative, is neither good nor bad. Energy simply is.

Dr. Stone maintained that a dynamic relationship of polar charge characterizes every level of organization, both animate and inanimate, in the universe. In the case of the human being, for instance, the head represents a positive pole, the feet a negative pole. Between the two, there are various zones of negative and positive charge throughout the body. Life energy pulsates out from its source in its positive, expansive phase and back in toward the source in its negative, contractive phase. This pulsation between two oppositely charged poles forms the basis of life. Dr. Stone called this pulsation the Polarity Principle.[2] The art of Polarity Therapy lies in balancing the rhythmic flow of energy between poles of positive and negative charge in the body.

Dr. Stone believed that vital life energy permeates the universe in unseen, subtle energetic currents that comprise the electromagnetic fields that surround us. These currents envelop us in a three-dimensional interplay like the currents of the ocean, intersecting and interacting in the dynamic dance of life. Energy achieves material expression within our physical bodies. In common with Eastern thinkers, Dr. Stone maintained that we are a microcosm of the greater macrocosm, which he encapsulated in the maxims "As above, so below" and "As within, so without."[3]

Dr. Stone believed that the original energy of the universe further expresses itself through differentiation into the Ayurvedic system of five elements. These elements are ether, air, fire, water, and earth. They are correlated with the lower five of the seven energy centers known as chakras in the Eastern metaphysical tradition. Subtle energy enters the body through the sixth, or brow, chakra located in the middle of the forehead in the area referred to as the third eye. It assumes increasingly dense material form as it descends lower in the body, passing through each successive chakra, or energy center. Each of the lower five chakras through which it passes is associated with one of the five elements. Each element is associated with emotions, mental states of consciousness and attitudes, physical organs and body functions, and even types of food. The five elements are interrelated in a dynamic system. This system provides a comprehensive and elegant representation of man's relation to the cosmos at large. Anyone interested in learning more about this fascinating system is encouraged to consult Franklyn Sills's excellent account in *The Polarity Process.*

Energy manifests in the body in three forms. The first and most subtle is the energy that flows through the chakras. As this energy becomes denser, it next condenses into the energy associated with the nervous system. The nervous system then acts as a kind of intermediary in directing this energy to its final and most material manifestation as the physical body with all its organs, muscles, and bones. Interconnecting currents of energy flow through the body, weaving a three-dimensional field. Some currents move in spiral formations while others intersect horizontally or longitudinally. Dr. Stone described this network as the "wireless anatomy of man." Blockage in any of these currents can cause disturbances that interrupt balanced functioning and lay the groundwork for illness and disease. By balancing the energy currents, the Polarity Therapist facilitates the free-flowing movement essential to health and well-being.

THE TYPICAL FORMAT OF A POLARITY THERAPY SESSION

The Polarity Therapist has at her disposal a variety of means to balance energy. First and foremost is bodywork.

A Polarity bodywork session typically lasts thirty to ninety minutes. The client lies on a padded massage table, on either his stomach or his back. The client is dressed in underwear or additional clothing. The practitioner drapes the client with a sheet. No lotion or oil is used.

Using both hands, the Polarity Therapist uses a series of gentle to vigorous holding, rocking, and vibrating movements to balance energy throughout the body. A Polarity Therapist draws on a repertoire of three types of touch whose names are derived from the Ayurvedic tradition. Rajasic touch is stimulating and can be gentle or deep; sattvic touch is a balancing, light touch; and tamasic touch is deep and dispersing. Polarity sessions utilizing sattvic touch can feel so light that clients may barely be aware of any movement or pressure—until they get up from the table, that is, and realize how relaxed or energized they are. At the other extreme, a tamasic touch used by a practitioner to penetrate deep into body tissue so as to effect releases of congested energy might feel painful. In addition, there may be some muscle soreness afterward.

Hands-on touch is used to harmonize the positive and negative charges of energy in the body. The practitioner's hands act as a kind of magnetic transmitter of energy to stimulate and amplify the client's own energy. A beginning practitioner frequently uses a protocol of twenty-two different hand positions to provide a complete Polarity session. Some of these positions are derived from CranioSacral Therapy.

As a practitioner gains in experience, she treats more intuitively. She uses technique as a starting point, but trusts her feeling for energy itself. She often finds herself drawn to areas of blocked energy and focuses on releasing them. As in nearly all bodywork, the loving intentionality of the practitioner to effect healing is a prime ingredient in Polarity Therapy. Beverly Kitts, a Polarity practitioner, reinforces this: "The foremost principle espoused in Polarity Therapy is the importance of working with love. Pannetier used to say that love was the most vital element of the whole session. He would say, 'If you don't know what to do, just put your hands on the person and love them.'"[4]

Polarity Therapy is self-empowering. The practitioner educates the client in how better to take care of himself. In addition to bodywork, the Polarity Therapist may offer advice on proper diet, which can be used to cleanse the body of harmful toxins and help build health by establishing a balanced internal chemical environment. Dr. Stone believed that food possesses energetic qualities. Because the quality of each type of food is related to one of the five elements, eating certain types of food can help redress energetic imbalances. Often, in the initial stage of treatment, a client undertakes a cleansing diet. He begins the day with a drink called a liver flush, composed of olive oil, lemon, citrus juice, and garlic, followed by cleansing teas throughout the day. Gradually, raw fruits and vegetables are added to build health. In general, the diet recommended by Dr. Stone is a vegetarian diet, which forms the basis of nutrition in the Ayurvedic tradition.

Between sessions, a client may be given exercises to do, referred to as Polarity yoga or Polarenergetics. Originally, these exercises were drawn from traditional yoga practice, but over time practitioners have developed or added their own exercises. These exercises, which involve squats and various stretches, are often accompanied by deep breathing, rhythmic movements, and vocalization of the grunt sound "Ha!"—all designed to release restrictions and encourage the free flow of energy.

Finally, some Polarity Therapists may provide counseling as Polarity theory views the mind and body as one. Emphasis is placed on positive thinking, which is considered essential to promoting sound health. Deepak Chopra, who was trained in both Western and Ayurvedic medicine and is an authority on bridging the gap between Western and Eastern approaches to healing, echoes this underlying attitude in his belief that happy thoughts make happy cells.[5]

Counseling is also important because releases in the physical body may sometimes be accompanied by psychological and emotional releases. Traditionally, Polarity Therapists receive some type of training in psychological counseling, such as Gestalt therapy, although the level of this training, as well as individual skill, varies widely.

THE EXPERIENCE: MY ENERGY CURRENTS GET BALANCED

I arrive at the office of Reese Williams, a registered Polarity practitioner, to experience a Polarity treatment. In addition to maintaining a private practice, he offers a series of courses to train and certify other Polarity practitioners. Reese, who is a native Californian with a background in art, literature, mythology, and the healing arts, has been a student and practitioner of Polarity Therapy for more than ten years. He came highly recommended to me by my friend Freda, who is also a colleague. (Freda and I both trained with the same shiatsu master.)

Reese's office is a spacious loft suite in a lower Manhattan commercial building. A receptionist greets me warmly when I arrive. Because I am a few minutes early, I wait for Reese in a large, open, classroom space painted starkly, serenely white; its gray carpeted floor is accented with a colorful pastel Oriental carpet. The sun streams through windows tinted with the warm amber glow of a late Indian summer afternoon while the soothing smell of sandalwood incense lulls my senses.

Reese comes out to greet me. He is average height and is dressed casually in a blue Shetland sweater, khaki trousers, and sneakers. His slightly graying hair, cut short, frames an open and bright face, which radiates peace, calm, and gentleness. Reese's manner is low-key and caring; it is easy for me to warm to him.

He escorts me into his studio. It is a small but comfortable office with a padded massage table standing in the center, two large quartz crystals arranged beneath it. Two chairs occupy the farther end of the room. His workspace is decorated with framed prints of East Indian motifs, and potted plants abound.

To begin the session, Reese invites me to sit down as he joins me to ask a few questions. He asks me why I have come. How am I feeling, both physically and emotionally? What can he do to help me?

I explain that I am writing a book and would like to experience a Polarity session. I tell Reese I tend to carry my tension in my back and shoulders, although they're feeling okay today. Emotionally, I'm also feeling pretty good. I'm finishing the last chapter of the book and I feel relief, pride, and exhilaration at completing the first draft of the manuscript as well as excitement at the prospect of freeing my time to entertain new projects and pursuits.

I, in turn, ask Reese for a little information. In particular, I ask if his sessions incorporate primarily bodywork or other aspects of Polarity as well, such as diet, exercise, and counseling.

In response, Reese shares a little of the history of the development of Polarity Therapy with me. "Originally, when he taught, Dr. Stone emphasized theory and principle in his teaching. This means that practitioners interpret his work in many ways, and the nature of a Polarity session can vary a great deal according to the practitioner you consult."

As a general rule, most practitioners emphasize the bodywork aspect of Polarity. Reese explains that he primarily uses bodywork with some counseling; other practitioners, however, particularly those who come to Polarity Therapy with backgrounds in naturopathy or natural healing methods, often do incorporate more guidance on diet and exercise in their work.

Having exchanged this preliminary information, Reese asks me to remove my shoes and socks, then lie down, face up, on the massage table. I remain dressed in my loose-fitting sweatpants, T-shirt, and sweatshirt. Reese places a light sheet over my body, covering me, from my ankles to my shoulders. He encourages me to let him know if I should become cool during the session.

Reese establishes his first physical contact with me by reading my right, then my left, pulse. To do this, he stands first at one side, then at the other, and lightly holds my wrist with his fingers. He is feeling for rhythm, amplitude, and strength of a number of discrete pulsations, which reflect the subtle flow of energy through the body. These will help draw his attention to areas of potential imbalance. In my case, he notes that there may be issues going on regarding the liver, spleen, and heart, although this is only a preliminary feeling. The rest of the session will provide more information.

"I think of the practitioner as a kind of mirror," Reese confides. "I believe that health is the free flow of energy. Part of what I do is become aware of areas of holding where energy is not flowing so freely. By focusing my attention there, I can become like a mirror, allowing the client, sometimes on a very subtle, even unconscious level, to become aware of that imbalance and to change the pattern to greater flow, if he so chooses."

Reese then seats himself comfortably on a chair at the head of the table. He cradles his hands gently, lightly, unobtrusively around the base of my skull. I can feel the energy throughout my whole body coming to life—my hip feels as though it is opening, and my legs, particularly my calves, vibrate with a heightened sense of awareness and aliveness. Reese's touch is very light. He explains that he is "just kind of hanging out," listening to my cranial rhythm and getting a feel for my energy.

He explains that Polarity practitioners weave a session based on the use of a repertoire of three qualities of touch. The practitioner's intention as well as the depth of an energy blockage determine which type of touch is used. Gentle, or sattvic touch, like the kind Reese is using now, is used when the practitioner wants to listen and gather information or when an energy blockage is slight. Tamasic, or deep touch, is used to stimulate or when an energy disturbance is more deeply embedded. Rajasic, or moderate touch, is used as a middle ground in between the two.

Having assessed my cranial rhythm and pulse, much as a CranioSacral practitioner might do, Reese feels for constriction in the soft tissue surrounding the base of my skull at the junction of the occiput and the upper vertebrae of the neck. He then uses a rajasic touch to stretch and free the muscles as he found a moderate amount of tension there. I feel the muscles in my neck relaxing as I become particularly aware of tension I am holding on my right side.

Reese stands up and moves down the table to work on my torso. He places the fingers of his hands one at the top of my pubic bone, the other at the bottom of my breastbone. His touch is again rajasic; it feels firm and moderately deep; it is neither light nor painfully intrusive either. He is selecting areas in such a way that by holding two points simultaneously he can balance the overall flow of energy. He continues to hold various areas of my torso and arms, using both hands to make connections between two points. This aspect of the work strikes me as particularly unique, because rather than emphasizing one problem area or point of tension, the focus is on balance and connecting whole energetic areas of the body with one another. I find this both unifying and energizing; a feeling of release and openness spreads not only in the areas that lie between his two hands, but also in the adjoining areas that radiate from them. I also feel my breath growing longer and deeper; my sinuses open, and my nose begins to run a little. I become aware that my nose had been stuffed up without my having been conscious of it.

Reese places one hand on my right shoulder and the other on my left hip. He gently rolls the hand on my hip back and forth, which initiates a rocking movement in my hip. It is a pleasurable, novel sensation. It is more than just a jostling or compression stroke used in other practices like Swedish massage or shiatsu to open up an area before deeper work. Rather, this stroke seems to be an end in itself, designed to awaken a whole region of the body and not just a particular muscle or point. I am reminded of friction strokes in Swedish massage, which move one layer of tissue over another, with the difference that here I feel as though whole planes of energy are being rolled about. I experience this rocking as a vibration that penetrates to the inner core of my tissue, and then pulsates outward with vibrant life.

Reese explains that he is helping to unwind the tension that is pulling between my shoulder and hip, and passing through my liver in its line of torque. He chose this rocking motion because it is associated with the water element, which he felt would help this area to expand and open.

Reese proceeds to work on my shoulders and upper back. He holds the fingers of one hand under the border of my right shoulder blade (an area that always seems a special treasure trove of hidden tension) and with his other hand he rotates my right arm in a slow circle over my head. The pressure of his touch is stronger; the area feels tender, bordering on painful. This is tamasic touch: Reese is approaching a tense area with an equal measure of resistance. As he holds his fingers under my shoulder for a few minutes, I feel my shoulder and back opening up. When he repeats this sequence on my left side, I feel a complete opening.

Reese moves to the foot of the table, where he pulls gently on the toes of my right foot and presses their tips. He places the fingers of one hand around my ankle, pressing firmly on the middle of both the inside and outside depressions in the middle of my heel. The touch is strong, slightly painful; again, this is tamasic touch. Not so much because this area is tense, but because it needs stimulating, and tamasic touch can be deeply stimulating. The points Reese is holding are associated with the water element. He stimulates them in order to support the flow of energy all the way to my feet and also because he feels my water element could use a little boost.

Reese returns to my torso and positions one hand lightly over the middle of my chest; his other hand, mirroring it, supports the middle of my back. He holds gently for several minutes, seemingly motionless. I can feel my heart, how tense the area around it feels, how much I have been holding there—sadness from my childhood; compassion and grief for the problems of my clients, some of whom are dying; how good it feels for this area to be touched—and how it seems to open up merely by virtue of the presence of a caring touch.

As if understanding the feelings I'm experiencing, Reese tells me that he felt my heart was very active at the beginning of the session and represented an area of possible concern. My heart has calmed down and is much more relaxed and balanced now. As further counseling, Reese explains to me that I have a tendency toward the characteristics of the air element, which predisposes me to holding tension in my upper body. Since the air element is associated with mental activity, this is not surprising. It accounts in part for my attraction to writing and intellectual understanding. Reese can also relate to this because he shares this tendency. He counsels me that as much as I can do to exercise my upper body to remove tension will be of value to me. He also tells me that my future development will involve my incorporating more of the other elements, particularly water and earth, into my way of being as I come to ground myself more. This is, in fact, why he incorporated a lot of water element movements into my treatment.

Do I understand what Reese is saying? To my rational mind, some of his explanation seems a little vague because I'm not conversant in the system that forms the theoretical construct for his method of evaluation. Yet I am willing to trust enough to believe that within this system it does make sense, just as I trust that two foreigners conversing on the street corner in a language I don't understand are making sense to one another.

On a deeper, intuitive level, I feel as though Reese has read my mind—or should I say body/mind? I feel as though I have spent the last year exercising my mind in doing the research, study, and reflection needed to write this book. I am excited about the prospect of entering the next phase of my work—having the time to practice all of the wonderful techniques and theories I've learned, to ground in day-to-day experience the mind-expanding ideas I've been acquiring.

Reese returns to my head. Again he cradles its base. While I've been chatting with him throughout the session, asking the questions I felt a good investigator ought to ask, I've completely surrendered to his touch. I drift, afloat in a place of quiet stillness.

As my analytic mind begins to relinquish its grasping to rationally understand everything that's happening, I become profoundly aware of something that is so obvious it has eluded me all this time, something I knew once but forgot along the way: Beyond the technique, there is the touch.

No matter how much we may try to intellectually understand and define techniques, strokes, and modalities, in the end, the body/mind surrenders in awe and amazement to the healing and inscrutable power of caring touch. When you experience this power, you know it. It is real and immediate. This is a knowing on the deepest level; it is not a thinking or a believing based on what others have reported. It is an undeniably palpable experience.

Reese, like the other gifted healers presented in this book, has the gift of touch. I am no longer aware of any particular stroke or manipulation he is ministering. I am silent, calm, blissful. Waves of violet color, which I associate with deep healing harmony, wash across the inner eye of my mind. I luxuriate in the realm of peace and wholeness that is my birthright.

I am aware in the very core of my being that the process of healing seems to flow from a mysterious, apparently unfathomable yet purposeful, orderly, and dynamic flow of energy. I rise from Reese's table and return to the reception area. As if to underscore this insight into the mystery of healing, there, waiting to see Reese next, is my friend Freda, whom I have not seen or spoken with for months.

As I greet Freda fondly, I am reminded of the words of Ohashi, our mutual shiatsu master. In characteristically Eastern terms, he had described to us the unknowable quality of the power that informs healing touch communication: "By accident, you and I meet and come together. By accident, we exchange touch with one another. By accident, you may get better. By accident, you may get worse."

Did Freda and I meet Ohashi, and one another, by accident? Did she refer Reese to me by accident? Did we meet today during this my only visit to Reese by accident? Can two fields of energy continue to influence one another, even when placed at opposite ends of a city of seven million people? I muse to myself as I reenter the bustling pace of rush-hour New York City.

These questions seem somehow to flow perfectly in synch with my experience of polarity Therapy, which deals with the realm of subtle energy flows that interweave and interconnect all of creation.

On what better note to end the experiential accounts in this book than to pose the provocative and unanswerable questions that spur me on in my continuing exploration of the unending possibilities afforded by the rich world of bodywork?

THE BENEFITS OF POLARITY THERAPY

"Polarity Therapy deals with energetic imbalances, not physical diseases," says Phil Young, a Polarity Therapy teacher and author of *The Art of Polarity Therapy*.[6] Proponents maintain that by balancing energy on the subtle plane before imbalance manifests on the physical plane, they can help to prevent the onset of physical illness and disease. In the case of physical illness, eradicating energy blockages and balancing energy can allow the body's self-healing mechanisms to assert themselves. Phil Young further explains: "Our energy system is self-regulating and will manage to rebalance itself very well as long as you simply maintain an overall impetus."[7]

Polarity Therapists report success in alleviating the pain and discomfort associated with both acute and chronic conditions, including low back pain; muscle cramps; migraine headaches; digestive disorders, such as indigestion and constipation; and emotional problems related to stress and tension.

Recipients of Polarity Therapy often report a sense of deep relaxation plus a heightened feeling of energy and vitality following a session. They may also feel better balanced emotionally and mentally.

CONTRAINDICATIONS TO POLARITY THERAPY

Because Polarity Therapy has at its disposal such a wide range of techniques, including gentle touch, dietary suggestions, exercises, and counseling, a therapist should be able to offer support for nearly any problem. However, because

Polarity Therapy can involve body manipulation, anyone with a serious medical condition should consult a physician before treatment.

BACKGROUND AND TRAINING OF PRACTITIONERS

The American Polarity Therapy Association (APTA) was established to set standards for the practice of Polarity Therapy and requires a minimum of 155 hours of training for associate practitioner and 520 hours for registered practitioner, for 675 hours total. As with all types of bodywork, check the background of any practitioner you're thinking of consulting.

FOR FURTHER INFORMATION

The APTA is the primary professional organization of Polarity practitioners in the United States. It has established a code of ethics for practitioners and set standards for registration, and it sponsors educational conferences in alternating years. Additionally, it serves as a clearinghouse for information on Polarity Therapy, providing educational material and a listing of schools offering Polarity training, and maintaining a registry of practitioners. You can contact the APTA at:

American Polarity Therapy Association
P.O. Box 19858
Boulder, CO 80308
Tel: (303) 545-2080
Fax: (303) 545-2161
Website: www.polaritytherapy.org
E-mail: hq@polaritytherapy.org

SUGGESTED FURTHER READING

I am indebted to the following books, which formed the basis for the material presented in this chapter:

Franklyn Sills, *The Polarity Process: Energy as a Healing Art* (Berkeley, CA: North Atlantic Books, 2002). This is an excellent introduction by a master Polarity teacher. It synthesizes the principles of Polarity Therapy with various systems of Eastern thought as well as current quantum physics theory.

Phil Young, *The Art of Polarity Therapy: A Practitioner's Perspective* (Dorset, England: Prism Press, 2000). Particularly recommended for practitioners of bodywork, this book contains insight into the practice of bodywork as well as an introduction to Polarity Therapy.

Dr. Stone's collected writings are available from CRSC Publications:

Randolph Stone, D.C., D.O., N.D., *Polarity Therapy: The Complete Collected Works on This Revolutionary Healing Art by the Originator of the·System* (2 volumes) (Sebastopol, CA: CRCS Publications, 1986).

The following are written by Polarity practitioners:

John Beaulieu, N.D., *Polarity Therapy Workbook* (New York: BioSonic Enterprises Ltd., 1994). This book by a skilled teacher presents clear, detailed information on the protocol of a Polarity Therapy session, complete with helpful photographs.

Beverly Kitts, "Polarity Therapy," *in Healing Massage Techniques: Holistic, Classic, and Emerging Methods* (East Norwalk, CT: Appleton & Lange, 1988). This is a brief, heartfelt introduction to Polarity Therapy.

PART VI

SUPPLEMENTAL INFORMATION: SIMPLE TOOLS

In the following section, you'll find helpful information to supplement your knowledge of the world of massage and bodywork.

CHAPTER 17

THE SPA EXPERIENCE: PAMPERING YOURSELF WHILE YOUR BODY WORKS

Health requires this relaxation, this aimless life.
This life in the present.[1]

—HENRY DAVID THOREAU

THE SPA EXPERIENCE: TOTAL IMMERSION

If you've become hooked on the idea of bodywork and would like to experience a variety of bodywork modalities, pamper yourself, and get away from it all at the same time, you might want to consider visiting a spa resort. More and more people are discovering the healthy joys of an escape that can combine massage, fitness exercise, healthy eating, and perhaps some instruction in relaxation and other self-healing techniques. Many spas are located in breathtaking physical settings, near water, woods, or mountains, with luxurious, attractive state-of-the-art fitness facilities. Complementing bodywork with an extended stay in a harmonious setting can be conducive to balancing body and mind. It can help you achieve a level of relaxation and wholeness beyond that of a single bodywork session.

With increasing interest in holistic and preventive health care, the appeal of spas has grown dramatically in recent years. According to the International SPA Association (ISPA) 2004 Spa Industry Study, there are estimated to be more than 12,000 spas throughout the United States and over 2,000 in Canada. Spas offer a variety of programs in diverse geographical settings.

Recognizing the key role played by stress in contributing to illness, spas have designed environments and programs specifically geared to destress you. Gone are the days of the fat farm pampering overweight socialites. The goal of today's spas is to make you feel beautiful on the inside as well as on the outside.

Spas range widely in their programs and offerings. Chances are you can find a program with an emphasis in an area of particular interest to you. Some, like the spa I visited in Tuscany, Spa'Deus, offer fitness classes and healthy cuisine (that is, low caloric, low fat, no caffeine, and no alcohol) along with bodywork treatments. Others can indulge your penchant for rich food and alcohol while providing luxuriously relaxing body treatments. Some retreat centers provide a spiritual framework where you can enjoy the gift of touch. Also gaining in popularity are urban spas, which offer programs from an hour of massage with spa amenities to a full day of bodywork and beauty treatments.

ORGANIZATIONS THAT SPECIALIZE IN SPA VACATIONS

The number of spas and the programs they offer is constantly expanding.

The following travel agency specializes in spa vacations:

Spa Trek Travel
475 Park Avenue South, 34th Floor
New York, NY 10016
Tel: (800) 272-3480 or (212) 717-7666
Fax: (212) 717-7668
Website: www.spatrek.com
E-mail: info@spatrek.com

While not a travel agency, the following organization is a valuable source of information on spas and spa vacations:

Spa Finder
257 Park Avenue South, 10th Floor
New York, NY 10010
Tel: (800) ALL-SPAS (255-7727) or (212) 924-6800
Fax: (212) 924-7240
Website: www.spafinder.com
E-mail: info@spafinder.com

Spa Finder publishes *The Luxury SpaFinder Magazine* and an annual Spa Finder *Worldwide Directory of Spas.*

Hannelore Levy is the founder and executive director of two trade organizations that can provide further information on day spas and medical spas:

The Day Spa Association
310-17th Street
Union City, NJ 07087
Tel: (201) 865-2065
Fax: (201) 865-3961
Website: www.dayspaassociation.com
E-mail: info@dayspaassociation.com

The International Medical Spa Association
310-17th Street
Union City, NJ 07087
Tel: (201) 865-2065
Fax: (201) 865-3961
Website: www.medicalspaassociation.org
E-mail: info@medicalspaassociation.org

The International SPA Association (ISPA) is the leading professional organization and voice of the spa industry. Founded in 1991, ISPA's membership is comprised of approximately 2,000 health and wellness facilities and providers from nearly seventy countries. ISPA strives to advance the professionalism of the spa industry by providing educational and networking opportunities, to promote the value of the spa experience to society, and to be the authoritative voice of the spa industry:

International SPA Association (ISPA)
2365 Harrodsburg Road, Suite A325
Lexington, KY 40504
Tel: (888) 651-ISPA (651-4772) or (859) 226-4326 (international)
Fax: (859) 226-4445
Website: www.experienceispa.com & www.ispaconference.com
E-mail: ispa@ispastaff.com

SUGGESTED FURTHER READING

Bernard Burt and Pamela Price, *100 Best Spas of the World* (Guilford, CT: Globe Pequot, 2003). Written by a team of award-winning travel writers, this is a well-written and handsomely illustrated guidebook to the world's best spas.

Christine Swiac, Editor, *Fodor's Healthy Escapes: 288 Spas, Resorts & Retreats Where You Can Relax, Recharge, Get Fit & Get Away From It All* (New York: Random House, 2003). This is a comprehensive guide to hundreds of spas throughout the United States, Canada, Mexico, and the Caribbean. It's updated regularly and features the concise, easy-to-follow format that characterizes the *Fodor* series of travel guides.

Zagat Top U.S. Hotels, Resorts & Spas (New York, Zagat Survey, updated annually).

Bernard Burt publishes a quarterly spa newsletter, and each issue contains information on bodywork. For further information, contact:

Bernard Burt's SpaGoer Newsletter
2400 Virginia Avenue, C-715
Washington, DC 20037
Fax: (202) 331-0036
Website: www.SpaGoer.com

CHAPTER 18

RESOURCES FOR
FURTHER EXPLORATION

Networking: Holistic Learning Centers

One of the best ways to learn more about, and experience, massage and bodywork is to enroll in a short course or workshop in a bodywork modality that appeals to you. A network of holistic learning centers is emerging across the country. Their mission is to provide education and experience in a wide spectrum of approaches to the body and mind. Since complementary healing practices are typically not included in the curriculum of many conventional educational institutions, these learning centers provide an opportunity for further exploration.

Most learning networks are nonprofit organizations, often manned by volunteers like you. The cost of taking a course, which could range from an introductory lecture to a weekend workshop or longer course, is generally kept as low as possible. Many networks are willing to consider providing scholarships to those in financial hardship and/or provide credit toward courses for work performed at the center under work-study programs.

Holistic learning centers are a valuable resource for learning more about all kinds of interesting approaches to healing. Many centers offer courses in massage and bodywork practices. In addition to supplying the learning experience of the course itself, they can provide a supportive environment for meeting other people with similar interests. A number of networks also offer individual bodywork sessions at a reasonable fee.

The learning centers that follow are presented because they offer courses in several types of bodywork and body awareness during their seasons of operation. The Glossary contains descriptions of many bodywork practices that are not described in detail in the text and whose meaning may be unclear. For other resources in your area, you might check with your local learning exchange, massage school, health food store, or metaphysical bookstore. For those of you interested in pursuing professional training, the American Massage Therapy

Association (AMTA) and Associated Bodywork & Massage Professionals (ABMP) can provide information on professional training programs. Their publications, as well as *Massage* magazine, also present helpful resource information. See Resources for Further Reading later in this chapter for addresses, phone numbers, and websites.

UNITED STATES

Esalen Institute
55500 Highway 1
Big Sur, CA 93920-9616
Tel: (831) 667-3000 (general information)
or (831) 667-3005 (reservations)
Fax: (831) 667-2724 (exclusively for reservations)
Website: www.esalen.org
E-mail: info@esalen.org

Purpose: to encourage work in the humanities and sciences that promotes human values and potentials. Its activities consist of public seminars, residential work-study programs, invitational conferences, research, and semiautonomous projects.
Location: once the home of a Native American tribe known as the Esalen, situated on a property that boasts hot springs and a commanding view of the Pacific Ocean. Located 300 miles north of Los Angeles and 175 miles south of San Francisco.
Bodywork courses/services: As a leader in the human potential movement, Esalen fostered the development of many well-known bodywork therapies as well as pioneered its own Esalen massage. Course offerings have included Esalen massage, Feldenkrais Method, massage in African tradition, Polarity Therapy, pressure-point massage, Rubenfeld Synergy, sports massage, Swedish massage, and Zero Balancing. Individual bodywork sessions available.
Accommodations: available; limited access for disabled; nudity (optional) in hot springs, swimming pool, and massage area

Himalayan Institute
952 Bethany Turnpike
Honesdale, PA 18431-9706
Tel: (800) 822-4547 or (570) 253-5551
Fax: (570) 253-9078
Website: www.himalayaninstitute.org
E-mail: info@himalayaninstitute. org

Purpose: founded by Sri Swami Rama of the Himalayas in 1971 to help individuals develop themselves physically, mentally, and spiritually as well as contribute to the transformation of society

Location: 400-acre campus in Pocono Mountains in northeastern Pennsylvania; three hours by car from New York City, and four hours from Philadelphia

Bodywork courses/services: emphasizes yoga science as a way of life with classes in Ayurveda, biofeedback, diet, homeopathy, movement yoga, and other courses in healing. Offers individual holistic medical services, therapeutic massage, and biofeedback by appointment as well as pancha karma and Ayurvedic rejuvenation programs.

Special notes: publishes *Yoga International* magazine and has excellent mail-order book selection. Branches and affiliates throughout the United States, Canada, the Caribbean, Western Europe, and India.

Accommodations: available

Kripalu Center for Yoga & Health
P.O. Box 793
Lenox, MA 01240
Tel: (800) 741-7353 or (413) 448-3152 (international and local calls)
Fax: (413) 448-3384
Website: www.kripalu.org
E-mail: reserve@kripalu.org (for general questions or to request a catalog)

Purpose: Kripalu Center is a secular institution where people can come to discover what it means to be fully human and fully alive through a nonsectarian and nondogmatic approach to yoga. Kripalu is dedicated to the honest and unfettered inquiry into, and pursuit of, all philosophies, techniques, and approaches that produce thriving in the individual, the family, the institution, the business, the community, the society, and the planet—all at the same time. The mission is to promote the art and science of yoga as a foundation for a revitalized society.

Location: modern residential facility located in Lenox, Massachusetts, in the Berkshire Mountains

Bodywork courses/services: pioneered own form of massage, Kripalu Bodywork, which combines compassionate, intuitive touch with technical expertise. Offers 200- and 500-hour residential training in Kripalu Bodywork. Healing Arts center offers private sessions in full range of touch therapies, energy work, self-discovery consultations, face and body care, and Ayurvedic treatments.

Accommodations: simple, retreat-style housing

The Learning Annex/Open U, Inc.
706 North First Street
Minneapolis, MN 55401
Tel: (800) 872-6639 or (612) 349-9273
Fax: (612) 349-9247
Website: www.learningannex.com
E-mail: openu@aol.com

Purpose: for-profit noncredit teaching/learning center committed to empower-
ing adults to realize and share their potential; offers low-cost courses
Location: warehouse district of Minneapolis
Bodywork courses/services: courses have included back and neck massage,
chakra balancing, shiatsu, tai chi, and tune-up massage. Visit the Learning
Annex's website (www.learningannex.com) for programs in other cities.

Mount Madonna Center
445 Summit Road
Watsonville, CA 95076
Tel: (408) 847-0406
Fax: (408) 847-2683
Website: www.mountmadonna.org
E-mail: programs@mountmadonna.org

Purpose: Sponsored by the Hanuman Fellowship, Mount Madonna is a community designed to nurture the creative arts and health sciences within a context of spiritual growth.
Location: 355 mountaintop acres of redwood forest and grassland overlooking
Monterey Bay; one and a quarter hours from San Jose Airport and two hours
from San Francisco Airport; Greyhound bus service available to Watsonville or
Gilroy; taxi service from there to center
Bodywork courses/services: Kaya Kalpa Wellness Center features Ayurvedic
bodywork, as well as more traditional massage. Mount Madonna also offers a
variety of yoga programs. Individual massage and herbal steam bath sessions
available by appointment.
Accommodations: campground facilities and indoor accommodations available

New York Open Center, Inc.
83 Spring Street
New York, NY 10012
Tel: (212) 219-2527 (main number); (212) 274-1829 (Wellness Service Center)
Fax: (212) 219-1347
Website: www.opencenter.org
E-mail: info@opencenter.org

Purpose: nonprofit holistic learning center offering broad range of educational courses for the body, mind, and spirit. Its course selection is one of the largest in the country.
Location: New York City, historic SoHo district of lower Manhattan
Bodywork courses/services: courses have included the Alexander Technique, Ayurvedic lymphatic massage, body balancing, connective tissue massage, CranioSacral Therapy, Feldenkrais Method, Jin Shin Do Bodymind Acupressure, Phoenix Rising Yoga Therapy, Rubenfeld Synergy, shiatsu, Swedish massage, Therapeutic Touch, and Touch for Health. Private Wellness Service sessions available in CranioSacral Therapy, Jin Shin Do Bodymind Acupressure, Polarity Therapy, reflexology, shiatsu, and Swedish massage. Certification programs available in Polarity Therapy and reflexology.

Omega Institute for Holistic Studies
150 Lake Drive
Rhinebeck, NY 12572
Tel: (800) 944-1001 (registration) or (845) 266-4444
Fax: (845) 266-3769
Website: www.eomega.org
E-mail: registration@eomega.org

Purpose: nonprofit holistic learning center offering broad range of educational courses for the body, mind, and spirit
Location: converted summer camp located on eighty acres of rolling hills in Hudson Valley, a two-and-a-half-hour drive north of New York City. Offers shuttle service to New York City and neighboring public transportation. Omega has been described as a summer camp for adults.
Bodywork courses/services: courses have featured the Alexander Technique, body logic, couples massage, Feldenkrais Method, neuromuscular therapy, Rosen Method, somatic therapy (advanced), and Zero Balancing. Individual sessions offered in a variety of bodywork modalities.

Special notes: Rhinebeck campus operates May through October; offsite programs available throughout the year
Accommodations: available

Pumpkin Hollow Farm
1184 Route 11
Craryville, NY 12521
Tel: (877) 325-3583 or (518) 325-3583
Fax: (518) 325-5633
Website: www.pumpkinhollow.org
E-mail: pumpkin@taconic.net

Purpose: retreat center for the Theosophical Society offering a broad range of courses in metaphysics and healing. This is the place where Therapeutic Touch was born.
Location: rustic, residential retreat on 130 acres of open fields and variegated forest in Hudson Valley, two and a half hours by car from New York City
Bodywork courses/services: program emphasizes Therapeutic Touch, with all levels of instruction from beginner to teacher certification
Special notes: full season of operation is April through November; limited operation January to mid-March. Pets discouraged.
Accommodations: available

Wainwright House
260 Stuyvesant Avenue
Rye, NY 10580
Tel: (914) 967-6080
Fax: (914) 967-6114
Website: www.wainwright.org
E-mail: registrar@wainwright.org

Purpose: not-for-profit learning center dedicated to awakening consciousness in mind, body, and spirit
Location: three houses (main home is French provincial mansion) on five acres overlooking oceanfront of Long Island Sound, an hour north of New York City
Bodywork courses/services: recent catalog offers courses in Reiki, shiatsu, Swedish massage, Therapeutic Touch, and yoga
Accommodations: available

FOREIGN LEARNING CENTERS

Maybe you'd like to expand your knowledge of bodywork while you expand your knowledge of the world. The following overseas learning centers offer a broad range of courses and programs in bodywork and healing.

CANADA

Hollyhock Retreat Center
P.O. Box 127
Manson's Landing
Cortes Island, B.C.
Canada V0P 1K0
Tel: (800) 933-6339 or (250) 935-6576 (outside North America)
Fax: (250) 935-6424
Website: www.hollyhock.ca
E-mail: registration@hollyhock.ca

Purpose: to inspire, nourish, and support people who are making the world better. The Hollyhock experience includes organic garden, naturalist-guided activities, and morning yoga.
Location: southern tip of Cortes Island, between mainland British Columbia and Vancouver Island
Bodywork courses/services: A staff of experienced practitioners offers an array of massage, body care, and specialty bodywork. Hollyhock's program includes workshops on body disciplines and practices, as well as health and healing.
Special notes: season runs May through October
Accommodations: rooms and cabins situated throughout the grounds

GERMANY

Frankfurter Ring e.V.
Oeder Weg 43
60318 Frankfurt
Germany
Tel: (0) 69 51 15 55
Fax: (0) 69 51 22 20
Website: www.frankfurter-ring.org
E-mail: info@frankfurter-ring.org

Purpose: holistic education for life, offering broad range of courses in alternative healing, taught by instructors with strong backgrounds in advanced techniques

Location: Frankfurt, Germany; accessible to airport and train stations
Bodywork courses/services: Energy Psychology, Feldenkrais Method, kinesiology, Pilates, qigong, Taoist massage, and yoga
Special notes: offers personal counseling

GREAT BRITAIN (SCOTLAND)

Findhorn Foundation
The Park
Forres
Scotland IV36 3TZ
Tel: (0) 1309 690311
Fax: (0) 1309 691301
Website: www.findhorn.org
E-mail: enquiries@findhorn.org

Purpose: part of the Findhorn Community, a charitable trust and spiritual community
Location: a holistic community situated in the beautiful, remote seaside of northeast Scotland, 25 miles east of Inverness airport
Bodywork courses/services: offerings have included a varied program in body/mind healing arts: Alexander Technique; aromatherapy; breath, movement, and perception; CranioSacral Therapy; creative anatomy; Egyptian belly dancing; Reiki; shiatsu; and Unwinding the Body from Within
Accommodations: inexpensive bed and breakfasts are located nearby

GREECE AND THAILAND

Skyros Holistic Holidays (on the island of Skyros, Greece
    and Ko Samet, Thailand)
92 Prince of Wales Road
London NW5 3NE
Great Britain
Tel: (0) 20 7267 4424 or (0) 20 7284 3065 (24 hours)
Fax: (0) 20 7284 3063
Website: www.skyros.com
E-mail: office@skyros.com

Purpose: Skyros offers holiday programs in personal development, on the Greek Island of Skyros, through two holistic learning centers: Skyros Centre and Atsitsa; and in Thailand on Ko Samet Island. Skyros's philosophy is founded on the hope that it is possible to renew our connection with other people, the environment, our bodies, and ultimately our deepest selves; and faith in our ability to rediscover our sense of common purpose.

Location: Skyros Centre is located in a picturesque villa with magnificent views in the heart of the village of Skyros Island, a ten-minute walk from the Aegean Sea. Atsitsa is situated on the secluded Atsitsa Bay, surrounded by pine forests. Skyros Island is accessible from Athens by plane (Olympic Airways) or ferry. Courses in Ko Samet are offered in luxury-style hotels.

Bodywork courses/services: Alexander Technique, body/mind massage, holistic massage, Pilates exercise, reflexology, Reiki, Swedish massage, tai chi, and yoga in every session; in Ko Samet, Thailand, courses are offered at a luxury resort.

Special notes: season of operation in Greece is generally April through October; no pets; no children under five; limited access for disabled; season of operation in Thailand is during the winter months

Accommodations: in Skyros, specially constructed accommodations in Skyros village; in Atsitsa, cabins or rooms; in Thailand, luxury chalets

NATIONAL CERTIFICATION BOARD FOR THERAPEUTIC MASSAGE AND BODYWORK (NCBTMB)

The National Certification Board for Therapeutic Massage and Bodywork (NCBTMB) certifies massage and bodywork therapy practitioners based upon a minimum of 500 hours of formal training, which can be comprised of a combination of approved professional education and experience, plus successful completion of a nationally administered examination. It can furnish local referrals of practitioners it has certified, as well as provide information on its certification procedures. Certification by this board is voluntary and does not necessarily indicate that practitioners have met state and/or local credentialing requirements.

Beginning in 2005, the NCBTMB introduced two additional certifications in addition to that previously offered, for a total of three options: the current exam, the National Certification Exam for Therapeutic Massage and Bodywork (NCETMB); the National Certification Exam for Massage Therapy (NCETM), a therapeutic-massage only certification; and the NCMT-A, an advanced credential for massage therapists.

The NCBTMB produces three publications, two of which are hosted online: *Connection,* a publication targeted to certified practitioners; *InfoLine,* a publication targeted to schools; and *Approved Provider News,* a publication targeted to approved continuing-education providers. The NCBTMB website has a page that lists states that utilize/recognize the NCETMB either by statute or rule. It also lists states that do not currently regulate massage and bodywork, but wherein large cities and counties often utilize the NCETMB in their local ordinances. For further information, contact:

National Certification Board for Therapeutic Massage and Bodywork
1901 S. Myers Road, Suite 240
Oakbrook Terrace, IL 60181
Tel: (800) 296-0664 (customer service) or (630) 627-8000
Fax: (630) 627-1122
Website: www.ncbtmb.com
E-mail: info@ncbtmb.com

GRADUATE DEGREE PROGRAMS

The following institutions offer accredited postgraduate degree programs in somatic education (body-oriented psychotherapy):

California Institute of Integral Studies
1453 Mission Street
San Francisco, CA 94103
Tel: (415) 575-1000
Fax: (415) 575-1268
Website: www.ciis.edu
E-mail: admissions@ciis.edu (admissions and all academic programs)

An independent graduate school integrating the intellectual and spiritual insights of Western and Eastern traditions in study and practice. Offers master's and doctoral degree programs.

Naropa University
2130 Arapahoe Avenue
Boulder, CO 80302
Tel: (800) 772-6951 or (303) 444-0202
Fax: (303) 444-0410
www.naropa.edu
E-mail: admissions@naropa.edu

Naropa University is a private, nonprofit, non-sectarian liberal arts institution dedicated to advancing contemplative education. Contemplative education is an approach to learning that integrates the best of Eastern and Western educational traditions, helping students know themselves more deeply and engage constructively with others. Offers master's degree program in somatic psychology, with specializations in body psychotherapy and dance/movement therapy.

SUPPORT GROUPS

Many people turn to various forms of complementary health care when faced with life-challenging illnesses that orthodox medicine is unable to resolve. Consequently, many support organizations that have been set up to help people deal with such challenges provide bodywork services or have lists of referrals of low-cost providers that you or your loved ones might try if faced with such a situation. Consult your local community organizations for information.

The American Self-Help Clearinghouse serves as a source of information on national self-help groups and local self-help clearinghouses. To find or form a self-help group for stressful life problems, contact:

American Self-Help Clearinghouse
St. Clare's Hospital
25 Pocono Road
Denville, NJ 07834
Tel: (973) 326-6789
Website: www.selfhelpgroups.org
E-mail: asha@cybernex.net

RESOURCES FOR FURTHER READING

PERIODICALS

The following periodicals are related to massage and bodywork.
Massage Therapy Journal is published four times a year by the American Massage Therapy Association. In addition, the AMTA has an online monthly publication, *e-touch, a massage newsletter.* For further information contact:

The American Massage Therapy Association
500 Davis Street, Suite 900
Evanston, IL 60201-4695
Tel: (877) 905-2700 or (847) 864-0123
Fax: (847) 708-1178
Website: www.amtamassage.org
E-mail: info@amtamassage.org

Massage & Bodywork Quarterly is published six times a year by Associated Bodywork & Massage Professionals. Contact:

Associated Bodywork & Massage Professionals
1271 Sugarbrush Drive
Evergreen, CO 80439
Tel: (800) 458-2267 or (303) 674-8478

Fax: (800) 667-8260
Website: www.massageandbodywork.com
E-mail: expectmore@abmp.com

MASSAGE Magazine is an independent publication devoted to the field of massage and bodywork, in publication since 1985. Articles published in *MASSAGE Magazine* include in-depth technique articles, business tips, profiles of innovative therapists, and updates on developments in the field. *MASSAGE Magazine* appears six times a year. Address inquiries to:

MASSAGE Magazine
5150 Palm Valley Road, Suite 103
Ponte Vedra Beach, FL 32082
Tel: (800) 533-4263 or (904) 285-6020
Fax: (904) 285-9944
Website: www.massagemag.com
E-mail: kmenehan@massagemag.com

BOOK RETAILERS/BOOK PUBLISHERS

If you're interested in pursuing any of the suggested further reading in this book, the following two retail book companies have a wide selection of books on bodywork and complementary health practices. They can ship the books they carry.

East West Books (Affiliated with the Himalayan Institute)
78 Fifth Avenue
New York, NY 10011
Tel: (212) 243-5995
Fax: (212) 243-7591
Website: www.eastwestnyc.com
E-mail: info@eastwestnyc.com

Redwing Book Company
202 Bendix Street
Taos, NM 87571
Tel: (800) 873-3946 (United States), (888) 873-3947 (Canada),
  or (505) 758-7758 (worldwide)
Fax: (505) 758-7768
Website: www.redwingbooks.com
E-mail: info@redwingbooks.com

The following two companies regularly publish books of interest on bodywork:

Inner Traditions • Bear and Company
One Park Street
Rochester, VT 05767
Tel: (800) 246-8648 or (802) 767-3174
Fax: (802) 767-3726
Website: www.innertraditions.com
E-mail: info@innertraditions.com

In addition to publishing original books on bodywork and complementary health practices, Inner Traditions reprints a number of classic texts on bodywork that the original publishers let go out of print.

North Atlantic Books
1435A Fourth Street
Berkeley, CA 94710
Tel: (800) 337-2665 or (510) 559-8277
Fax: (510) 559-8279
Website: www.northatlanticbooks.com
E-mail: visit website for links to contact via e-mail

If you have difficulty locating any recommended books, you might also try contacting the corresponding professional bodywork association. Often, it carries books related to its practice.

PROFESSIONAL ASSOCIATIONS OF ADDITIONAL BODYWORK PRACTICES

Each chapter of this book contains information on professional associations that can provide you with further information on the individual practice profiled.

Following is a list of organizations that can give you information on other bodywork practices (see the Glossary for a description of these practices). In addition to information regarding training, books, audio- and videotapes, they can often supply practitioner referrals.

Applied Kinesiology/Energy Kinesiology

Topping International Institute, Inc.
2505 Cedarwood Avenue, Suite 3
Bellingham, WA 98225
Tel: (888) 783-2711 or (360) 647-2703
Fax: (360) 647-0164
Website: wwww.wellnesskinesiology.com
E-mail: topping@wellnesskinesiology.com

International College of Applied
   Kinesiology, U.S.A.
6405 Metcalf Avenue, Suite 503
Shawnee Mission, KS 66202-3929
Tel: (913) 384-5336
Fax: (913) 384-5112
Website: www.icakusa.com
E-mail: info@icakusa.com

Ayurveda

American Institute of Vedic Studies
P.O. Box 8357
Santa Fe, NM 87504-8357
Tel: (505) 983-9385
Website: www.vedanet.com
E-mail: info@vedanet.com

Ayurvedic Institute
P.O. Box 23445
Albuquerque, NM 87192-1445
Tel: (505) 291-9698
Fax: (505) 294-7572
Website: www.ayurveda.com
E-mail: wwerner@ayurveda.com

Himalayan Institute
952 Bethany Turnpike
Honesdale, PA 18431-9706
Tel: (800) 822-4547 or
   (570) 253-5551
Fax: (570) 253-9078
Website: www.himalayaninstitute.org
E-mail: info@himalayaninstitute.org

Energetic Healing
(other approaches to healing
  with energy)
Barbara Brennan School of Healing
500 N.E. Spanish River Boulevard,
  Suite 108
Boca Raton, FL 33431

Tel: (800) 924-2564 or
  (561) 620-8767
Fax: (561) 620-9028
Website: www.barbarabrennan.com
E-mail:
  bbsh.office@barbarabrennan.com

Laying on of Hands:
Rev. Rosalyn L. Bruyere
Healing Light Center Church
261 East Alegria Avenue, #12
Sierra Madre, CA 91024
Tel: (626) 306-2170
Fax: (626) 355-0996
Website: www.rosalynbruyere.org

Multi Incarnational Recall and
  Emotional Body Balancing:
The Light Institute of Galisteo
66 Avenida Vieja
Galisteo, NM 87540
Tel: (505) 466-1975
Fax: (505) 466-7217
Website: www.lightinstitute.com
E-mail: thelight@lightinstitute.com

Esalen Massage
Esalen Institute
55500 Highway 1
Big Sur, CA 93920-9616
Tel: (831) 667-3000
  (general information) or
  (831) 667-3005 (reservations)
Fax: (831) 667-2724
Website: www.esalen.org
E-mail: info@esalen.org

Hakomi for Bodyworkers

Hakomi Institute
P.O. Box 1873
Boulder, CO 80306
Tel: (888) 421-6699 or
     (303) 499-6699
Website: www.hakomiinstitute.com
E-mail: hakomihq@aol.com

Infant Massage

International Association of Infant
     Massage
1891 Goodyear Avenue, Suite 622
Ventura, CA 93003
Tel: (800) 248-5432 or
     (805) 644-8524
Fax: (805) 644-7699
Website: www.iaim-us.com
E-mail: iaim4us@aol.com

Jin Shin Jyutsu Physio-Philosophy

Jin Shin Jyutsu, Inc.
8719 East San Alberto Drive
Scottsdale, AZ 85258
Tel: (480) 998-9331
Fax: (480) 998-9335
Website: www.jinshinjyutsu.com
E-mail: info@jsjinc.com

KURED

Kurashova Institute
P.O. Box 6246
Rock Island, IL 61204
Tel: (800) 791-9248 or
     (309) 786-4888
Fax: (309) 786-8687
Website: www.kurashova.com
E-mail: info@kurashova.com

Lomilomi Massage

Hawaiian Lomilomi
P.O. Box 221
Captain Cook, HI 96704
Tel: (808) 323-2416
Website: www.hawaiian.net/~kea/
     aunty.html
E-mail: kea@hawaiian.net

Manual Lymph Drainage (MLD)

North American Vodder Association
     of Lymphatic Therapy (NAVALT)
833 Independence Drive
Longmont, CO 80501
Tel: (888) 462-8258 or
     (303) 702-0557
Fax: (303) 776-1891
Website: www.navalt.org
E-mail: info@navalt.org

Ortho-Bionomy

Society of Ortho-Bionomy
     International
5335 North Tacoma Street,
     Suite 21G
Indianapolis, IN 46220
Tel: (800) 809-3747 or
     (317) 536-0064
Fax: (317) 536-0065
Website: www.ortho-bionomy.org
E-mail: office@ortho-bionomy.org

Pfrimmer Deep Muscle Therapy

Thérèse C. Pfrimmer International
    Association of Deep Muscle
    Therapists, Inc.
c/o Pfrimmer Institute for Corrective
    Muscle Therapy
1173 Egypt Road
P.O. Box 151
Oaks, PA 19456
Tel: (888) 355-2698
Fax: (610) 666-9553
Website: www.pfrimmer.com
E-mail: info@piforcmt.com

The Radiance Technique

The Radiance Technique
    Association International, Inc.
    (TRTAI)
P.O. Box 40570
St. Petersburg, FL 33743-0570
Tel: (727) 347-2106
Website: www.trtai.org
E-mail: TRTAI@aol.com

Tellington TTouch

Tellington TTouch Equine
    Awareness Method &
    TTouch Training USA
P.O. Box 3793
Santa Fe, NM 87501
Tel: (800) 854-8326 or
    (505) 455-2945
Fax: (505) 455-7233
Website:
    www.TellingtonTTouch.com
E-mail: info@TTouch.com

Touch for Health

Touch for Health Kinesiology
    Association
P.O. Box 392
New Carlisle, OH 45344
Tel: (800) 466-8342 or
    (937) 845-3404
Fax: (937) 845-3909
Website: www.tfhka.org
E-mail: admin@tfhka.org

GLOSSARY

BODYWORK
FROM A TO Z

This glossary is a descriptive guide to the major forms of massage and bodywork practiced today. In addition to those therapies presented individually in the text of this book, other interesting approaches—which constraints of time and space did not permit to be included in the text—are presented. (Information on how to find out more about some of these practices is included in Resources for Further Exploration.) Terms describing other complementary health practices, about which there is frequently confusion or misunderstanding (such as chiropractic, osteopathy, and naturopathy), are also included here to clarify the role of massage and bodywork in relation to other allied health practices.

ACUPRESSURE—See "shiatsu."

ACUPUNCTURE—Literally meaning "needle piercing," acupuncture is a nearly five-thousand-year-old Chinese system of inserting fine needles into specified points lying along channels in the body known as meridians. The meridians are believed to be the pathways by which ch'i, qi, or ki, a vital life force, or energy, circulates. All illness is believed to result from an imbalance in the flow of ki. Acupuncture modulates the flow of this vital energy so as to prevent the onset of illness or to redress imbalances that have resulted in pain and disease. Most states and foreign countries have licensing laws that regulate the practice of acupuncturists, whose training differs from that of massage therapists.

ALEXANDER TECHNIQUE—Developed by the Australian actor F. Matthias Alexander (1869–1955) at the turn of the twentieth century, the Alexander Technique is a method that teaches how to improve the alignment of the head, neck, and torso. Improper use of the body is believed to be the source of stress, physical discomfort, and impaired performance.

Practitioners of the Alexander Technique, called teachers, assist clients, called students, to inhibit inefficient habits and learn improved ways of moving through a combination of gentle hands-on guidance and verbal instructions aimed at both conscious and kinesthetic awareness. The emphasis in the Alexander Technique is on releasing the head up off the spine, lengthening the neck and torso, and widening the back. This results in a feeling of lightness and ease. Lessons in the Alexander Technique form part of the training of many performing artists whose livelihoods depend upon proper use of the body.

AMMA (ANMA)—The traditional massage of Japan, and a precursor to shiatsu, amma is based on the principles of traditional Chinese medicine. Amma uses stroking and pressure on the points along the energy pathways (meridians) in addition to specialized stretching, kneading, and percussion.

AMMA MASSAGE—Developed by Korean-born Tina Sohn and taught at the New York College of Health Sciences in Syosset, New York, Amma massage is a unique synthesis of traditional Eastern and Western medical and manipulative principles. Amma massage also incorporates guidance regarding diet and the use of herbs and vitamins.

APPLIED KINESIOLOGY—Applied kinesiology uses muscle testing (testing for strength and mobility of a given muscle) as well as analysis of posture, gait, and lifestyle to evaluate the elements that may contribute to an individual's dysfunction. It then employs a broad range of techniques, including joint mobilization, soft tissue manipulation, stimulation of acupressure points, Cranio-Sacral techniques, and counseling in diet, vitamins, and herbs, to correct imbalances. Applied kinesiology is properly used exclusively by healthcare professionals such as medical doctors, osteopaths, chiropractors, and dentists, who are authorized to diagnose illness by virtue of their license. During the past forty years, applied kinesiology and Touch for Health (see "Touch for Health") have given rise to many other kinesiologies, which could be collectively described as energy kinesiology.

AROMATHERAPY—Aromatherapy, which traces its origins to ancient Egypt, India, Babylon, Greece, Rome, and the Arab empire, uses essential oils extracted from plants and flowers to heal. Essential oils are a highly concentrated, volatile mixture of potent chemicals that possess antibiotic, antiseptic, and other therapeutic properties. While these oils can be ingested in any number of ways, including diffusion into the air, aromatic baths, the application of fragrant waters, and even taken orally (but *only* under medical supervision), they are most frequently mixed with oil and applied to the skin in the form of aromatherapy massage. Long practiced in Europe, aromatherapy has become increasingly popular in the United States and Canada in recent years.

ASTON-PATTERNING—Aston-Patterning is a form of movement reeducation developed by Judith Aston. A former teacher of dance, physical education, and theater movement, Aston studied with Ida Rolf and developed a system of education to incorporate Rolf's principles of balance and alignment, which were taught in static positions, into well-ordered, efficient patterns of dynamic movement. This work later became known as Rolf Movement Integration. Aston-Patterning grew, as Aston's own work developed beyond the scope of Rolf Movement Integration, to include fitness training, bodywork, ergonomics, and product design.

AURA BALANCING—See "energy balancing."

AYURVEDA—Meaning "the science of life" in Sanskrit, Ayurveda is a five-thousand-year-old system of healing based on the teachings codified in the sacred Vedic literature of India. Generally considered the earliest system of health care based upon scientific principles, it maintains that all life is composed of five elements. Imbalances in the relationship of the five elements within us are the cause of illness and disease. Ayurvedic treatments use combinations of diet, nutrition, herbs, aromatic essences, massage, crystals, visualization, and meditation, among other healing measures, to restore balance.

Ayurvedic medicine, which is recognized by the World Health Organization (WHO), is a thriving practice in India. One of the most famous practitioners of Ayurvedic medicine in the West is Deepak Chopra, M.D., who through a series of books has done much to educate Westerners in Ayurvedic medicine. Dr. Chopra's contributions include delineating the parallels between Western thought, especially quantum physics, and Ayurvedic principles.

BACH FLOWER REMEDIES—This modality was developed beginning in the 1920s by Dr. Edward Bach (1886–1936), a British physician, who believed that illness is caused by negative emotions. He further maintained that certain flower essences have the capability to overcome specific negative emotions, thereby restoring mental and physical balance. Bach Flower Remedies represent the extraction of one or a combination of these flower essences, which are ingested orally in small doses.

BINDEGEWBSMASSAGE—See "connective tissue massage."

BIOENERGETICS—This is a form of psychotherapeutic work developed by doctors Alexander Lowen and John Pierrakos and is based on the work of psychiatrist Wilhelm Reich (1897–1957). Reich believed that illness results from psychological and emotional trauma. This trauma results in the blockage of energy in the body, which is reflected in muscle tension, or armoring. Bioenergetics works to free trapped energy through a combination of psychotherapy, breathing, and releasing bodywork. Reich coined the term "orgone" to describe the energy that permeates the universe.

BIOFEEDBACK—Developed in the 1960s, biofeedback is a relaxation technique that uses electronic instruments to give feedback on physiological responses related to stress. Biofeedback equipment measures such indicators as muscle tension, skin temperature, and breathing and heart rates. Through guided relaxation exercises conducted by trained facilitators, clients can learn to control these processes, formerly considered involuntary, so as to reduce tension and stress. Biofeedback therapy is frequently offered by psychotherapists and physicians as a means of reducing stress and therefore helping to alleviate stress-related illness.

CHAIR MASSAGE—See "on-site massage."

CHAKRA—Literally meaning "wheel" in Sanskrit, a chakra is one of seven centers of subtle energy that Eastern metaphysical systems believe regulate the flow of energy within the body/mind. A chakra is a kind of energy transformer, taking in high vibratory energy from outside the body. Through a process of conversion, the chakras transform subtle energy into denser form that can be used by the body. Considered centers of consciousness in both the Hindu and Buddhist traditions, chakras play an important role in many types of energy-based bodywork, which is directed at balancing and amplifying the flow of energy through the chakras.

CHIROPRACTIC—Developed in the late nineteenth century by Daniel Palmer (1845–1913), a self-schooled Iowan, chiropractic ("to do by hand") is a system of healing that holds that disease is caused by subluxations, or misalignments, of the vertebrae of the spinal column. Subluxations can affect nerves, resulting in physical dysfunction. Chiropractors focus on adjusting the bones that form the spine, generally through physical manipulation or electrical stimulation. Chiropractors are licensed to practice in all fifty of the United States under the title "Doctor of Chiropractic," designated by the initials "D.C." after their names.

CONNECTIVE TISSUE MASSAGE—Developed in Germany (where it is known as *Bindegewebsmassage*) in the 1930s by physiotherapist Elisabeth Dicke, and later elaborated on by physicians, this therapy massages the layer of tissue between skin and muscle known as connective tissue. Plagued by infection and pain in her right leg, which was so severe that doctors advised her to have it amputated, Dicke embarked on a journey of experimentation on her own body that resulted in her self-healing. Her method posits a powerful association between particular areas of connective tissue and specific paths of the nervous system and internal organs, so that massaging one area of the body can have powerful effects upon other areas of the body. While connective tissue massage has traditionally been practiced mainly in Germany, more and more American massage therapists are incorporating it into their work.

CRANIOSACRAL THERAPY—CranioSacral Therapy is a recently developed hands-on approach to healing that applies gentle, noninvasive pressure to balance what is known as the craniosacral system. An offshoot of the teachings of Dr. William Sutherland, an osteopath, this form of bodywork aims to ease restrictions in the bones and soft tissue forming the skull, mouth, and face (cranium); the vertebral column; and the bones at the base of the spine (sacrum).

Circulating through a semiclosed system (the body's craniosacral system) is a clear, colorless liquid known as cerebrospinal fluid (CSF). CranioSacral Therapy balances the rhythmic flow of the cerebrospinal fluid to restore balance to the central nervous system and the entire body, for which it is the master control. John Upledger, D.O., O.M.M., an osteopath by training, has done much to expand and popularize CranioSacral Therapy through the teaching and clinical experience afforded at the Upledger Institute. He coined the term "CranioSacral Therapy."

DEEP TISSUE MASSAGE—Deep tissue massage, or bodywork, is a general category that includes a number of approaches to freeing the body's system of myofascial connective tissue through deep manipulation. Many of these approaches owe their origins to Rolfing.

DO-IN—This is a system of exercises developed by Michio Kushi, a leading proponent of macrobiotics and founder of the Kushi Institute in Becket, Massachusetts. Based on ancient Eastern healing practices, Do-In exercises resemble yoga postures and are meant to balance the flow of energy through the meridian system that forms the basis for the practices of shiatsu and acupuncture.

DREAMBODY WORK—Developed by Arnold Mindell, Ph.D., an American psychotherapist at the Jung Institute in Zurich, Switzerland, this approach to healing represents a synthesis of the fields of dreams and bodywork.

Recognizing that the patterns of an individual's physical disease reflect patterns in his dreams, Dreambody Work uses a combination of counseling and bodywork to explore and heal the source of illness as it manifests in the unconscious.

EFFLEURAGE—This is the principal stroke of Swedish massage (see "Swedish massage").

ENERGY BALANCING—A general term used to describe a variety of practices whose aim is to balance the flow of energy in and around the body, which is known as the human energy field. The human energy field is sometimes referred to as the subtle, or etheric, body, as well as the human aura. Practitioners generally attempt to remove blockages in and balance and amplify the flow of this energy. Some practitioners balance energy without even touching the body while others incorporate the use of crystals, flower essences, herbs, and visualizations as aids to balance, focus, and amplify energy.

ESALEN MASSAGE—Named after the Esalen Institute in Big Sur, California, Esalen massage is a unique blend of Swedish massage enriched with the sensory awareness principles of Charlotte Selver. Esalen massage incorporates the long, lengthening strokes of Swedish massage with light rocking, passive joint movement, and deeper tissue work within a caring, supportive, and nurturing environment.

FELDENKRAIS METHOD—Developed by Russian-born Israeli physicist Moshe Feldenkrais, D.Sc. (1904–1984), the Feldenkrais Method is a comprehensive approach to movement reeducation that aims to restore and optimize full range of human function. The practitioner helps the client become aware of habitual and limited patterns and provides the context for learning new skills. This results in greater ease and flexibility of movement as well as reduction of pain and increased levels of vital energy. The Feldenkrais Method is taught in two formats: one-on-one private lessons in Functional Integration (FI) and group lessons in Awareness Through Movement (ATM) classes.

FRICTION—This is a principal stroke of Swedish massage (see "Swedish massage").

HAKOMI FOR BODYWORKERS—An outgrowth of Hakomi, a body-centered, experiential psychotherapeutic method developed by Ron Kurtz in the early 1980s, Hakomi for Bodyworkers draws from body therapies, psychotherapy, and Eastern philosophies, which form the foundation of its use of Mindfulness and Non-Violence in therapy. Hakomi psychotherapists help clients access and process the core beliefs that unconsciously shape their lives, relationships, and self-images.

Hakomi for Bodyworkers retains the intent of bodywork—to facilitate change and healing in the body—while centering on the client's somatic experience and incorporating Hakomi's fundamental approach, principles, and verbal skills. The techniques of Hakomi for Bodyworkers guide the client's attention to their embodied experience. From somatic experiences, unconscious emotions, images, and even memories may emerge. As the interplay of these elements becomes conscious, held energy can be released, the tissue yields, and structure and alignment are affected. Psychological material released into awareness can be safely reintegrated, which can result in profound and lasting change, both in the client's psyche and physical body.

HELLERWORK—Developed by Joseph Heller, an aerospace engineer and first president of the Rolf Institute, Hellerwork combines deep tissue manipulative techniques (see "Rolfing") with movement education and interactive dialogue regarding emotional issues that may arise during treatment. A complete Hellerwork treatment consists of a series of eleven to twenty ninety-minute sessions that address eleven thematic sections of the body.

HOLOTROPIC BREATHWORK—Developed by Czech-born psychiatrist Stanislav Grof with his wife, Christina, Holotropic Breathwork is a powerful form of self-exploratory experiential work that uses highly evocative music, played at high volume, coupled with deep, accelerated breathing to promote transformation and healing. Holotropic Breathwork, which combines insights from modern consciousness research, depth psychology (the psychology of unconscious behavior), and various spiritual practices, facilitates the attainment of nonordinary states of consciousness in which spontaneous healing of the body and mind can occur. As appropriate, focused bodywork is applied by trained facilitators to release areas of blockage encountered during Breathwork sessions.

HOMEOPATHY—A healthcare practice developed by Dr. Samuel Hahnemann (1755–1843), a German physician, homeopathy is based on the principle of "like cures like." Disease is treated by the administration of minute doses of natural substances that in a healthy individual would cause the same illness (the practice of vaccination exhibits parallels to homeopathy). The goal of homeopathy is to rid the body of toxins and restore balance of mind and body. Homeopathy is most frequently practiced by physicians, chiropractors, and naturopaths. Some states, such as Arizona, Connecticut, and Nevada, regulate the practice of homeopathy with special licensing laws. Homeopathy is a well-accepted practice in Europe: The Royal Family of Great Britain are well-known proponents.

HYDROTHERAPY—Literally meaning "water therapy," hydrotherapy harnesses the healing properties of water. Hydrotherapy can take many forms, including massage in or under water; aerobic or stretching exercises performed in water; soaking in hot springs; use of steam vapors; and revitalizing hot, cold, or alternating shower sprays. Some massage therapists are trained in specific applications of hydrotherapy. It has long been part of European healing traditions, where it has formed the core of spa cures. Increasingly, many American resorts and spas are incorporating various forms of hydrotherapy into their menu of offerings.

HYPNOTHERAPY—Hypnotherapy is the therapeutic use of hypnosis—an altered state lying somewhere between sleep and unconsciousness and resembling that attained during meditation or trance—to help an individual achieve greater clarity and allow her self-healing powers to emerge more fully. Because this state is associated with relaxation, it is conducive to relieving stress-related disorders as well as promoting more positive attitudes and habits. Many people spontaneously enter states associated with hypnosis as they drift off in the relaxing realm of massage. Some massage therapists and bodyworkers are specifically trained in techniques of hypnotherapy, which they incorporate as adjuncts to their practice.

INFANT MASSAGE—A form of massage based largely on the techniques of Swedish massage, infant massage is taught to parents so they can massage their newborns. Infant massage can help to improve circulation in newborns and relieve some common infant ailments, such as gas, constipation, and colic. In addition, it promotes the formation of strong nurturing bonds and helps relax both parents and newborn. Recent studies performed on infants born prematurely have demonstrated that massage can result in significant weight gain and developmental improvements.

IRIDOLOGY—This is a practice used by some physicians, chiropractors, naturopaths, and natural healers to evaluate the state of a client's health based on visual analysis of the iris, or colored portion, of the eye. Iridologists believe that every organ of the body relates to a specific area of either the right or left iris and that the state of tissues, organs, body parts, and physiological systems can be observed in an individual's eyes. Using the information gleaned from this noninvasive technique, counseling regarding preventive healthcare practices, such as nutrition and lifestyle, can be given.

JIN SHIN DO BODYMIND ACUPRESSURE—Jin Shin Do (literally, "way of the compassionate spirit") Bodymind Acupressure was developed by psychotherapist Iona Marsaa Teeguarden. It is an approach to healing that combines gentle yet deep finger pressure on the acupoints with verbal body focusing and emotional processing techniques to help release physical and emotional tension and armoring. Jin Shin Do is a unique synthesis of traditional Japanese acupressure, classic Chinese acupuncture theory, Taoist philosophy, qigong (breathing and execise techniques), Reichian segmental theory, and principles of Ericksonian hypnotherapy.

JIN SHIN JYUTSU PHYSIO-PHILOSOPHY—Literally meaning "the creator's art through knowing and compassionate man," Jin Shin Jyutsu is a Japanese healing art that aims to balance the flow of energy through the body. Jin Shin Jyutsu does not involve physical manipulation of muscles, but rather the gentle application of the hands along energy pathways, facilitating relaxation, increased circulation, and the harmonization of body, mind, and spirit.

KINESIOLOGY—See "applied kinesiology."

KRIPALU BODYWORK—Kripalu bodywork is a unique, soothing form of meditative bodywork using techniques drawn from Swedish massage, Polarity Therapy, and energy balancing, joined with intuitive awareness and breathing practices. It derives its name from the Kripalu Center for Yoga and Health in Lenox, Massachusetts, where this form of bodywork was developed and is practiced and taught.

KURED—This is a form of Russian medical and sports massage introduced to the United States by Zhenya Kurashova Wine. Wine was trained in Russia as a physiotherapist, where massage is one of the major forms of medical treatment, used in hospitals, clinics, and wellness resorts. KURED employs a repertoire of more than one hundred strokes that evolved from traditional massage. These strokes enable the practitioner to work as deeply or gently as necessary, in accordance with the physiological basis of a client's condition. Treatments are pain-free in order to encourage the body's innate healing mechanism. KURED is used to treat a wide variety of physical dysfunctions, enhance athletic performance, induce relaxation, and reenergize weary bodies. KURED is taught at sites throughout the United States by the Kurashova Institute, which is headquartered in Rock Island, Illinois.

LOMILOMI—A form of Hawaiian massage derived from a spiritual massage practiced by the kahunas, or the shamans of the Hawaiian Islands, lomilomi emphasizes use of the forearms and elbows. Lomilomi can use deep pressure strokes as well as rhythmical rocking movements.

LOOYENWORK—Developed by counselor Ted Looyen, who was born in Holland and educated in Australia, LooyenWork represents a synthesis of various techniques of deep tissue therapy and postural integration. It is a noninvasive approach to releasing and separating adhesions in the muscles and fascia of the body. Using pain-free deep pressure techniques, LooyenWork aims to release habitual patterns of holding (resulting from such factors as postural imbalances and emotional and physical trauma) and achieve permanent structural realignment.

LYMPH DRAINAGE—See "manual lymph drainage."

MACROBIOTICS—Literally meaning "long-lived," macrobiotics is an approach to eating based loosely on the concepts of traditional Chinese medicine, which aims for appropriate balance in one's diet. Generally, it involves eating foods cultivated locally and avoiding processed foods. Macrobiotic diets emphasize whole grains, beans, seeds, nuts, vegetables, fruits, and fish while eschewing red meat, sugar, and dairy products. The most well-known advocate of macrobiotics is Michio Kushi, who established the Kushi Institute at Becket, Massachusetts, in the Berkshire Mountains.

MANUAL LYMPH DRAINAGE (MLD)—This massage practice was developed in the 1930s by the Danish couple Dr. Emil Vodder and his wife, Estrid, while working as massage therapists on the French Riviera. MLD is a form of massage that assists the function of the lymphatic system, which is crucial to the effective functioning of the immune system. Lymph is a clear, colorless fluid that flows throughout the body in a system of vessels similar to those of the blood system. The lymphatic system is responsible for identifying, containing, and destroying disease-producing microorganisms in the body. Lymph circulates much more slowly than blood. Manual Lymph Drainage uses light, slow, repetitive strokes specifically designed to boost the circulation of the lymphatic system, which facilitates the removal of excess water, wastes, toxins, and foreign substances from body tissues. Also known as Vodder Lymph Drainage, or simply lymph drainage, MLD therapy has long been widely practiced in Europe, particularly in Germany and Austria, and is now becoming more popular in North America. The Dr. Vodder School in Walchsee, Austria, emphasizes use of MLD in postmastectomy therapy to relieve pain, edema, and fibrosis.

MARIEL—Developed and taught by Ethel Lombardi, a Reiki Master (see "Reiki"), MariEL ("beloved of God") uses a gentle laying on of hands to release emotional blockages that lead to pain, illness, and stress; balance the overall energy of the body; and aid in spiritual transformation. Emphasis is placed on transforming repressed emotional energy from past trauma into positive energy that can be used to foster personal growth. A MariEL session often involves interactive dialogue between practitioner and client.

MEDICAL MASSAGE—Medical massage is a form of Swedish massage that has developed specific techniques for treating injuries and a wide variety of illnesses as well as aiding in physical rehabilitation. Massage therapists who practice medical massage work under a prescription provided by a physician or chiropractor directing them in their course of treatment. Medical massage treatments are frequently shorter than full-body massages as they are directed toward local problem areas in the body. Common conditions treated in medical massage include spinal deformities; brachial neuralgia (shoulder pain); various forms of tendinitis (such as tennis elbow) and muscle pain; chondromalacia patellae (a common source of knee pain); sciatica; TMJ disorder; repetitive stress disorders; and sprained ankles.

MULTI INCARNATIONAL RECALL AND EMOTIONAL BODY BALANCING—A therapeutic approach developed by energetic healer and bestselling author Chris Griscom, multi incarnational recall and emotional body balancing utilizes gentle touch and energy balancing techniques from Windows to the Sky acupressure to remove blockages and facilitate the recall of multi incarnations. Multi incarnational recall and emotional body balancing is offered at the Light Institute of Galisteo, New Mexico (with branches in Europe and Latin America), founded and directed by Chris Griscom.

MYOFASCIAL RELEASE—Most frequently associated with the pioneering work of John Barnes, a physical therapist, Myofascial Release aims specifically to release tension in the fascia, which is the connective tissue that surrounds and supports the muscles, organs, and bones in the body, in order to restore balance to the entire body. Myofascial Release integrates a variety of techniques designed to manipulate and facilitate movement in the fascia and muscular structure of the body as well as CranioSacral Therapy (see "CranioSacral Therapy"). The practitioner uses the surfaces of her body, such as the fingers, palms, forearms, and elbows, in long, slow, gliding strokes to stretch and mobilize the fascia. Many massage therapists have studied Myofascial Release techniques and incorporate them into their practice.

MYOTHERAPY—See "trigger point therapy."

NATUROPATHY—Naturopathic medicine developed in the late nineteenth century as an alternative to then common medical approaches, which included the use of toxic drugs and surgery. In 1900, Benedict Lust, a German-born medical doctor, introduced naturopathy in the United States to promote the use of natural substances and therapies to assist our own innate natural healing abilities. Naturopathic doctors, known by the initials "N.D." after their names, treat their patients with therapies drawn from the fields of nutrition, herbal remedies, homeopathy, physical exercise and therapy, acupuncture, hydrotherapy, and a variety of bodywork techniques.

NEUROMUSCULAR THERAPY—See "trigger point therapy."

OHASHIATSU—A form of shiatsu developed by Wataru Ohashi, Ohashiatsu incorporates a view of the Eastern energy system refined by Masunaga, a psychiatrist and teacher of shiatsu, with the insights of Ohashi to integrate body, mind, and spirit. The emphasis of Ohashiatsu is on the communication and synergy between giver and receiver; the self-development of the giver, as well as the receiver; and on physical, psychological, and spiritual harmony for both. Ohashiatsu in particular among bodywork practices aims to maintain and improve the giver's posture, movement, and well-being. This form of shiatsu is taught at the Ohashi Institute as well as in its branches in the United States and other countries throughout the world.

ON-SITE MASSAGE—One of the fastest-growing forms of massage therapy, on-site massage, sometimes known as chair massage, involves the massage therapist's coming to the client's location, most frequently the workplace but also shopping malls, airports, and even the park on a sunny day. Generally, the client remains fully clothed while sitting in a comfortable, custom-designed padded massage chair, which permits the back to be exposed. On-site massage typically focuses on the back, shoulders, neck, and face. A session is usually short and provides a quick pick-me-up in the middle of a busy day.

ORTHO-BIONOMY—Developed by Arthur Lincoln Pauls, D.C., a British osteopath (see "osteopathy"), Ortho-Bionomy aims to enhance a sense of balance and well-being. It uses gentle, noninvasive touch, dialogue, and movement education in such common activities as sitting, standing, and walking.

OSTEOPATHY—Osteopathy is a branch of medicine developed by Dr. Andrew Taylor Still, a nineteenth-century surgeon. After his three children died from an epidemic of meningitis, he became discouraged with the invasive approach of the medicine of his day. He developed an alternative approach to healing that emphasized looking at our bodies as complete systems, not as isolated symptoms; seeking the cause of illness, not only its manifestation; encouraging the body's own self-healing abilities; and treating primarily with physical manipulation, exercises, and lifestyle advice rather than drugs.

Today, doctors of osteopathy, recognized by the initials "D.O." after their names, undergo a seven-year training program not unlike that of medical doctors. They are licensed to practice in all fifty states, where they have many of the privileges associated with M.D.s, such as dispensing drugs, performing surgery, and admitting patients to major hospitals. They differ in their focus, however, which is to stimulate the body's own healing powers.

PÉTRISSAGE—This is a principal stroke in Swedish massage (see "Swedish massage").

PFRIMMER DEEP MUSCLE THERAPY—Developed by Thérèse C. Pfrimmer, a registered massage therapist and physiotherapist from Ontario, Canada, in the 1940s, Pfrimmer Deep Muscle Therapy is a highly refined system of corrective treatment designed to aid in the restoration of damaged muscles and soft tissue in the entire body. Using the specific theories of cross tissue movements applied to the muscles, a fully trained Pfrimmer Deep Muscle Therapist concentrates on all layers of muscle that have become depleted of their normal blood and lymphatic flow. This specific therapy helps restore the circulation with its natural healing properties.

PHYSIATRICS—This is the branch of medicine that deals with physical therapy. Physiatrists, who are M.D.s, are specialized in physical medicine to treat muscular pain and facilitate physical rehabilitation using a variety of means, including stretching, massage, application of heat and cold, physical exercises, and high-tech electronic equipment.

PHYSICAL THERAPY—Physical therapy is a healthcare profession aimed at helping individuals promote health and recover from disabling conditions, such as accidents, surgery, sprains, fractures, neurological disorders, strokes, and other trauma. Physical therapists undertake a four- or five-year course of study in such areas as anatomy, physiology, biomechanics, exercise, rehabilitation, prosthetics, and orthotics. They must then pass a state licensing exam before using the initials "P.T." after their names. In many states, you must be referred to a physical therapist by a doctor.

Physical therapists use a broad range of therapeutic modalities, including massage, exercise, and electrical stimulation, with their principal goal being to facilitate movement. Some physical therapists specialize in particular areas, such as occupationally related disorders, sports injuries, or pediatric therapy.

PILATES METHOD—This is a series of movement exercises developed by German-born Joseph Pilates (1880–1967) in the 1920s. The Pilates Method aims to make people more aware of their bodies and to use them more efficiently. Pilates exercises are designed to stretch and strengthen muscles, open joints, and release tension. They are used in physical rehabilitation and fitness training, and by performing artists, especially dancers.

POLARITY THERAPY—Developed by Dr. Randolph Stone (1890–1981) a Viennese-born chiropractor, osteopath, and naturopath, in the mid-1900s, Polarity Therapy aims to restore balance to currents of energy that are believed to flow through and around the body. Drawing on principles that inform both Western medicine and Eastern healing arts, Polarity Therapy integrates many approaches to healing as it seeks to balance negative and positive poles of energy in the body. Polarity Therapists use a combination of four methods that form the foundation of a Polarity treatment: gentle hands-on bodywork to guide and conduct energy; counseling on diet and nutrition; guidance in Polarity yoga exercises; and psychological counseling that emphasizes the importance of positive thinking.

PSYCHONEUROIMMUNOLOGY—Psychoneuroimmunology (PNI; literally, "mind nervous system immunology") is an exciting new field of scientific exploration of the relation between the mind and illness. Spurred by the pioneering work of experimental psychologist Robert Ader in the 1970s, PNI investigates the connection between the nervous system and the immune system. While the two systems have traditionally been considered independent of one another, recent research has suggested that they are intricately interconnected by neural pathways. The way we think or feel, therefore, may be able to influence the functioning of our immune system and our state of health. Researchers from such disparate fields as psychology, immunology, anatomy, neurology, biology, epidemiology, and oncology are joining this fascinating field, hoping to unlock the mystery of the connection of the mind and the body in healing.

RADIANCE TECHNIQUE—The Radiance Technique is a system that teaches individuals how to access and use natural universal energy for stress management and personal growth. This seven-level technique can be learned by anyone, children as well as adults. The Radiance Technique is nonmanipulative. It works with or without touch, as appropriate, to balance and align the energy field of the body and the self. The Radiance Technique addresses the whole self, viewing each person as an entire physical, emotional, mental, and spiritual dynamic.

REBIRTHING—Rebirthing uses a simple technique of conscious breathing in order to facilitate access to greater awareness of physical, emotional, and mental feelings and sensations. During this process, undertaken with the guidance of a trained rebirther, an individual may become consciously aware of blockages relating to previously suppressed feelings. Rebirthers report that trauma experienced in the birth process often surfaces during a rebirthing session as the birth process is a powerful source of many of our later feelings of pain and rejection. The process of rebirthing is designed to allow suppressed feelings to emerge in a safe environment so that healing, balance, and acceptance may take place.

REFLEXOLOGY—Reflexology is a technique of manipulating the feet (and, less frequently, the hands) in order to improve circulation, ease pain, and increase relaxation in the body. Reflexology is based on the theory that all body parts, organs, and glands are associated with specific areas, called reflex zones, in the hands and feet, which serve as a kind of mini map, of the whole body. By manipulating the associated zone, changes can be effected in the corresponding body part. For this reason, reflexology is sometimes called zone therapy.

REIKI—Reiki (pronounced "ray-key"), literally meaning "universal life energy," is an energetic healing technique based on ancient Tibetan healing practices that utilizes the laying on of hands. Reiki practitioners tap into life force energy for healing purposes. They place their hands gently on areas of a client's body for several minutes at a time to energize and balance body, mind, and spirit. The areas covered correspond to the chakras of Eastern metaphysics and the major organs and glands of Western anatomy. To become a Reiki practitioner, a series of attunements, or initiations, to activate the practitioner's healing power are required. There are three levels, called degrees, of initiation into traditional Reiki practice; the higher levels teach healing at remote distances, using visualization. Reiki is designed to align universal energy with individual energy. In addition to treating acute and chronic physical problems by promoting balance and health in the body, it is a useful tool to heal emotional crises and foster personal transformation.

ROLFING—The Rolfing Method of Structural Integration, more commonly known as Rolfing, was developed by Ida P. Rolf, Ph.D. (1896–1979), a biochemist. It aims to reorganize or restructure the body through deep manipulation of the body's myofascial system, which is comprised of the muscles and soft connective tissue known as fascia that intertwines the muscles and forms a continuous web throughout the body. Rolf maintained that over time, the fascia is pulled out of alignment through a history of trauma, which includes poor postural habits, accidents, and emotional stress. Rolfing aims, through a series of ten sessions, to reorganize the body completely, from outer to inner layers, to achieve proper alignment. Only practitioners trained and certified by the Rolf Institute in Boulder, Colorado, are authorized to call themselves Rolfers.

ROSEN METHOD—Developed by German-bom physical therapist Marion Rosen, Rosen Method is a simple, noninvasive approach that utilizes gentle touch and verbal communication. Touch is used to detect areas of muscular contraction; attention is focused on the client's breath as a sign of inner change; and verbal communication is used to explore areas of physical and emotional holding. This combination can result in relaxation, amelioration of pain, and enhanced self-awareness. Because it is concerned with emotional release and heightened awareness, Rosen Method can also be used as a powerful tool for personal growth.

RUBENFELD SYNERGY METHOD—Ilana Rubenfeld developed Rubenfeld Synergy as an educational approach to healing that combines touch and verbal expression. Refined over a period of more than forty-five years, it integrates Rubenfeld's eclectic background, which includes certification as a teacher of the Alexander Technique and the Feldenkrais Method, and training in Gestalt practice and Ericksonian hypnosis. Rubenfeld Synergy treats each individual as a whole being and searches for the cause of a problem, rather than its manifestation. The Synergist, as a practitioner is called, uses gentle touch and movement to detect areas of emotional holding and tension. The Synergist then dialogues with the client to evoke, and release, the unconscious emotional issues that are vested in that holding. Additional techniques address breathing patterns and postural habits and incorporate visualizations as well as ample doses of humor.

SHIATSU—Shiatsu, literally meaning "finger pressure" in Japanese and also known as acupressure, is a Japanese system of healing that is derived from the precepts of traditional Chinese medicine originating thousands of years ago. Practitioners apply pressure from the fingers, hands, elbows, or knees to pressure points along invisible channels of energy called meridians. (These points are the same ones into which an acupuncturist inserts needles; see "acupuncture.") The goal of shiatsu is to balance the flow of vital life energy, or ki, in the body. Since all disease is seen as a disturbance in the flow of ki, shiatsu is used to prevent illness as well as to relieve acute and chronic physical problems. In addition to pressure along the lines of meridians, shiatsu can also involve gentle stretching.

SOMATOEMOTIONAL RELEASE (SER)—Developed by John Upledger, D.O., O.M.M., SomatoEmotional Release is based on the principle that our bodies hold the energy of past traumas, both physical and emotional, in the form of memories in the physical tissues of the body. Upledger coined the expression "energy cysts" for these areas of congestion, which disrupt the normal functioning of the body. SomatoEmotional Release seeks to find and discharge the energy that has become embedded in these cysts.

SPORTS MASSAGE—Sports massage is a specialization of Swedish massage that aids the body to achieve maximum physical performance. Administered before physical activity, it can help protect against pain and injuries while boosting performance. Following physical exertion, it helps remove lactic acid and restore normal muscle tone and range of motion. Sports massage is used by professional athletes, dancers, and performers as well as by weekend warriors and anyone who wishes to use his body at peak efficiency.

STRUCTURAL INTEGRATION—Structural Integration was the original name that Ida P. Rolf gave her work. It is now a general term that refers to a number of bodywork therapies that aim to integrate the structure of the body, particularly in respect to gravity. (See "deep tissue massage" and "Rolfing.")

SWEDISH MASSAGE—Probably the most commonly practiced form of massage in the West, Swedish massage is a system of movements and exercises developed by the Swede Per Heinrik Ling (1776–1839). A massage therapist applies oil to the body and gradually administers a series of strokes designed to induce relaxation, enhance circulation, and increase range of motion. The main strokes of Swedish massage are *effleurage* (gliding), *pétrissage* (kneading), *friction* (rubbing), *tapotement* (tapping), and *vibration* (shaking) movements. Swedish massage can help the body remove toxins, deliver nutrients to tissues and cells more efficiently, and recover from strains and trauma more quickly. In addition to using the standard strokes of Swedish massage, some therapists also apply hot and cold packs, instruct in exercises, and incorporate hydrotherapy into their practice.

TAI CHI CHUAN—Tai chi is an ancient Chinese Taoist martial arts practice used to unite body and mind. Sometimes referred to as "meditation in motion," tai chi integrates mental focus, awareness of breath, and slow, graceful, flowing movements. This practice is frequently used to induce relaxation and promote good health.

TAPOTEMENT—This is a principal stroke of Swedish massage (see "Swedish massage").

TELLINGTON TTOUCH (TTOUCH)—TTouch is a gentle system of bodywork developed by Linda Tellington-Jones. It is based on the application of a circular touch performed with a light pressure on the skin. The intent of TTouch is to provide information to the nervous system, affecting the entire body even to the level of cellular function. Linda Tellington-Jones envisions the purpose of TTouch "to activate the function of the cells and awaken cellular intelligence—a little like turning on the electric lights of the body." TTouch has been used successfully with horses and other animals, as well as people. Underlying the TTouch method is a profound respect for all beings, human and animal, and the desire to awaken the perfection in each of us.

THAI MASSAGE—The traditional massage of Thailand, Thai Massage traces its roots to India some twenty-five hundred years ago. Influenced by both Chinese and Indian healing arts, the techniques used in Thai Massage resemble those used in shiatsu, with the practitioner applying pressure with the palms and fingers to release blockages and balance the energy along specified pathways in the body. The network of energy followed, however, is more closely related to the Hindu energetic system of nadis than to the Chinese system of meridians. In addition to pressure strokes, Thai Massage uses a series of passive stretching exercises to energize and increase range of motion. As more foreign massage therapists have the opportunity to visit and train in Thailand, Thai Massage is becoming increasingly more popular in the West.

THERAPEUTIC TOUCH—Therapeutic Touch (TT) is a contemporary interpretation of several ancient healing practices, one of which is the laying on of hands. Developed by Dora Kunz, a spiritual healer, and Dolores Krieger, Ph.D., R.N., professor emerita at New York University's Division of Nursing, TT is based on the principle that we represent an open energy system and that illness is the result of imbalance, or blockage, in our energy field. TT aims to balance and energize the body by modulating the energy in the human energy field that surrounds and interpenetrates the body.

The term "Therapeutic Touch" is in a way a misnomer because most frequently the TT practitioner does not physically touch the body. Instead, she centers herself and assesses the receiver's field. Then, through a series of gentle hand movements, she balances the energy in the field. The practitioner does not do the healing but rather unblocks congestion in the receiver's field so that the individual's own innate healing capacities can function better. TT has been shown to induce the relaxation response, reduce pain, speed recovery from such trauma as fractures and sprains, and alleviate certain psychosomatic conditions such as anxiety. While TT has largely been taught to nurses (through programs at more than eighty colleges in the United States as well as being taught in more than seventy foreign countries), a number of massage therapists are learning TT to incorporate into their practice.

TOUCH FOR HEALTH—Developed by chiropractor John Thie, Touch for Health draws upon the principles of traditional Chinese medicine, chiropractic, and applied kinesiology (see "applied kinesiology"). A practical guide to natural health, Touch for Health uses muscle testing and monitoring to locate blockages in the muscle and meridian systems of the body; it then applies acupressure, massage, and metaphor to improve postural balance and reduce physical and mental pain and tension. Touch for Health is taught to laypersons and health professionals alike through the Touch for Health School of the International Kinesiology College, which certifies instructors worldwide from its international headquarters in Queensland, Australia. Training programs are taught through Kinesiology Institutes around the world ranging from short programs to full professional training as a health professional kinesiologist. The Touch for Health School of the International Kinesiology College is a nonprofit, member-run organization devoted to empowering people to improve their health through simple self-help techniques.

TRAGER APPROACH—Developed by Milton Trager, M.D., who recognized his gift for bodywork as a teenager in the 1920s, the Trager Approach is a method of psychophysical integration that utilizes nonintrusive pain-free hands-on touch (tablework) and a program of do-it-yourself exercises (Mentastics, short for "mental gymnastics"), to release areas of holding and blockage in the body.

Trager teaches that the source of tension and pain lies in the mind, which, through the nervous and neurochemical communicating systems, maintains muscles in chronically tense positions. The practitioner enters a meditative state that Trager terms hook-up in which he centers himself to attune to the flow of energy all around him. Then through gentle, rhythmic rocking, kneading, shaking, vibrating, and stretching movements, he works to increase range of motion, induce relaxation, and reeducate the client as to what it feels like to have a free and open body. Movement exercises in his series of Mentastics, which is also called mindfulness in motion, are taught in classes and workshops, and to clients to perform at home to reinforce the feeling of freedom imparted during a Trager session.

TRIGGER POINT THERAPY—Trigger point therapy is a general term applied to a variety of methods used to release trigger points, which are tender areas, usually found in tight bands of muscle, that may radiate pain to other areas of the body. The individual generally credited with introducing trigger point therapy is Janet Travell, M.D., former White House physician to Presidents Kennedy and Johnson. As practiced by massage therapists, trigger point therapy uses deep, sustained finger pressure to release trigger points. Variations of trigger point therapy include myotherapy, popularized by Bonnie Prudden (Bonnie Prudden Myotherapy), and neuromuscular therapy.

TUINA—Tuina (pronounced "t-weigh na") is an ancient Chinese system of manual therapeutics, which is based on the theoretical precepts of traditional Chinese medicine. It aims to facilitate healing by regulating the circulation of blood and ki, which controls body function and enhances resistance to disease. Tuina encompasses an extremely wide range of indications and techniques; principal strokes include pressing, rubbing, waving, shaking, percussion, and manipulating. Refined over a period of two thousand years, Tuina is routinely offered to patients in Chinese hospitals. Knowledge and practice of Tuina are expanding in the West as professional exchanges with the People's Republic of China grow.

VIBRATION—This is a principal stroke of Swedish massage (see "Swedish massage").

VIBRATIONAL MEDICINE—Vibrational medicine is a name given to an approach to healing that aims to treat the whole person by addressing and balancing the unifying energy system that underlies mind, body, and spirit. (See "energy balancing.")

VISUALIZATION THERAPY—This is an approach to healing that uses visualizations, or relaxed, guided meditations, to help an individual image a desired condition, such as optimum health.

YOGA—Literally meaning "yoking" or "union," the term "yoga" describes a variety of practices developed in ancient India to unify the body and mind. Most commonly involving a series of stretching postures (called asanas), breathing exercises, and meditative practices, yoga attempts to calm the mind and tone the body so as to create a state of balance in which higher aspects of consciousness can be accessed. Feelings of both mental and physical well-being often accompany these practices.

ZEN SHIATSU—Originated by Ohashi (see "Ohashiatsu") in 1975, the term "Zen shiatsu" refers to a particularly meditative, flowing form of shiatsu, which aims to unify body, mind, and spirit.

ZERO BALANCING (ZB)—Developed by Fritz Smith, M.D., who also trained in osteopathic medicine and acupuncture, this hands-on approach integrates Western manipulative techniques with the Eastern energy system. Gentle touch is used to balance the body's deep energy currents with the structural components of bone, skeleton, and joints. Zero Balancing is one of a variety of practices included in the course offerings of the Upledger Institute (see "Cranio-Sacral Therapy").

COMPARATIVE SUMMARY OF BODYWORK PRACTICES

The comparative table on this and the following pages highlights the key features of the various bodywork practices profiled in *Bodywork*.

Bodywork Practice	Goals	Setting	Length of Session
Swedish (traditional Western) massage	Increase relaxation, circulation, range of movement	Client disrobed and draped on massage table; oil used	30–60 minutes
Structural/Functional/Movement Integration: Somatic Education			
Rolfing Method of Structural Integration	Realign structural components of body for enhanced function	Client disrobed to underwear; relaxes on massage table; no oil used; deep pressure	60 minutes
Alexander Technique	Educate client (student) in proper use of self: head forward; neck up; torso long and wide	Client comfortably dressed; lies on table, sits, stands, or walks; teacher uses light touch and verbal directions	45 minutes
Feldenkrais Method	Reeducate body to optimize range of function; make unconscious movement conscious	Client comfortably dressed; Two formats: Functional Integration—private lesson, gentle touch, on table; Awareness Through Movement (group class)—teacher leads gentle exercises to increase awareness	Both formats: 45–60 minutes
Other Contemporary Western Bodywork Practices			
Myofascial Release	Release myofascial constriction for pain relief and improved function	Client undressed to underwear, on table; no oil; long, deliberate stretching strokes	30–90 minutes
Trager Approach	Release psychophysiological areas of holding to relieve pain and improve function	Two formats: Tablework—private session, disrobe to underwear or additional clothing, on table, no oil; Mentastics—exercises to do at home or in class	60–90 minutes; 30–60 minutes
Rubenfeld Synergy	Combine touch and talk therapy to explore cause of problem and help unfold its resolution	Client comfortably dressed; lies on firm, padded table	45 minutes

Recommended Frequency of Sessions

As a general rule, in most cases where the number of sessions depends upon condition, many therapists would recommend that in the case of particular complaints, sessions initially be frequent until the condition improves. In cases where the end is relaxation or health maintenance, sessions once a week or every few weeks may be adequate.

Contraindications

As with any health practice, individuals with a particular medical condition or history should seek the advice of their physician before beginning any massage or bodywork therapy.

Fee	Recommended Frequency of Sessions	Benefits	Contraindications
$30–$120/ hour	Relaxation: as often as you like Remedial: determined by severity of complaint	Reduce stress; relieve pain; promote healing; optimize physical, mental, and emotional well-being	Fever; nausea; jaundice; cancer; infection; bleeding; circulatory and skin disorders; varicose veins
$75–$125/ session	Basic series = 10 sessions; interval of 1–2 weeks between each	Optimize well-being; relieve chronic pain	As above; prolonged addiction; acute pain
$45–$100/ lesson	Number of lessons varies; average = 20 to 30 lessons, spaced once or twice a week	Become aware of and release inefficient patterns of use; improve function; gain sense of lightness and ease	None standard; check with practitioner
Private Lesson: $50–$90 Class: $10–$15	Recommended number of classes and lessons varies	Optimize full physical function and awareness	None standard; check with practitioner
$100–$150/ session	Several sessions to begin; practitioner then reassesses	Provide long-term relief for chronic pain; promote well-being	Total contraindication; malignancy, aneurysm, rheumatoid arthritis Local: bruises, wounds, fractures
$45–$120/ session	Begin with series; practitioner then reassesses	Help wide variety of muscular and other psychophysiological conditions; promote lightness and ease	Broken bones; blood clots; joint, bone, and disk disorders; recent surgery or hospitalization; problem pregnancies; drugs that alter perception
$10–$15/ class	Can be done as frequently as desired		
$50–$150/ session	Entails gradual unfolding process—average time varies; consult practitioner	Promote healing by unifying body, mind, and spirit	None standard; check with practitioner

Bodywork Practice	Goals	Setting	Length of Session
Rosen Method	Use gentle touch and verbal support to unlock old memories and promote self-growth and well-being	Client undressed to underwear on massage table; no oil	60 minutes
Asian Bodywork			
Shiatsu: Asian acupressure	Balance flow of energy (ki) through channels (meridians) by pressing acupuncture points	Client comfortably dressed; lies on futon on floor, or on table; therapist applies pressure with fingers, hands, elbows, knees	30–90 minutes
Reflexology	Improve circulation; ease pain; increase relaxation	Client comfortably dressed on table; shoes and socks removed; practitioner applies pressure to reflex zones in feet associated with body parts, organs, and glands	30–60 minutes
Aromatherapy massage	Use essential oils extracted from plants and flowers to heal	Aromatherapy massage uses essential oils in conjunction with a particular modality; see individual bodywork practices	
Energetic Bodywork			
Therapeutic Touch (TT)	Balance and amplify flow of energy through human energy field	Client fully clothed, seated in chair; practitioner centers and modulates energy around client; hands do not need to come into physical contact with client	20–25 minutes
CranioSacral Therapy	Balance flow of cerebrospinal fluid through craniosacral system (from head to sacrum)	Client clothed, on table; therapist uses light touch to release constriction in soft tissue and craniosacral system	45–60 minutes
Reiki	Use gentle hands-on touch and visualizations to access universal life energy for healing	Client comfortably dressed on table; practitioner gently places his hands for several minutes at a time over key areas corresponding to chakras/endocrine glands	60–90 minutes
Holotropic Breathwork	Utilize evocative music and deep accelerated breathing to access nonordinary states of consciousness	Partners pair up; one lies on floor, comfortably dressed, music played at loud volume for several hours while he or she breathes; partner available to assist	Group workshops of one to six days; individual sessions also available
Polarity Therapy	Restore energetic balance through gentle touch, advice on diet and exercise, and psychological counseling	Client comfortably clothed, on massage table; practitioner uses her two hands to balance poles of energy in body	30–90 minutes

Fee	Recommended Frequency of Sessions	Benefits	Contraindications
$50–$110/ hour	Practitioner appraises	Prevent onset of illness; foster self-transformation	Individuals with serious emotional or psychological problems should consult with practitioner
$30–$120/ hour	Number of sessions varies by need and complaint	Optimize health; prevent disease; relieve pain	Fever; infection; cancer; brittle bones; some heart conditions; some individuals on cortisone treatment
$30–$120/ hour	Number of sessions varies by need and complaint	Help relieve stress and stress-related conditions (e.g., back pain; digestion) for optimum well-being	Trauma to foot; severe systemic illnesses
Often sliding scale based on ability to pay	Number of sessions varies by need and complaint	Induce relaxation; alleviate pain; accelerate healing process	As with any bodywork, treatment of the elderly, very young, or seriously ill should be short
$40–$150/ session	Number of sessions varies by need and complaint	Alleviate pain; reduce stress; aid brain and spinal dysfunction; promote well-being	Recent, acute conditions of stroke, illness, and trauma to head
$30–$100/ session	Number of sessions varies by need and complaint	Balance mental, emotional, and spiritual energies; encourage spiritual transformation	None standard; check with practitioner
$150–$300 for two-day workshop	This work is deeply experiential; number of sessions varies by individual	Promote greater psychological unfoldment and personal transformation; spontaneously resolve psychosomatic conditions	Pregnancy; cardiovascular problems; breathing disorders; systemic debilitating disease; epilepsy; glaucoma; history of mental illness
$30–$100/ 30–90 minute session	Number of sessions varies by need and complaint	Redress imbalances in vital energy to prevent illness and promote health and well-being	None standard; check with practitioner; consult physician in case of serious illness

NOTES

Getting Started: How to Use This Book

1. Malcolm W. Browne, "A Museum Hall That Celebrates Human Evolution," *The New York Times,* April 23, 1993, p. C1.

Introduction

1. Mary Ann D'Urso, "Massage for the Masses," *Health,* (April 1987): 63.

2. Ashley Montagu, Ph.D., *Touching: The Human Significance of the Skin* (New York: Harper & Row, 1986), pp. 23, 238–39.

3. Ibid., p. 97.

4. Charles R. Halpern, "Mind vs. Medicine," *The New York Times,* January 30, 1993, p. 21.

5. David M. Eisenberg, M.D., et al., "Unconventional Medicine in the United States: Prevalence, Costs, and Patterns of Use," *The New England Journal of Medicine,* (28 January 1993): 246–52.

6. Tiffany Field, Ph.D., "Tactile/Kinesthetic Stimulation Effects on Pre-term Neonates," *Pediatrics,* Vol. 7, No. 55, (May 1986): 654–58.

7. David Villano, "Just the Right Touch," *Miami Magazine,* (Fall 1992): 32.

8. Mirka Knaster, "A New Dimension in Intensive Care: Premature Infants Grow with Massage—Dr. Tiffany Field's Research," *Massage Therapy Journal,* Vol. 30, No. 3, (Summer 1991): 50.

9. Leslie Miller, "Healthful Benefits of Massage Gaining Attention," *USA Today,* October 15, 1992, p. 6D.

10. Field quoted in ibid.

Part I: Traditional Western Massage

1. Friedrich Nietzsche, *Thus Spake Zarathustra* in *The Portable Nietzsche,* trans. and ed. Walter Kaufmann (New York: Viking Press, 1959). Quoted in *Parabola,* Vol. X No. 3, August 1985, p. 34.

Chapter 1: Swedish Massage and Its Variations

1. Elizabeth C. Wood and Paul D. Becker, *Beard's Massage* (Philadelphia, PA: W. B. Saunders, 1981), p. 11.

2. Herbert Benson, M.D., *The Relaxation Response* (New York: William Morrow, 1975).

3. John E. Upledger, D.O., O.M.M., "The Facilitated Segment," *Massage Therapy Journal*, (Summer 1989): 25.

4. Leslie Miller, "Healthful Benefits of Massage Gaining Attention," *USA Today*, October 15, 1992, p. 6D.

5. Frances M. Tappan, *Healing Massage Techniques: Holistic, Classic, and Emerging Methods* (Norwalk, CT: Appleton & Lange, 1988), p. 3.

6. John Carey, "The Message About Massage," *Newsweek*, November 15, 1984, p.110.

7. Ellen Markowitz, "Massage Therapy," *New York Runner*, July 1986, p. 8.

8. "Medical Notes," *Health* (January 1990): 21.

9. Miller, op. cit.

10. Tiffany Field, Ph.D., "Massage Reduces Anxiety in Child and Adolescent Psychiatric Patients," *Journal of the American Academy of Children and Adolescent Psychiatry*, (January 1992): 125–31.

11. Elliot Greene, "Capital Conference Features Massage," *Massage Therapy Journal*, Vol. 32, No. 3, (Summer 1993): 85.

12. Miller, op. cit.

13. Jack Meagher with Pat Boughton, *SportsMassage: A Complete Program for Increasing Performance and Endurance in 15 Popular Sports* (Barrytown, NY: Station Hill Press, 1990), p. xv.

14. Ibid.

15. John Zlatic, "Trigger Point Therapy: The Technique That Helped JFK's Back," *Back to Health*, (June 1989): 23–26.

16. Ibid.

PART II: STRUCTURAL/FUNCTIONAL/MOVEMENT INTEGRATION: SOMATIC EDUCATION

1. Rolf quoted in Jeffrey Maitland, *Rolfing & Rolfing Movement Integration: The Whole–Body Approach to Well–Being* (Boulder, CO: Rolf Institute, 1991).

Chapter 2: The Rolfing Method of Structural Integration

1. Ida P. Rolf, Ph.D., *Rolfing: Reestablishing the Natural Alignment and Structural Integration of the Human Body for Vitality and Well–Being* (Rochester, VT: Healing Arts Press, 1989; first published 1977), p. 27.

2. Ibid., p. 17.

3. Ida P. Rolf, Ph.D., "Structure—A New Factor in Understanding the Human Condition." Address presented at the Explorers of Humankind Conference, June 10, 1978.

4. Ida P. Rolf, Ph.D., "Structural Integration: A Contribution to the Understanding of Stress," *Confinia Psychiatrica*, 16, (1973): 69–79.

5. Ida P. Rolf, Ph.D., *Rolfing and Physical Reality,* ed. Rosemary Feitis (Rochester, VT: Healing Arts Press, 1990; first published 1978), p. 194.

6. In a fascinating bit of speculation, Rolf ventured that areas of habitual tension may correspond to pressure points, trigger points, and the reflex zones of reflexology. See Rolf, *Rolfing: Reestablishing the Natural Alignment,* p. 39.

7. Rolf, *Rolfing and Physical Reality,* p. 31.

8. Lisa Connolly, "Ida Rolf," *Human Behavior,* (May 1977): 19.

9. Jeffrey Maitland, *Rolfing & Rolfing Movement Integration: The Whole–Body Approach to Well–Being* (Boulder, CO: Rolf Institute, 1991).

10. Rolf, *Rolfing and Physical Reality,* p. 186.

11. Kalen Hammann, Ph.D., "What Structural Integration (Rolfing) Is and Why It Works," *The Osteopathic Physician,* (March 1972).

12. Rolf, *Rolfing and Physical Reality,* p. 27.

13. Valerie V. Hunt, Ph.D., et al., "A Study of Structural Integration from Neuromuscular, Energy Field, and Emotional Approaches." Study sponsored by the Rolf Institute (Boulder, CO, 1977).

14. Julian Silverman, Ph.D., et al., "Stress, Stimulus Intensity Control, and the Structural Integration Technique," *Confinia Psychiatrica,* 16 (1973): 201–19.

15. John T. Cottingham, Stephen W. Porges, Ph.D., and Todd Lyon, "Effects of Soft Tissue Mobilization (Rolfing Pelvic Lift) on Parasympathetic Tone in Two Age Groups," *The Journal of American Physical Therapy Association,* Vol. 68, No. 3, (March 1988): 352–56; and John T. Cottingham, Stephen W. Porges, Ph.D., and Kent Richmond, "Shifts in Pelvic Inclination Angle and Parasympathetic Tone Produced by Rolfing Soft Tissue Manipulation," *The Journal of American Physical Therapy Association,* Vol. 68, No. 9, (September 1988): 1364–70.

Chapter 3: The Alexander Technique: Aligning the Spine

1. Alexander quoted in Eleanor Rosenthal, "The Alexander Technique: What It Is and How It Works," *American Music Teacher,* (October/November 1989): 25.

2. John Dewey, Introduction to F. M. Alexander *Constructive Conscious Control of the Individual* (New York: E. P. Dutton, 1923); reprinted in *John Dewey and F. M. Alexander* (Champaign, IL: North American Society of Teachers of the Alexander Technique, n.d.), p. 11.

3. Wilfred Barlow, M.D., *The Alexander Technique: How to Use Your Body Without Stress* (Rochester, VT: Healing Arts Press, 1990), pp. vii–viii.

4. Edward Maisel, ed., *The Alexander Technique: The Essential Writings of F. Matthias Alexander* (New York: Lyle Stuart, 1990), pp. xxii–xxiii.

5. Rosenthal, op. cit., pp. 26–27.

6. Hillary Mayers and Linda Babits, "A Balanced Approach: The Alexander Technique," *Music Educators Journal,* (November 1987): 52.

7. Frank Pierce Jones, Ph.D., "Awareness, Freedom & Muscular Control," *Musical America,* (January 1949); reprinted in Frank Pierce Jones, Ph.D., *A Technique for Musicians* (Champaign, IL: North American Society of Teachers of the Alexander Technique, n.d.).

8. Barlow, op. cit., pp. 17–18.

9. Ibid., p. 52.

10. Ibid., p. 18.

11. Maisel, op. cit., p. xxvi.

12. Karen H. Siegal, Ph.D., "The Alexander Technique: An Innovative Approach to Reducing Physical Tension and Stress," *Behavioral Medicine* (November–December 1981): 29.

13. Maisel, op. cit., p. x.

14. Ibid., pp. xliii–xliv and 197–99.

15. Nikolaas Tinbergen, "Ethology & Stress Diseases: An Examination of the Alexander Technique." Nobel Prize acceptance address, Stockholm, Sweden, 1974.

Chapter 4: The Feldenkrais Method: Awareness Through Movement

1. Feldenkrais quoted in Feldenkrais Learning Center *Program Catalogue* (New York).

2. Moshe Feldenkrais, D.Sc., *The Potent Self: A Guide to Spontaneity* (San Francisco: HarperCollins, 1985), p. 155.

3. Albert Rosenfeld, "Teaching the Body How to Program the Brain Is Moshe's 'Miracle,' " *Smithsonian,* January 1981.

4. Margaret McIntyre, "Unlock the Trunk!" *Skiing* (October 1992): 141.

PART III: OTHER CONTEMPORARY WESTERN BODYWORK PRACTICES

1. Milton Trager, M.D., "Trager Psychophysical Integration and Mentastics," *The Trager Journal,* Vol. 1, (Fall 1982): 6.

Chapter 5: Myofascial Release: Physical Therapy Joins Hands With Massage Therapy

1. John F. Barnes, P.T., *Myofascial Release: The Search for Excellence, a Comprehensive Evaluatory and Treatment Approach* (Paoli, PA: Myofascial Release Seminars, 1990), p. 29.

2. Ibid., p. 2.

Chapter 6: The Trager Approach: Meditation In Motion

1. Trager quoted in Carol Cavanaugh, "Beyond Relaxation: The Work of Milton Trager," *The Trager Journal,* Vol. 1, (Fall 1982): 3.

2. Ibid., p. 6.

3. Milton Trager, M.D., with Cathy Guadagno, Ph.D., *Trager Mentastics: Movement as a Way to Agelessness* (Barrytown, NY: Station Hill Press, 1987), p. 101.

4. Cavanaugh, op. cit., p. 1.

Chapter 7: Rubenfeld Synergy Method: Touch Therapy Meets Talk

1. Ilana Rubenfeld, "Ushering in a Century of Integration," *Somatics,* (Autumn–Winter 1990–1991): 60.

2. Moshe Feldenkrais, D.Sc., *The Potent Self: A Guide to Spontaneity* (San Francisco: HarperCollins, 1985), p. 3.

Chapter 8: Rosen Method: Listening to the Body

1. Rosen quoted in Bevalyn Crawford, "The Healing Touch of Rosenwork," *Yoga Journal,* (March–April 1990): 13.

2. Ibid., p. 13.

PART IV: ASIAN BODYWORK: PRACTICES WITH EASTERN ROOTS

1. Chuang–tzu, *Texts of Taoism,* trans. James Legge (New York: Dover Publications, Inc., 1891). Quoted in *Parabola,* Vol. X, No. 3, (August 1985): 40.

Chapter 9: Shiatsu: Oriental Acupressure and Other Bodywork Practices

1. Michael I. Weintraub, M.D., FACP, "Alternative Medical Care: Shiatsu, Swedish Muscle Massage, and Trigger Point Suppression in Spinal Pain Syndrome," *American Journal of Pain Management,* Vol. 2, No. 2, (April 1992): 74–78.

2. Hal Rudnianin and Maggie Glasser, "Traditional Chinese Medicine in the People's Republic of China: Studying Massage Therapy in China," *Massage Therapy Journal,* Vol. 31, No. 4, (Fall 1992): 50.

Chapter 10: Reflexology: Baring Your Sole

1. Eunice D. Ingham, *Stories the Feet Can Tell Thru Reflexology, in The Original Works of Eunice D. Ingham* (St. Petersburg, FL: Ingham Publishing, Inc., 1984), pp. 13, 104.

2. Frances M. Tappan, *Healing Massage Techniques: Holistic, Classic and Emerging Methods* (East Norwalk, CT: Appleton & Lange, 1988), p. 255.

3. Dwight C. Byers, *Better Health with Foot Reflexology: The Original Ingham Method* (St. Petersburg, FL: Ingham Publishing, Inc., 1991), p. 1.

4. Anika Bergson and Vladimir Tuchak, *Zone Therapy* (Los Angeles: Pinnacle Books, 1974), p. 11.

5. Byers, op. cit., pp. 2–3.

6. Laura Norman with Tom Cowan, *Feet First: A Guide to Foot Reflexology* (New York: Simon & Schuster 1988), p. 17.

7. Louise Klein, "Reflexology, the Healing Art of 'Sole' Searching," *Massage,* 40, (November/December 1992): 62.

8. Byers, op. cit., p. 56.

9. Judith Togut, "Reflexology: No Mean Feat for Aches and Pains," *New York Post,* August 6, 1987.

Chapter 11: Aromatherapy Massage: Appealing to the "Scentses"

1. Robert B. Tisserand, *The Art of Aromatherapy: The Healing and Beautifying Properties of the Essential Oils of Flowers and Herbs* (Rochester, VT: Healing Arts Press, 1977).

2. Jerry E. Bishop, "New Research Suggests That Romance Begins by Falling Nose Over Heels in Love," *The Wall Street Journal,* April 7, 1993, pp. B1, B6.

3. Mitchell Pacelle, "Many People Refuse to Check in if a Hotel Has Odors in the Lobby," *The Wall Street Journal,* July 18, 1992, p. B1.

4. "Fragrance: Spirits That Soar," *Essence,* November 1991; and Tom Belden, "Use of Aromatherapy to Beat Jet Lag Makes 'Scents' to Airlines," *Journal of Commerce and Commercial,* (22 August 1991): 14ff.

5. C. Kallan, "Probing the Power of Common Scents," *Prevention* (October 1991): 38ff.

PART V: ENERGETIC BODYWORK: HEALING WITH THE HUMAN ENERGY FIELD

1. Einstein quoted in Barbara Ray, Ph.D., *The Reiki Factor in the Radiance Technique* (St. Petersburg, FL: Radiance Associates, 1992), p. 132.

2. Antoine de Saint–Exupéry, *The Little Prince,* trans. Katherine Woods (New York: Harcourt Brace, 1971), p. 87.

Chapter 12: Therapeutic Touch (TT): Modulating The Human Energy Field

1. Dolores Krieger, Ph.D., R.N., *Accepting Your Power to Heal: The Personal Practice of Therapeutic Touch* (Santa Fe, NM: Bear & Co., 1993), p. 8.

2. _____. *Living the Therapeutic Touch: Healing as a Lifestyle* (New York: Dodd, Mead, 1987), pp. 11–12.

3. David M. Rorvik, "The Healing Hand of Mr. E," *Esquire,* Vol. 81, No. 2 (February 1974): 70, 154, 156, 159–60.

4. Franklyn Sills, *The Polarity Process: Energy as a Healing Art* (Dorset, England: Element Books, 1990), p. 15.

5. Ibid., p. 13.

6. Dolores Krieger, Ph.D., R.N., "Healing by the 'Laying-on' of Hands as a Facilitator of Bioenergetic Exchange: The Response of In-Vivo Human Hemoglobin," *International Journal of Psychoenergetic Systems*, 1 (2), (1976): 121–29.

7. _____. *The Therapeutic Touch: How to Use Your Hands to Help or to Heal* (New York: Prentice Hall, 1986), pp. 74–76.

8. Ashley Montagu, Ph.D., "Therapeutic Touch," Appendix I to *Touching: The Human Significance of the Skin* (New York: Harper & Row, 1986), pp. 404–11.

9. Daniel P. Wirth, M.S., J.D., "The Effect of Non-Contact Therapeutic Touch on the Healing Rate of Full Thickness Dermal Wounds," *Subtle Energies*, Vol. 1, No. 1, (1990): 1–20.

Chapter 13: Craniosacral Therapy: The Skull Speaks

1. John E. Upledger, D.O., O.M.M., *Craniosacral Therapy, Somato-Emotional Release, Your Inner Physician and You* (Berkeley, CA: North Atlantic Books, and Palm Beach Gardens, FL: The Upledger Institute, 1991), p. 110.

2. _____. "The Relationship of Craniosacral Examination Findings in Grade School Children with Developmental Problems," *Journal of the American Osteopathic Association*, Vol. 77, (June 1978): 760–83.

3. _____. and Jon D. Vredevoogd, M.F.A., *Craniosacral Therapy* (Seattle, WA: Eastland Press, 1983), p. 6.

4. _____. *Craniosacral Therapy I–Study Guide* (Palm Beach Gardens, FL: The Upledger Institute, 1992), p. 10.

5. Michelle P. Pronsati, "Erb's Palsy: Once Considered Incurable, Now Helped with NDT, Craniosacral and Manual Therapy," *Advance for Occupational Therapists*, May 27, 1991.

6. Sharon Weiselfish, M.A., R.P.T., "Shannon—A Pictorial Case History Presenting Cranial Therapy for Cerebral Palsy," *Physical Therapy Forum*.

Chapter 14: Reiki: Universal Life Energy

1. Bodo J. Baginski and Shalila Sharamon, *Reiki: Universal Life Energy*, trans. Christopher Baker and Judith Harrison (Mendocino, CA: Life Rhythm, 1988), p. 29.

2. Ibid., pp. 22–27.

3. Clayton Lay Thomas, M.D., M.P.H., ed., *Taber's Cyclopedic Medical Dictionary*, 16th ed. (Philadelphia: F. A. Davis Company, 1989), p. 588.

4. Wendy S. Wetzel, M.S.N., R.N., "Reiki Healing: A Physiologic Perspective," *Journal of Holistic Nursing*, Vol. 7, No. 1, (1989): 51.

5. Phyllis Lei Furumoto, *The Usui System of Natural Healing* (Cataldo, ID: The Reiki Alliance).

6. Baginski and Sharamon, op. cit., p. 113.

Chapter 16: Polarity Therapy: Balancing Currents of Energy

1. Stone quoted in Franklyn Sills, *The Polarity Process: Energy as a Healing Art* (Dorset, England: Element Books, 1990), p. 1.

2. Ibid., pp. 8–10.

3. Phil Young, *The Art of Polarity Therapy: A Practitioner's Perspective* (Dorset, England: Prism Press, 1990), p. 43.

4. Beverly Kitts, "Polarity Therapy," *in Healing Massage Techniques: Holistic, Classic, and Emerging Methods* (East Norwalk, CT: Appleton & Lange, 1988), p. 201.

5. Deepak Chopra, M.D., *Perfect Health: The Complete Mind/Body Guide* (New York: Crown, 1991) pp. 109–110.

6. Young, op. cit., p. 14.

7. Ibid., p. 123.

PART VI: SUPPLEMENTAL INFORMATION: SIMPLE TOOLS

Chapter 17: The Spa Experience: Pampering Yourself While Your Body Works

1. Thoreau quoted in Deborah Vajde, "Meditation Medication," *Utne Reader,* (July–August 1992): 32.

BIBLIOGRAPHY

ORGANIZATION OF THE BIBLIOGRAPHY

The following bibliography attempts to pay homage to the many fine writers who have cogently and eloquently presented the subject of bodywork and to whom I am deeply indebted. It is organized in three sections: (1) reference books that are recommended as good sequels on the overall field of bodywork; (2) a general bibliography on the field of bodywork and healing; and (3) a listing of reference sources unique to each bodywork practice in the order of chapter presentation.

RECOMMENDED REFERENCE BOOKS

Ashley, Martin, J.D., L.M.T. *Massage: A Career at Your Fingertips,* 4th edition. (Carmel, NY: Enterprise Publishing, 2003). (Answers many questions you might have about choosing bodywork as a career; served as the source of much useful information regarding professional and political issues that are presented in this book.)

Cottingham, John T. *Healing Through Touch: A History and a Review of the Physiological Evidence.* (Boulder, CO: Rolf Institute, 1985). (Explores the relationship between various bodywork practices and the underlying physiological functioning of the body. Also contains a great deal of information on the history of various practices, which served as a basis for some of the historical information presented in this text, particularly the Introduction.)

Juhan, Deane. *Job's Body: A Handbook for Bodywork.* (Barrytown, NY: Station Hill Press, 1987). (Recommended for the bodywork professional; a comprehensive reference on the workings of the body/mind by a master teacher.)

McIntosh, Nina. *The Educated Heart: Professional Guidelines for Massage Therapists, Bodyworkers, and Movement Teachers.* (Memphis, TN: Decatur Bainbridge Press, 1999).

Montagu, Ashley, Ph.D. *Touching: The Human Significance of the Skin,* 3rd edition. (New York: Harper & Row, 1986). (The authoritative reference on the physiological, psychological, and sociological effects of touch.)

Tappan, Frances M. *Healing Massage Techniques: Holistic, Classic, and Emerging Methods.* (Upper Saddle River, NJ: Pearson Education, 2005). (An educational text that describes techniques for performing a variety of methods of massage.)

Thompson, Diana L. *Hands Heal: Communication, Documentation, and Insurance Billing for Manual Therapists,* 2nd edition. (Philadelphia, PA: Lippincott Williams & Wilkins, 2002).

GENERAL BIBLIOGRAPHY

Ajaya, Swami, Ph.D. *Yoga Psychology: A Practical Guide to Meditation.* (Honesdale, PA: The Himalayan International Institute of Yoga Science and Philosophy of the U.S.A., 1976).

Arya, Pandit Usharbudh, D. Litt. *Superconscious Meditation.* (Honesdale, PA: The Himalayan International Institute of Yoga Science and Philosophy of the U.S.A., 1978).

Ballentine, Rudolph M. *The Theory and Practice of Meditation.* (Honesdale, PA: The Himalayan International Institute of Yoga Science and Philosophy of the U.S.A., 1986).

Beck, Mark. *Theory and Practice of Therapeutic Massage,* 3rd edition. (Albany, NY: Milady Publishing Company, 1999).

Benson, Herbert, M.D. *The Relaxation Response.* (New York: William Morrow, 1975).

Berkow, Robert, M.D., ed. *The Merck Manual of Diagnosis and Therapy,* 16th ed. (Rahway, NJ: Merck & Co., Inc., 1992).

Bertherat, Thérèse, and Carol Bernstein. *The Body Has Its Reasons: Anti-Exercises and Self-Awareness.* (New York: Random House, 1977).

Campbell, Joseph. *The Inner Reaches of Outer Space: Metaphor as Myth and as Religion.* (New York: Harper & Row, 1986).

Carlson, Richard, Ph.D., and Benjamin Shield. *Healers on Healing.* (Los Angeles: Jeremy P. Tarcher, 1989).

Chopra, Deepak, M.D. *Quantum Healing: Exploring the Frontiers of Mind/Body Medicine.* (New York: Bantam Books, 1990).

Dychtwald, Ken. *Bodymind.* (Los Angeles: Jeremy P. Tarcher/Perigee, 1986).

Goleman, Daniel, Ph.D., and Joel Gurin, eds. *Mind Body Medicine: How to Use Your Mind for Better Health.* (Yonkers, NY: Consumer Report Books, 1993).

Haich, Elisabeth. *Initiation.* (Palo Alto, CA: Seed Center, 1974).

Hamilton, Clarence H. *Buddhism: A Religion of Infinite Compassion.* (Indianapolis: Bobbs–Merrill, 1952).

Hay, Louise L. *You Can Heal Your Life.* (Santa Monica, CA: Hay House, 1987).

Healing and the Mind with Bill Moyers: A Resource Guide for the Field of Mind Body Health. (Kalamazoo, MI: Fetzer Institute, 1993).

Hoff, Benjamin. *The Tao of Pooh.* (New York: Penguin, 1982).

Houston, Jean, Ph.D. *The Possible Human: A Course in Enhancing Your Physical, Mental, and Creative Abilities.* (Los Angeles: Jeremy P. Tarcher, 1982).

Joy, W. Brugh, M.D. *Avalanche: Heretical Reflections on the Dark and the Light.* (New York: Ballantine Books, 1990).

Jung, Carl G. *The Basic Writings of C. G. Jung.* Ed. Violet S. de Laszlo. (New York: Random House, 1959).

Kapit, Wynn, and Lawrence M. Elson. *The Anatomy Coloring Book.* (New York: HarperCollins, 1977).

Kastner, Mark, L.Ac., Dipl.Ac., and Hugh Burroughs. *Alternative Healing: The Complete A–Z Guide to Over 160 Different Alternative Therapies.* (La Mesa, CA: Halcyon Publishing, 1993).

Krishna, Gopi. *Kundalini: The Evolutionary Energy in Man.* (Boston: Shambhala, 1985).

Kurtz, Ron, and Hector Prestera, M.D. *The Body Reveals: What Your Body Says About You.* (San Francisco: Harper & Row, 1984).

Levine, Stephen. *Healing into Life and Death.* (New York: Doubleday, 1987).

Liberman, Jacob, O.D., Ph.D. *Light Medicine of the Future: How We Can Use It to Heal Ourselves Now.* (Santa Fe, NM: Bear & Company, 1991).

Locke, Steven, M.D., and Douglas Colligan. *The Healer Within: The New Medicine of Mind and Body.* (New York: E. P. Dutton, 1986).

Maharishi Mahesh Yogi. *Science of Being and Art of Living: Transcendental Meditation.* (New York: New American Library, 1968).

Masters, Robert, Ph.D., and Jean Houston, Ph.D. *Listening to the Body: The Psychophysical Way to Health and Awareness.* (New York: Dell Publishing, 1978).

Meyer, Marvin W., trans. *The Secret Teachings of Jesus: Four Gnostic Gospels.* (New York: Random House, 1984).

Mindell, Arnold, M.S., Ph.D. *Dreambody: The Body's Role in Revealing the Self.* (Boston: Sigo Press, 1982).

Morse, Melvin L., M.D., with Paul J. Perry. *Closer to the Light: Learning from the Near-Death Experiences of Children.* (New York: Ballantine Books, 1990).

Moyers, Bill. *Healing and the Mind.* (New York: Doubleday, 1993).

Muktananda, Swami. *Play of Consciousness: A Spiritual Autobiography.* (South Fallsburg, NY: SYDA Foundation, 1990).

Nelson, Dawn. *Compassionate Touch: Hands-on Caregiving for the Elderly, the Ill, and the Dying.* (Barrytown, NY: Station Hill Press, 1994).

Neihardt, John G. *Black Elk Speaks: Being the Life Story of a Holy Man of the Oglala Sioux*. (Lincoln: University of Nebraska Press, 1972).

Olsen, Andrea. *Body Stories: A Guide to Experiential Anatomy*. (Barrytown, NY: Station Hill Press, 1991).

Parabola, The Magazine of Myth and Tradition: The Body. New York: Society for the Study of Myth and Tradition, Vol. X, No. 3, August 1985. (Issue devoted to the body; diverse contributors.)

Prevention Magazine: Hands-on-Healing: Massage Remedies for Hundreds of Health Problems. (Emmaus, PA: Rodale Press, 1989).

Rama, Swami, and Swami Ajaya. *Creative Use of Emotion*. (Honesdale, PA: The Himalayan International Institute of Yoga Science and Philosophy of the U.S.A., 1976).

_____. Rudolph Ballentine, M.D., and Alan Hymes, M.D. *Science of Breath: A Practical Guide*. (Honesdale, PA: The Himalayan International Institute of Yoga Science and Philosophy of the U.S.A., 1979).

Reader's Digest: Family Guide to Natural Medicine: How to Stay Healthy the Natural Way. (Pleasantville, NY: Reader's Digest, 1993).

Rinpoche, Sogyal. *The Tibetan Book of Living and Dying*. (San Francisco: Harper-Collins, 1992).

Rumi, Jelaluddin. *The Ruins of the Heart*. Trans. Edmund Helminski. (Putney, VT: Threshold Books, 1981).

Schwarz, Jack. *Voluntary Controls: Exercises for Creative Meditation and for Activating the Potential of the Chakras*. (New York: E. P. Dutton, 1978).

Sieg, Kay W., M.Ed., OTR, and Sandra P. Adams, M.O.T., OTR. *Illustrated Essentials of Musculoskeletal Anatomy*, 2d ed. (Gainesville, FL: Megabooks, Inc., 1985).

Siegel, Bernie S., M.D. *Love, Medicine & Miracles: Lessons Learned About Self-Healing from a Surgeon's Experience with Exceptional Patients*. (New York: Harper & Row, 1986).

Sohnen–Moe, Cherie. *Business Mastery: A Guide for Creating a Fulfilling, Thriving Business and Keeping It Successful (Designed for Healing Arts Professionals)*. (Tucson, AZ: Sohnen-Moe Associates, 1999).

Steinbrecher, Edwin C. *The Inner Guide Meditation: A Spiritual Technology for the 21st Century*. (York Beach, ME: Samuel Weiser, Inc., 1988).

Thomas, Clayton L., M.D., M.P.H., ed. *Taber's Cyclopedic Medical Dictionary*, 16th edition. (Philadelphia: F. A. Davis Company, 1989).

Todd, Mabel E. *The Thinking Body*. (Brooklyn, NY: Dance Horizons, Inc., 1979).

Tortora, Gerard J., and Nicholas P. Anagnostakos. *Principles of Anatomy and Physiology*, 6th ed. (New York: Harper & Row, 1990).

Wale, J. O. *Tidy's Massage and Remedial Exercises,* 11th ed. (Bristol, England: John Wright & Sons Ltd., 1968).

Weil, Andrew, M.D. *Natural Health, Natural Medicine: A Comprehensive Manual for Wellness and Self-Care.* (Boston: Houghton Mifflin, 1990).

Wood, Elizabeth C., and Paul D. Becker. *Beard's Massage.* (Philadelphia: W. B. Saunders Company, 1981).

REFERENCES BY CHAPTER

Getting Started: How to Use This Book

Dubitsky, Carl, O.B.T., L.M.T., et al. "Three Paradigms–Five Approaches: Diverse Practitioners Propose a Schema for Massage and Bodywork." *Massage Therapy Journal, Vol.* 30, No. 3, (Summer 1991): 21–23.

Rubenfeld, Ilana. "Ushering in a Century of Integration." *Somatics,* (Autumn–Winter 1990–91): 59–63.

Introduction

American Massage Therapy Association (AMTA). *A Guide to Massage Therapy in America.* (Evanston, IL: AMTA, 1993.)

"AMTA at the White House: Health Care Reform Meeting Includes Massage Therapy." *Massage Therapy Journal,* Vol. 32, No. 2 (Spring 1993): 11–13.

Angier, Natalie. "U.S. Opens the Door just a Crack to Alternative Forms of Medicine." *The New York Times,* January 10, 1993, pp. 1, 22.

_____. "Where the Unorthodox Gets a Hearing at N.I.H." *The New York Times,* March 16, 1993, pp. C1, C6.

Ashley, Martin, J.D., L.M.T. *Massage: A Career at Your Fingertips.* (Barrytown, NY: Station Hill Press, 1992).

D'Urso, Mary Ann. "Massage for the Masses." *Health,* (April 1987): 63–64, 66–67, 89.

Eisenberg, David M., M.D., et al. "Unconventional Medicine in the United States: Prevalence, Costs, and Patterns of Use." *The New England Journal of Medicine,* (28 January 1993): 246–52.

Field, Tiffany, Ph.D. "Tactile/Kinesthetic Stimulation Effects on Preterm Neonates." *Pediatrics,* Vol. 77, No. 5, (May 1986): 654–58.

Gallo, Nick. "The Benefits of Massage: Ancient Relief for Today's Stresses." *Better Homes and Gardens,* (April 1991): 55–56, 58.

Greene, Elliot. "Capitol Conference Features Massage." *Massage Therapy Journal,* Vol. 32, No. 3, (Summer 1993): 85–87.

_____. "Riding the Waves of Change to the Year 2000." *Massage Therapy Journal,* Vol. 31, No. 3, (Summer 1992): 27–28.

_____. "What Is Going on at NIH?" *Massage Therapy Journal,* Vol. 31, No. 4, (Fall 1992): 15–16.

Halpern, Charles R. "Mind vs. Medicine." *The New York Times,* January 30, 1993, p. 21.

"Harkin Hears You: AMTA Meets with U.S. Senator." *Hands On,* Vol. X, No. 1, (Spring 1994): 7, 14.

Kellogg, John H., M.D. *The Art of Massage: A Practical Manual for the Nurse.* (Battle Creek, MI: Modern Medicine Publishing Co., 1923).

Knaster, Mirka. "A New Dimension in Intensive Care: Premature Infants Grow with Massage—Dr. Tiffany Field's Research." *Massage Therapy Journal,* Vol. 30, No. 3, (Summer 1991): 50–51, 54.

Miller, Leslie. "Healthful Benefits of Massage Gaining Attention." *USA Today,* October 15, 1992, p. 6D.

Newsweek staff. "The Power to Heal: From Ancient Arts to Modern Medicine, a Photo Portfolio." *Newsweek,* September 24, 1990, pp. 38–41, 44–45, 48–49, 51, 54–55, 58.

"NIH Funds Massage Studies." *Hands On,* Vol. IX, No. 4, (Winter 1993): l.

Squires, Sally. "Medinews: News for Babies, a Touching Discovery." *Ladies' Home Journal,* (July 1988): 70.

State of New Mexico. *Professional and Occupational License Bulletin.* (1991 Supplement): 40–47.

State of New York. *Massage Handbook.* (Albany, NY: The State Education Department, 1992).

Van Why, Richard. "Father of Massage Therapy in the United States: Cornelius E. DePuy, M.D." *Massage Therapy Journal,* Vol. 30, No. 3, (Summer 1991): 31–32.

Villano, David. "Just the Right Touch." *Miami Magazine,* (Fall 1992): 31–32, 34–35.

Wallis, Claudia. "Why New Age Medicine Is Catching On." *Time,* November 4, 1991, pp. 68–72.

"Wellness Proposals Presented to National Health Care Reform Task Force." *Massage Therapy Journal,* Vol. 32, No. 2, (Spring 1993): 100–103.

Chapter 1: Swedish Massage and Its Variations

Ashley, Martin, J.D., L.M.T. *Massage: A Career at Your Fingertips.* (Barrytown, NY: Station Hill Press, 1992).

Field, Tiffany, Ph.D., et al. "Massage Reduces Anxiety in Child and Adolescent Psychiatric Patients." *Journal of the American Academy of Children and Adolescent Psychiatry,* January 1992, 125–31.

Greene, Elliot. "Capital Conference Features Massage." *Massage Therapy Journal,* Vol. 32, No. 3, (Summer 1993): 85–87.

Harrold, Fiona. *The Complete Body Massage: A Hands-on Manual.* (New York: Sterling Publishing Company, Inc., 1992).

Health magazine staff. "Medical Notes." *Health,* January 1990, 21

Inkeles, Gordon, et al. *The Art of Sensual Massage.* (New York: Simon & Schuster, 1972).

Lacroix, Nitya. *Massage for Total Stress Release: The Art of Relieving Tension Through Massage.* (New York: Random House, 1990).

Maxwell-Hudson, Clare. *The Complete Book of Massage: Fully Illustrated Step-by-Step Instructions for Sensuously Massaging the Whole Body.* (New York: Random House, 1988).

Miller, Leslie. "Healthful Benefits of Massage Gaining Attention." *USA Today,* October 15, 1992, p. 6D.

Upledger, John E., D.O., O.M.M. "Craniosacral Osteopathy, the Energy Cyst: Part II." *Caduceus,* No. 7, 1989.

_____. "The Facilitated Segment." *Massage Therapy Journal,* (Summer 1989), p. 22ff.

Zerinsky, Sidney, Ph.D., M.Th. *Basic Massage.* (New York: Swedish Institute, 1980).

Medical Massage

Zerinsky, Sidney, Ph.D. *Introduction to Pathology for the Massage Practitioner.* rev. and ed. Jill Thompson, B.A., M.Div. (New York: Swedish Institute, 1987).

Sports Massage

Carey, John, et al. "The Message about Massage." *Newsweek,* October 15, 1984, p. 110.

Meagher, Jack, with Pat Boughton. *Sportsmassage: A Complete Program for Increasing Performance and Endurance in 15 Popular Sports.* (Barrytown, NY: Station Hill Press, 1990).

Markowitz, Ellen. "Massage Therapy." *New York Runner,* July 1986, p. 8.

"The Runs of '91." *MetroSports Magazine,* (February 1991), pp. 16–17.

Trigger Point Therapies

Hackett, James. *Muscular Anatomy and Applied Techniques of Muscle Therapy.* (Chicago: Chicago School of Massage, 1991).

Prudden, Bonnie. *Myotherapy: Bonnie Prudden's Guide to Pain-Free Living.* (New York: Ballantine Books, 1985).

_____. *Pain Erasure: The Bonnie Prudden Way.* (New York: Ballantine Books, 1985).

Travell, Janet G., M.D., and David G. Simons, M.D. *Myofascial Pain and Dysfunction, the Trigger Point Manual.* (Baltimore: Williams and Wilkins, 1983).

Zlatic, John. "Trigger Point Therapy: The Technique That Helped JFK's Back." *Back to Health,* June 1989.

Chapter 2: The Rolfing Method of Structural Integration

Bernard, Randy. "Rolfing Handicapped Children." *Physical Therapy Forum,* Western Ed., Vol. V, No. 25, (18 June 1986).

Bond, Mary. *Rolfing Movement Integration: A Self-Help Approach to Balancing the Body.* (Rochester, VT: Healing Arts Press, 1993).

Boyce, James. "Understanding Rolfing." *Physical Therapy Forum,* Vol. VII, No. 49, (5 December 1988).

Connolly, Lisa. "Ida Rolf." *Human Behavior,* (May 1977): 17–23.

Cottingham, John T., Stephen W. Porges, Ph.D., and Todd Lyon. "Effects of Soft Tissue Mobilization (Rolfing Pelvic Lift) on Parasympathetic Tone in Two Age Groups." *The Journal of American Physical Therapy Association,* Vol. 68, No. 3, (March 1988): 352–56.

Cottingham, John T., Stephen W. Porges, Ph.D., and Kent Richmond. "Shifts in Pelvic Inclination Angle and Parasympathetic Tone Produced by Rolfing Soft Tissue Manipulation." *The Journal of American Physical Therapy Association,* Vol. 68, No. 9, (September 1988): 1364–70.

Fahey, Brian W., Ph.D. "Can Rolfing Help Your Running?" *Footnotes,* Vol. 12, No. 6, (Summer 1985).

Hamman, Kalen, Ph.D. "What Structural Integration (Rolfing) Is and Why It Works." *Osteopathic Physician,* (March 1972).

Hunt, Valerie V., Ph.D., et al. *A Study of Structural Integration from Neuromuscular, Energy Field, and Emotional Approaches.* (Boulder, CO: Rolf Institute, 1977).

Johnson, Don. *The Protean Body: A Rolfer's View of Human Flexibility.* (New York: Harper & Row, 1977).

Kirkby, Ron, Ph.D. *The Probable Reality Behind Structural Integration: How Gravity Supports the Body.* (Boulder, CO: Rolf Institute).

Knaster, Mirka M. "Heal Thyself: Massaging Out Bad Memories." *Natural Health,* Vol. 32, No. 2, (March–April 1993): 42–43.

_____. "Philosopher Turned Somatic Educator: An Interview with Jeffrey Maitland." *Massage Therapy Journal,* Vol. 31, No. 2, (Spring 1992): 56–63, 114, 116, 118, 120.

Maitland, Jeffrey. *Rolfing & Rolfing Movement Integration: The Whole Body Approach to Well-Being.* (Boulder, CO: Rolf Institute, September 1991).

Mixter, Jason. "Rolfing," in *Whole Body Healing.* (Emmaus, PA: Rodale Press, 1983): 351ff.

Olson, Eric. "Getting the Treatment." *The Runner,* 1984.

Robbie, David L., M.D. "Tensional Forces in the Human Body." *Orthopaedic Review,* Vol. VI, No. 11, (November 1977): 45–48.

Rolf, Ida P., Ph.D. *Rolfing and Physical Reality.* Ed. Rosemary Feitis. (Rochester, VT: Healing Arts Press, 1990).

_____. *Rolfing: Reestablishing the Natural Alignment and Structural Integration of the Human Body for Vitality and Well-Being.* (Rochester, VT: Healing Arts Press, 1989).

_____. *Rolfing: The Vertical-Experiential Side to Human Potential.* (Boulder, CO: Rolf Institute, March 1977).

_____. "Structure—a New Factor in Understanding the Human Condition." Address presented at the Explorers of Humankind Conference, June 10, 1978.

_____. "Structural Integration: A Contribution to the Understanding of Stress." *Confinia Psychiatrica,* 16 (1973): 69–79.

Rolf Institute. *The Rolfing Technique of Connective Tissue Manipulation.* (Boulder, CO: Rolf Institute, 1976).

Sant'Anna, Dorris, and Frank Hanenkrat, Ph.D. *The Rolfing Experience.* (Lynchburg, VA: The Rolfing Partnership, 1991).

Schutz, Will, and Evelyn Turner. *Evy: An Odyssey into BODYMIND.* (New York: Harper & Row, 1976).

Silverman, Julian, Ph.D., et al. "Stress, Stimulus Intensity Control, and the Structural Integration Technique." *Confinia Psychiatrica,* 16 (1973): 201–19.

Sise, Betsy. *Rolfing: Structural Balance Opens Potential.* (Boulder, CO: Rolf Institute, 1987).

Wing, Heather. *Rolfing Movement Integration: An Introduction.* (Boulder, CO: Rolf Institute).

Chapter 3: The Alexander Technique: Aligning the Spine

Alexander, F. Matthias. *Constructive Conscious Control of the Individual.* (Long Beach, CA: Centerline Press, 1985).

_____. *Man's Supreme Inheritance.* (Long Beach, CA: Centerline Press, 1989).

_____. *The Use of the Self.* (Long Beach, CA: Centerline Press, 1985).

_____. *The Universal Constant in Living.* (Long Beach, CA: Centerline Press, 1986).

Barlow, Wilfred, M.D. *The Alexander Technique: How to Use Your Body Without Stress.* (Rochester, VT: Healing Arts Press, 1990).

Brody, Jane E. "Personal Health: A Technique to Shed Muscle Tension Habits Helps People Suffering from Chronic Pain." *The New York Times,* June 21, 1990, p. B6.

Caplan, Deborah, P.T. *Back Trouble: A New Approach to Prevention and Recovery Based on the Alexander Technique.* (Gainesville, FL: Triad Publishing Company, 1987).

Connington, Bill. "The Alexander Technique: A Method for Psychophysical Change." *Massage & Bodywork Quarterly,* Vol. VIII, Issue 1, (Winter 1993): 9–10.

Dewey, John, and Frank Pierce Jones, Ph.D. *John Dewey and F. M. Alexander.* (Champaign, IL: North American Society of Teachers of the Alexander Technique).

Gelb, Michael. *Body Learning: An Introduction to the Alexander Technique.* (New York: Henry Holt, 1987).

Gray, John. *Your Guide to the Alexander Technique.* (New York: St. Martin's Press, 1990).

Jones, Frank Pierce, Ph.D. *A Technique for Musicians.* (Champaign, IL: North American Society of Teachers of the Alexander Technique). Contains "Awareness, Freedom and Muscular Control" reprinted from *Musical America,* (January 1949); and "The Organization of Awareness," a paper presented at Michigan State University, (May 1967).

_____. *Body Awareness in Action.* (New York: Shocken Books, 1976).

Liebowitz, Judith, and Bill Connington. *The Alexander Technique: The World-Famous Method for Enhancing Posture, Stamina, Health, and Well-being, and for Relieving Pain and Tension.* (New York: HarperCollins, 1990).

Maisel, Edward, ed. *The Alexander Technique: The Essential Writings of F. Matthias Alexander.* (New York: Lyle Stuart, 1990).

Mayers, Hilary, and Linda Babits. "A Balanced Approach: The Alexander Technique." *Music Educators Journal,* (November 1987): 51–54.

Rosenthal, Eleanor. "The Alexander Technique: What It Is and How It Works." *American Music Teacher,* (October–November 1989): 24–27, 57.

Siegal, Karen H., Ph.D. "The Alexander Technique: An Innovative Approach to Reducing Physical Tension and Stress." *Behavioral Medicine,* (November–December 1981): 27–29.

Tinbergen, Nikolaas. "Ethology & Stress Diseases: An Examination of the Alexander Technique." (Nobel Prize acceptance address, Stockholm, Sweden: Nobel Foundation, 1974).

Chapter 4: The Feldenkrais Method: Awareness Through Movement

Calvert, Robert. "The Feldenkrais Method: The Man, His Work and the Training." *Massage,* 47, (January–February 1994): 30, 32–34, 36.

Feldenkrais, Moshe, D.Sc. *Awareness Through Movement. Easy-to-Do Health Exercises to Improve Your Posture, Vision, Imagination, & Personal Awareness* (San Francisco: Harper & Row, 1972).

_____. *The Elusive Obvious or Basic Feldenkrais.* (Cupertino, CA: Meta Publications, 1981).

_____. *The Potent Self—A Guide to Spontaneity.* (San Francisco: HarperCollins, 1985).

Leri, Dennis. "Learning How to Learn: Rather Than 'Fixing' the Body, Moshe Feldenkrais Taught How to Expand Its Capacities and Range of Choice." *Gnosis,* (Fall 1993): 49–53.

McIntyre, Margaret. "Unlock the Trunk!" *Skiing,* (October 1992): 139–44.

Rosenfeld, Albert. "Teaching the Body How to Program the Brain Is Moshe's 'Miracle.'" *Smithsonian,* (January 1981).

Spire, Mary, M.M. "The Feldenkrais Method: An Interview with Anat Baniel." *Medical Problems of Performing Artists,* (December 1989): 159–62.

Williams, Kelly L. "Muscle Sense: A Moving Look at the Feldenkrais Method." *US Air Magazine,* (November 1991).

Zemach–Bersin, David, et al. *Relaxercise: Ten Effortless Techniques for a More Flexible, Energetic, Pain-Free, Stress-Free Body.* (San Francisco: HarperCollins, 1990).

Chapter 5: Myofascial Release: Physical Therapy Joins Hands with Massage Therapy

Barnes, John F., P.T. "The Myofascial Release Approach." *Massage,* 49, (May–June 1994): 36–38, 40–45; 50, (July–August 1994): 58, 60–64; 51, (September–October 1994): 84–88; and 52, (November–December 1994): 72–77.

_____. *Myofascial Release: The Search for Excellence, a Comprehensive Evaluatory and Treatment Approach.* (Paoli, PA: Myofascial Release Seminars, 1990.)

Calvert, Robert. "Exclusive Interview: John Barnes, P.T.: Founder of Myofascial Release." *Massage,* 41, (January–February 1993): 46, 48–53, 55; 42, (March–April 1993): 54–58, 60–61.

Heinrich, Steve, P.T. "Learning to Let Go–The Role of Somato Emotional Release in Clinical Treatment." *Physical Therapy Forum,* Vol. VIII, No. 24, (June 19, 1989): 1, 3–5.

Juett, Tim, P.T. "Myofascial Release–An Introduction for the Patient." *Physical Therapy Forum,* (October 3, 1988): 9–12.

Riemer, Jan. "I Became Unglued." *The Main Line Community Magazine,* (April 1989).

Chapter 6: The Trager Approach: Meditation in Motion

Convery, Ann. "Recuperation: Beyond the Depths of Massage." *Muscle & Fitness,* (December 1993): 60.

Grandinetti, Deborah. "Trager Psychophysical Integration: The Gentle Therapy." *Your Personal Bat,* (April 1991): 12–13.

Juhan, Deane, M.A. "The Physiology of Hook-up: How TRAGER Works." Keynote address at Sixth International Trager Conference, San Diego, California, Sept. 18, 1992.

_____. *An Introduction to Trager Psychophysical Integration and Mentastics Movement Education.* Mill Valley, CA: Trager Institute, 1989.

Laskin, Jack. "Milton Trager, M.D.: The Master at 86." *Massage,* 51, (September–October 1994): 26, 28–29.

Leviton, Richard. "Moving with Milton Trager: An *East West* Interview with a Bodywork Pioneer." *East West Journal,* (January 1988).

Trager, Milton, M.D., with Cathy Guadagno, Ph.D. *Trager Mentastics: Movement as a Way to Agelessness.* (Barrytown, NY: Station Hill Press, 1987).

Trager Journal, The. Mill Valley, CA: Trager Institute. Vol. 1, (Fall 1982); Vol. 11, (Fall 1987).

Chapter 7: Rubenfeld Synergy Method: Touch Therapy Meets Talk Therapy

Gallagher, Winifred. "The Healing Touch: Searches on the Mind-Body Coast." *American Health,* (October 1988): 49, 52–53.

Gustinella, M.K., M.S., MFCC. "A Touch of Synergy: Ilana Rubenfeld." *Beyond Survival,* Vol. 3, No. 2, (1992): 20–21.

Knaster, Mirka. "Ilana Rubenfeld: Our Lady of Synergy." *Massage Therapy Journal,* Vol. 30, No. 1, (Winter 1991): 36–45.

Mechner, Vicki. *Healing Journeys: The Power of Rubenfeld Synergy.* (Chappaqua, NY: Omniquest Press, 1998).

Rubenfeld, Ilana. "Beginner's Hands: Twenty-five Years of Simple Rubenfeld Synergy–the Birth of a Therapy." *Somatics,* (Spring–Summer 1988).

_____. "Gestalt Therapy and the BodyMind: An Overview of the Rubenfeld Synergy Method," in *Gestalt Therapy: Perspectives and Applications.* ed. Edwin C. Nevis. (New York: Gardner Press, Inc., 1992): 147–77.

_____. *The Listening Hand: Self-Healing Through the Rubenfeld Synergy Method of Talk and Touch.* (New York: Bantam, 2000).

_____. "Ushering in a Century of Integration." *Somatics,* (Autumn–Winter 1990–91): 59–63.

Schwarzbaum, Lisa. "All the Right Moves." *Daily News Magazine,* October 1, 1989.

Warrick, Sally. "A Touch for Survival." *Beyond Survival,* Vol. 3, No. 2, (1992): 7–10.

Chapter 8: Rosen Method: Listening to the Body

Calvert, Robert, and Judi Calvert. "Exclusive Interview: Marion Rosen." *Massage,* 32, (July–August 1991): 48–55.

Crawford, Bevalyn. "The Healing Touch of Rosenwork." *Yoga Journal,* (March–April 1990): 12ff.

Rosen, Marion, with Sue Brenner. *The Rosen Method of Movement.* (Berkeley, CA: North Atlantic Books, 1991).

Wooten, Sandra. "The Rosen Method." *Massage,* 44, (July–August 1993): 62, 64, 66, 67–69.

_____. "Rosen Method Bodywork." *Massage & Bodywork Quarterly,* Vol. VI, No. 3, (Summer 1992): 6–12.

Chapter 9: Shiatsu: Oriental Acupressure and Other Bodywork Practices

Shiatsu

Academy of Traditional Chinese Medicine, The. *An Outline of Chinese Acupuncture.* (Beijing: Foreign Languages Press, 1975).

Bienfield, Harriet, L.Ac., and Efrem Korngold, L.Ac., O.M.D. *Between Heaven and Earth: A Guide to Chinese Medicine.* (New York: Ballantine Books, 1991).

Calvert, Robert. "Exclusive Interview: Wataru Ohashi: Shiatsu Teacher, Author and Practitioner." *Massage,* 48, (March–April 1994): 60–68.

Connelly, Dianne M., Ph.D., M.Ac. *All Sickness is Home Sickness.* (Columbia, MD: The Centre for Traditional Acupuncture, Inc., 1986).

_____. *Traditional Acupuncture: The Law of the Five Elements.* (Columbia, MD: The Centre for Traditional Acupuncture, Inc., 1989).

Dubitsky, Carl, O.B.T., L.M.T., AOBTA. "History of Shiatsu/Anma." *Massage Therapy Journal,* Vol. 31, No. 4, (Fall 1992): 109–10, 112, 114.

Durckheim, Karlfried Graf. *Hara: The Vital Centre of Man.* (London: Unwin Hyman Limited, 1989).

Gach, Michael Reed. *The Bum Back Book: Acupressure Self-Help Back Care for Relieving Pain and Tension.* (Berkeley, CA: Celestial Arts, 1983).

Haas, Elson M., M.D. *Staying Healthy with the Seasons.* (Berkeley, CA: Celestial Arts, 1981).

Hammer, Leon, M.D. *Dragon Rises, Red Bird Flies: Psychology & Chinese Medicine.* (Barrytown, NY: Station Hill Press, 1990).

Hashimoto, Keizo, M.D., with Kawakami Yoshiaki, M.D. *Sôtai: Balance and Health Through Natural Movement.* (Tokyo: Japan Publications, Inc., 1983).

Jones, Marjorie, and Catherine Straffon. "A Biochemical Investigation of Meridian Energy." *Massage Therapy Journal,* Vol. 31, No. 4, (Fall 1992): 77–78, 80, 82–83.

Kaptchuk, Ted J. *The Web That Has No Weaver: Understanding Chinese Medicine.* (New York: Contemporary Books, 2001).

Koplewitz, Laura. "Ohashiatsu: The Healing Touch." *Yoga Journal,* (January–February 1989): 19ff.

Kushi, Michio. *Your Face Never Lies: An Introduction to Oriental Diagnosis.* (Wayne, NJ: Avery Publishing Group, 1983).

Larre, Claude, and Elisabeth Rochat de la Valle. *Rooted in Spirit: The Heart of Chinese Medicine.* (Barrytown, NY: Station Hill Press, 1995).

Maciocia, Giovanni. *The Foundations of Chinese Medicine: A Comprehensive Text for Acupuncturists and Herbalists.* (New York: Churchill Livingstone, 1989).

Masunaga, Shizuto. *Zen Imagery Exercises: Meridian Exercises for Wholesome Living.* (New York: Japan Publications, Inc., 1987).

_____. with Wataru Ohashi. *Zen Shiatsu: How to Harmonize Yin and Yang for Better Health.* (New York: Japan Publications, Inc., 1977).

Namikoshi, Toru. *Shiatsu Therapy: Theory and Practice.* (New York: Japan Publications, Inc., 1974).

"Now, a Report That Sleeping Can Bring On a Heart Attack." *The New York Times,* February 4, 1993, p. B8.

Ohashi, Wataru. *Do-It-Yourself Shiatsu: How to Perform the Ancient Japanese Art of "Acupuncture Without Needles."* (New York: E. P. Dutton, 1976).

_____. with Tom Monte. *Reading the Body: Ohashi's Book of Oriental Diagnosis.* (New York: Arkana, 1991).

Rudnianin, Hal, and Maggie Glasser. "Traditional Chinese Medicine in the People's Republic of China: Studying Massage Therapy in China." *Massage Therapy Journal,* Vol. 31, No. 4, (Fall 1992): 42–44, 46–50, 52, 54.

Sasaki, Pauline. "Shiatsu: An Overview," in *Healing Massage Techniques.* (Norwalk, CT: Appleton & Lange, 1988): 183–95.

Serizawa, Katsusuke, M.D. *Effective Tsubo Therapy: Simple and Natural Relief Without Drugs.* (New York: Japan Publications, Inc., 1984).

Swedish Institute. *Energetic Shiatsu: A Manual.* (New York: Swedish Institute, 1987).

Weintraub, Michael I., M.D., FACP. "Alternative Medical Care: Shiatsu, Swedish Muscle Massage, and Trigger Point Suppression in Spinal Pain Syndrome." *American Journal of Pain Management,* Vol. 2, No. 2, (April 1992): 74–78.

Amma Massage

Sohn, Tina. *AMMA Therapy: An Integration of Oriental Medical Principles, Bodywork, Nutrition, & Exercise.* (Rochester, VT: Inner Traditions, 1994).

_____. and Donna Finando. *Amma: The Ancient Art of Oriental Healing.* (Rochester, VT: Healing Arts Press, 1988).

Jin Shin Do Bodymind Acupressure

Teeguarden, Iona Marsaa, M.A., M.F.C.C. *Acupressure Way of Health: Jin Shin Do.* (New York: Japan Publications, Inc., 1978).

_____. *The Joy of Feeling: Bodymind Acupressure.* (New York: Japan Publications, Inc., 1987).

Tuina

Chinese Educational Travels, Ltd. *Tuina–Chinese Manual Therapy* (videotape). (Skokie, IL: Chinese Educational Travels, Ltd., 1989).

Lubowich, Ken, O.M.D. "An Introduction to Tuina." *AOBTA Bulletin,* Vol. 1, No. 1, (Spring 1991): 19.

Rudnianin, Hal, and Maggie Glasser. "Tuina: A Pictorial Walk through a Massage Department in China." *Massage Therapy Journal,* Vol. 32, No. 1, (Winter 1993): 55–58.

Zhengling, Kou. "The Blind: Making Contribution to Society." *Beijing Review,* Vol. 34, No. 35, (2 September 1991): 27–29.

Chapter 10: Reflexology: Baring Your Sole

Bergson, Anika, and Vladimir Tuchak. *Zone Therapy.* (Los Angeles: Pinnacle Books, 1974).

Berkolds, Andra. "Reflexology: Healing Through the Feet." *New Body,* (August 1992): 54.

Bloom, Marc. "A Therapy Based on Tapping Your Feet." *The New York Times,* July 16, 1990.

Byers, Dwight C. *Better Health with Foot Reflexology: The Original Ingham Method.* (St. Petersburg, FL: Ingham Publishing, Inc., 1991).

Ingham, Eunice D. *The Original Works of Eunice D. Ingham: Stories the Feet Can Tell Thru Reflexology and Stories the Feet Have Told Thru Reflexology* with revisions by Dwight C. Byers. (St. Petersburg, FL: Ingham Publishing, Inc., 1984).

Klein, Louise. "Reflexology, the Healing Art of 'Sole' Searching." *Massage,* 40, (November–December 1992): 60, 62, 64.

Michael, Jane Wilkens. "The Hip Way to Health." *Town & Country,* (February 1992): 44.

Norman, Laura, with Thomas Cowan. *Feet First: A Guide to Foot Reflexology.* (New York: Simon & Schuster, 1988).

Togut, Judith. "Reflexology: No Mean Feat for Aches & Pains." *New York Post,* August 6, 1987.

Chapter 11: Aromatherapy Massage: Appealing to the "Scentses"

Belden, Tom. "Use of Aromatherapy to Beat Jet Lag Makes 'Scents' to Airlines." *Journal of Commerce & Commercial,* (22 August 1991): 10A.

Bishop, Jerry E. "New Research Suggests That Romance Begins by Falling Nose over Heels in Love." *The Wall Street Journal,* April 7, 1993, pp. B1, B6.

"Fragrance: Spirits That Soar." *Essence,* November 1991, p. 14ff.

Kallan, Carla. "Probing the Power of Common Scents." *Prevention,* (October 1991): 38ff.

Lavabre, Marcel. *Aromatherapy Workbook.* (Rochester, VT: Healing Arts Press, 1990).

Moore, Kimberley A. "Applications of Aromatherapy & Herbal Remedies for Massage." *Massage Therapy Journal,* Vol. 31, No. 3, (Summer 1992): 56–58, 60, 62–63, 110, 112, 114.

Pacelle, Mitchell. "Many People Refuse to Check in if a Hotel Has Odors in the Lobby." *The Wall Street Journal,* July 18, 1992, p. B1.

Straley, Carol. "Aromatherapy: How to Relax Your Body and Renew Your Spirits with Scent." *Parents,* (November 1986): 193–96.

Strom, Stephanie. "Human Pheromones: His and Hers Fragrances with Chemicals That Drive the Libido? Would a Dozen Roses Smell So Sweet?" *The New York Times,* April 18, 1993, p. B1.

Tisserand, Robert B. *The Art of Aromatherapy: The Healing and Beautifying Properties of the Essential Oils of Flowers and Herbs.* (Rochester, VT: Healing Arts Press, 1977).

Valnet, Jean. *The Practice of Aromatherapy.* (Rochester, VT: Healing Arts Press, 1990).

Part V: Energetic Bodywork: Healing with the Human Energy Field

Becker, Robert O., M.D., and Gary Selden. *The Body Electric: Electromagnetism and the Foundation of Life.* (New York: William Morrow, 1985).

Brennan, Barbara Ann. *Hands of Light: A Guide to Healing Through the Human Energy Field.* (New York: Bantam Books, 1987).

Gerber, Richard, M.D. *Vibrational Medicine: New Choices for Healing Ourselves.* (Santa Fe, NM: Bear & Co., Inc., 1988).

Joy, W. Brugh, M.D. *Joy's Way: A Map for the Transformational Journey–An Introduction to the Potentials for Healing with Body Energies.* (Los Angeles: Jeremy P. Tarcher, 1979).

Karagulla, Shafika, M.D., and Dora Kunz. *The Chakras and the Human Energy Fields.* (Wheaton, IL: The Theosophical Publishing House, 1989).

Ray, Barbara, Ph.D. *The "Reiki" Factor in the Radiance Technique,* expanded edition (St. Petersburg, FL: Radiance Associates, 1992).

Saint-Exupéry, Antoine de. *The Little Prince.* Trans. Katherine Woods. (New York: Harcourt Brace, 1971).

Tansley, David V. *Subtle Body: Essence and Shadow.* (New York: Thames and Hudson, 1988).

Chapter 12: Therapeutic Touch (TT): Modulating the Human Energy Field

Calvert, Robert. "Exclusive Interview: Dolores Krieger, Ph.D. and Her Therapeutic Touch." *Massage,* Issue 47, (January–February 1994): 56–60.

Krieger, Dolores, Ph.D., R.N. *Accepting Your Power to Heal: The Personal Practice of Therapeutic Touch.* (Santa Fe, NM: Bear & Co., Inc., 1993).

_____. "Healing by the 'Laying-On' of Hands as a Facilitator of Bioenergetic Exchange: The Response of In-Vivo Human Hemoglobin." *International Journal of Psychoenergetic Systems* 1(2), (1976): 121–29.

_____. *Living the Therapeutic Touch: Healing as a Lifestyle.* (New York: Dodd, Mead, 1987).

_____. *The Therapeutic Touch: How to Use Your Hands to Help or to Heal.* (New York: Prentice Hall Press, 1979).

Macrae, Janet, Ph.D., R.N. *Therapeutic Touch: A Practical Guide.* (New York: Alfred A. Knopf, 1992).

Montagu, Ashley, Ph.D. *Touching: The Human Significance of the Skin.* (New York: Harper & Row, 1986).

Rorvik, David M. "The Healing Hand of Mr. E." *Esquire,* Vol. 81, No. 2, (February 1974): 70–71, 154, 156, 159–60.

Sandroff, Ronni, R.N. "A Skeptic's Guide to Therapeutic Touch: Practitioners Say It Relieves Suffering and Speeds Healing. Is It Really Something New . . . or Just Good Old TLC with Paranormal Airs?" *RN,* (January 1980): 25ff.

Williams, Gurney, III. "The Lowest-Tech Medicine Ever: Why a Growing Number of Doctors, Nurses and Hospitals Are Using Therapeutic Touch on Their Patients." *Longevity,* (January 1992): 60ff.

Wirth, Daniel P., M.S., J.D. "The Effect of Non-Contact Therapeutic Touch on the Healing Rate of Full Thickness Dermal Wounds." *Subtle Energies,* Vol. 1, No. 1, (1990): 1–19.

Chapter 13: CranioSacral Therapy: The Skull Speaks

Kotzsch, Ronald. "Craniosacral Therapy: Bodywork That Gets Results with Pressure as Light as the Weight of a Nickel." *Natural Health,* Vol. 23, No. 4, (July–August 1993): 42, 44.

Lauterstein, David. "What Is Zero-Balancing?" *Massage Therapy Journal,* Vol. 33, No. 1, (Winter 1994): 28–30, 32, 34.

Magoun, Harold Ives, A.B., D.O., O.M.M. *Osteopathy in the Cranial Field,* 3rd ed. (Kirksville, MD: Journal Printing Co., 1976).

Pronsati, Michelle P. "Erb's Palsy: Once Considered Incurable, Now Helped with NDT, Craniosacral and Manual Therapy." *Advance for Occupational Therapists,* (27 May 1991).

Smith, Fritz F., M.D. *Inner Bridges: A Guide to Energy Movement and Body Structure.* (Atlanta, GA: Humanics New Age, 1986).

Upledger, John E., D.O., O.M.M. *A Brain Is Born.* (Palm Beach Gardens, FL: The Upledger Institute, 1995).

_____. *CranioSacral Therapy I Study Guide.* (Palm Beach Gardens, FL: The Upledger Institute, 1992).

_____. *CranioSacral Therapy II, Beyond the Dura.* (Seattle, WA: Eastland Press, 1987).

_____. *CranioSacral Therapy, SomatoEmotional Release, Your Inner Physician and You.* (Berkeley, CA: North Atlantic Books, and Palm Beach Gardens, FL: The Upledger Institute, 1991).

_____. "The Relationship of Craniosacral Examination Findings in Grade School Children with Developmental Problems." *Journal of the American Osteopathic Association,* Vol. 77, (June 1978): 760–83.

_____. and Jon D. Vredegvoogd, M.F.A. *Craniosacral Therapy.* (Seattle, WA: Eastland Press, 1988).

Weiselfish, Sharon, M.A., R.P.T, and Jay Kain, M.S., P.T., A.T.C. "Introduction to Developmental Manual Therapy–an Integrated Systems Approach for Structural and Functional Rehabilitation." *Physical Therapy Forum,* northeast ed., Vol. IX, No. 6, (12 February 1990): 1, 3–5.

_____. "TOS—an Introduction to the Evaluation and Treatment of Complex Neuro-musculoskeletal. Dysfunction with Manual and Craniosacral Therapy: Parts I & II." *Physical Therapy Forum,* (21 June 1991): 9–13; and (28 June 1991): 11–12.

_____. "An Overview of Erb's Palsy with Case History Documenting Treatment with Manual and Craniosacral Therapy." *Physical Therapy Forum,* western ed., Vol. IX, No. 12, (26 March 1990): 1, 3–6.

_____. "Shannon—a Pictorial Case History Presenting Cranial Therapy for Cerebral Palsy." *Physical Therapy Forum.*

Chapter 14: Reiki: Universal Life Energy

Baginski, Bodo J., and Shalila Sharamon. *Reiki: Universal Life Energy.* Trans. Christopher Baker and Judith Harrison. (Mendocino, CA: Life Rhythm, 1988).

Furumoto, Phyllis Lei. *The Usui System of Natural Healing.* (Cataldo, ID: The Reiki Alliance).

Horan, Paula. *Empowerment Through Reiki: The Path to Personal and Global Transformation.* (Wilmot, WI: Lotus Light Publications, 1992).

Rand, William Lee. "Reiki Energy: What Is It? How Does It Heal?" *Massage,* 50, (July–August 1994): 86, 88.

Rosenstiel, Léonie, Ph.D. *Reiki: First Degree Manual* (Rainbow Empowerment Series). (New York: Dayspring Resources, 1991).

_____. *Reiki: Second Degree Manual* (Rainbow Empowerment Series), (New York: Dayspring Resources, 1991).

Verheijden, Bernard. "Reiki: The Healing Touch." *Massage,* 50, (July–August 1994): 84–89.

Wetzel, Wendy S., M.S.N., R.N. "Reiki Healing: A Physiologic Perspective." *Journal of Holistic Nursing,* Vol. 7, No. 1, (1989): 47–54.

Chapter 15: Holotropic Breathwork: The Music of Breath

Grof, Christina. *The Stormy Search for the Self.* (Los Angeles: Jeremy P. Tarcher, 1990).

_____. *Spiritual Emergency.* (Los Angeles: Jeremy P. Tarcher, 1989).

_____.and Stanislav Grof. *Beyond Death: The Gates of Consciousness.* (London: Thames & Hudson, 1980).

_____. "Spiritual Emergency: The Understanding and Treatment of Transpersonal Crises." *Re-Vision,* Vol. 8, No. 2, (Winter–Spring 1986): 7–20.

Grof, Stanislav, M.D. *The Adventure of Self-Discovery: Dimensions of Consciousness and New Perspectives in Psychotherapy and Inner Exploration.* (Albany, NY: State University of New York Press, 1988).

_____. *Ancient Wisdom and Modern Science.* (Albany, NY: State University of New York Press, 1984).

_____. *Beyond the Brain: Birth, Death, and Transcendence in Psychotherapy.* (Albany, NY: State University of New York Press, 1985).

_____. *East & West: Ancient Wisdom & Modern Science.* (Lake Oswego, OR: Robert Briggs, 1985).

_____. *Frontiers of the Hidden Mind.* (Alameda, CA: Hunter House, 1992).

_____. *Human Survival and Unconscious Evolution*. (Albany, NY: State University of New York Press, 1988).

LSD Psychotherapy. (Alameda, CA: Hunter House, 1980).

Realms of the Human Unconscious: Observations from LSD Research. (New York: Viking Press, 1975).

_____. with Hal Z. Bennett. *The Holotropic Mind: The Three Levels of Human Consciousness and How They Shape Our Lives*. (San Francisco: HarperCollins, 1993).

_____. and Joan Halifax. *The Human Encounter with Death: Dimensions of Consciousness & New Perspectives in Psychotherapy & Inner Exploration*. (New York: E. P. Dutton, 1977).

Taylor, Kylea. *The Breathwork Experience: Exploration and Healing in Nonordinary States of Consciousness*. (Santa Cruz, CA: Hanford Mead, 1994).

Chapter 16: Polarity Therapy: Balancing Currents of Energy

Beaulieu, John, N.D. *Music and Sound in the Healing Arts*. (Barrytown, NY: Station Hill Press, 1987).

_____. *Polarity Therapy Workbook*. (New York: BioSonic Enterprises Ltd., 1994).

Calvert, Robert. "Exclusive Interviews: Franklyn Sills & Will Leichnitz." *Massage*, 43, (May–June 1993): 33, 36, 38, 40, 44–45.

Chitty, John, R.P.P. "Introduction to Polarity Therapy." *Massage & Bodywork Quarterly*, Vol. VIII, Issue 1, (Winter 1993): 42, 44, 45, 47.

Chopra, Deepak, M.D. *Perfect Health: The Complete Mind/Body Guide*. (New York: Crown, 1991).

Eabry, Martha, and Steve Eabry. "Dr. Randolph Stone, Polarity Therapy and the Chakras." *Massage Therapy Journal*, Vol. 32, No. 3, (Spring 1993): 64–66.

Hall, Robert K., M.D. "Polarity: Remembering Uncle Randolph." *Massage*, 43, (May–June 1993): 32, 34, 42, 44.

Kitts, Beverly, R.P.T. "Polarity Therapy," in *Healing Massage Techniques: Holistic, Classic, and Emerging Methods*. (East Norwalk, CT: Appleton & Lange, 1988): 197–218.

Siegel, Alan, N.D. *Polarity Therapy: The Power That Heals*. (Dorset, England: Prism Press, 1987).

Sills, Franklyn. *The Polarity Process: Energy as a Healing Art*. (Dorset, England: Element Books, 1990).

Stone, Randolph, D.C., D.O., N.D. *Polarity Therapy: The Complete Collected Works on This Revolutionary Healing Art by the Originator of the System*. (Sebastopol, CA: CRCS Publications, 1986).

Young, Phil. *The Art of Polarity Therapy: A Practitioner's Perspective*. (Dorset, England: Prism Press, 1990).

Chapter 17: The Spa Experience: Pampering Yourself While Your Body Works

Burt, Bernard. *Fodor's Healthy Escapes: 243 Resorts and Retreats Where You Can Get Fit, Feel Good, Find Yourself, and Get Away from It All.* 4th ed. (New York: Fodor's Travel Publications, 1995).

_____. *The Best Spas with Learning Programs.* (New York: Random House, 1994).

"The Spa Spell." *Self,* (December 1991): 90–102.

Vajde, Deborah. "Meditation Medication." *Utne Reader,* (July–August 1992): 32.

Van Itallie, Theodore B., M.D., and Leila Hadley. *The Best Spas: Where to Go for Weight Loss, Fitness Programs and Pure Pleasure in the U.S. and Around the World.* (New York: Harper & Row, 1988).

Zagat U.S. Hotel, Resort and Spa Survey. (New York: Zagat Survey, 1992).

Chapter 18: Resources for Further Exploration

Goldman, Caren. "Enrich Yourself. A Guide to 19 Leading Centers for Personal Growth." *Natural Health,* Vol. 23, No. 3, (May–June 1993): 98–110.

Glossary: Bodywork from A to Z

New York Naturally. (New York: City Spirit Publications, Winter–Spring 1994).

1992–1993 Holistic Health Directory. (Brighton, MA: New Age Journal, 1992–1993).

UNLEARNING

The instructess
appeared to me
in a dream

and counseled

me my body
is a shell

hard
and
empty

at the
same time;

the life
inside
resides

in unlearning
everything
I've ever
learned,

the suppleness
there
where flow

the poems
and dreams

yet to be
written.

—THOMAS CLAIRE

INDEX

ABOUT THE AUTHOR

Thomas Claire is a New York State licensed massage therapist, writer, body/mind practitioner, and personal development facilitator. The first edition of *Bodywork: What Type of Massage to Get—and How to Make the Most of It* was hailed as a trustworthy, comprehensive, and highly readable guide to massage and bodywork. His most recent book, *Yoga for Men: Postures for Healthy, Stress-Free Living* (Career Press/New Page Books, 2004) was also critically acclaimed for its contribution to the field of yoga.

Thomas is a former Assistant Professor of Healing Arts at Queensborough Community College City University of New York, where he was program coordinator for a new degree program in massage therapy that he helped design and implement. He practices a variety of bodywork techniques, including Swedish massage, shiatsu, CranioSacral Therapy, Myofascial Release, and Therapeutic Touch, and is in addition a traditional Reiki Master. He lives and works in New York City.

Thomas has been practicing the healing arts for more than thirty years. His goal is to help each individual connect with his or her own inner source of well-being by presenting tools for health, transformation, and personal growth drawn from a wide range of traditions in as simple and clear a manner as possible. Thomas facilitates classes, workshops, and intensive private sessions in bodywork and other personal transformation practices around the world.

For further information on his work, you can visit him at his website: www.thomasclaire.com

You can also write to him at:

Thomas Claire
c/o Clairefontaine, Inc.
P.O. Box 1040
Grand Central Station
New York, NY 10163-1040